FOOD VALUES

Fats and Cholesterol

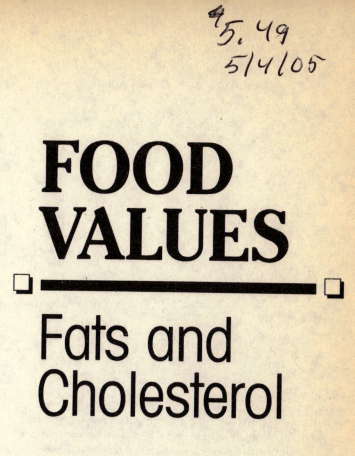

FOOD VALUES

Fats and Cholesterol

Patty Bryan

 HarperPerennial
A Division of HarperCollins*Publishers*

HarperCollins books may be purchased for educational, business, or sales promotional use. For information, please write: Special Markets Department, HarperCollins Publishers, Inc., 10 East 53rd Street, New York, NY 10022.

FIRST HARPERPERENNIAL EDITION

Designed by Alma Hochhauser Orenstein

LIBRARY OF CONGRESS CATALOG CARD NUMBER: 91-58287

ISBN 0-06-273125-4

92 93 94 95 96 PS / RRD 10 9 8 7 6 5 4 3 2 1

Contents

Introduction   ix
How to Use This Book   xv
Sources   xxiii
Abbreviations   xxiv

Baking Ingredients   1
Baking Mixes   3
Beef, Fresh & Cured   7
Beverages   18
Breadcrumbs, Croutons, Stuffings, & Seasoned
  Coatings   24
Breads, Rolls, Biscuits, & Muffins   27
Breakfast Cereals, Cold & Hot   35
Breakfast Foods, Prepared   43
Butter & Margarine Spreads   48
Candy   55
Cheese & Cheese Foods   58
Cookies, Bars, & Brownies   67
Crackers   74
Desserts: Cakes, Pastries, & Pies   77
Desserts: Custards, Gelatins, Puddings,
  & Pie Fillings   87

ozen: Ice Cream, Ice Milk, Ices & Sherbets,
Juice, Pudding, Tofu, & Yogurt   92

Dessert Sauces, Syrups, & Toppings   100

Dinners, Frozen   103

Eggs & Egg Substitutes   106

Entrees & Main Courses, Canned & Boxed   107

Entrees & Main Courses, Frozen   110

Fast Foods   120

Fats, Oils, & Shortenings   132

Flours & Cornmeals   135

Fruit, Fresh & Processed   138

Fruit Spreads   148

Infant & Toddler Foods   150

Lamb, Veal, & Miscellaneous Meats   167

Legumes & Legume Products   168

Milk, Milk Substitutes, & Milk Products: Cream,
Sour Cream, Cream Substitutes, Milk, Milk
Substitutes, Whey, & Yogurt   173

Noodles & Pasta, Plain   178

Nuts & Nut-based Butters, Flours, Meals, Milks,
Pastes, & Powders   179

Pickles, Olives, Relishes, & Chutneys   183

Pizza   185

Pork, Fresh & Cured   187

Poultry, Fresh & Processed   196

Processed Meat & Poultry Products: Sausages,
Frankfurters, Cold Cuts, Pâtés, & Spreads   206

Rice & Grains, Plain & Prepared   214

Salad Dressings, Mayonnaise, Vinegar, & Dips   218

Sauces, Gravies, & Condiments   224

Seafood & Seafood Products   229

Seasonings   238

Seeds & Seed-based Butters, Flours, & Meals   238

Snacks   240

Soups, Prepared   246

Soybeans & Soybean Products   259

Special Dietary Foods   261

Sugars & Sweeteners: Honey, Molasses, Sugar,
    Sugar Substitutes, Syrup, & Treacle   262

Vegetables, Plain & Prepared   264

Introduction

Americans consume the equivalent of three-quarters of a cup of oil every day. Of course, we don't drink a glassful for lunch. Some of the fat in our diet is a natural part of popular foods, like hard cheeses and the beloved hamburger, but much of it is "discretionary:" We add fats and oil to many foods to flavor them, make our chicken crisp by frying it in oil, drench our muffins with butter or margarine, soak salad greens in assorted oils, spoon sour cream on our baked potatoes and serve fish swimming in melted butter.

In the process, we increase our intake of *lipids*—the generic term for fats, oils and fatlike substances, including cholesterol, which make food more palatable and are a normal part of our diets. The lipids now supply an average of 37% of the food energy—calories—in the American diet. Much better would be 30%. The National Institute of Health, the American Cancer Society, and the American Heart Association are confident that the incidence of coronary heart disease and possibly some cancers would be lowered if we reduced our daily fat intake to that 30% level (10% each for saturated, monounsaturated, and polyunsaturated fat).

We are also urged to eat less than 300 milligrams of cholesterol and to have a total blood cholesterol level (TBC) of less than 200mg/dl. Americans now consume an average of 350–400 milligrams of cholesterol daily, and many of us have higher than desirable cholesterol levels.

This book provides you with the data you need to assess, and then adjust your consumption of fat and cholesterol.

Fats and Oils

Our bodies need some fat to insulate the body, sheath and protect internal organs, and provide us with a store of energy. We use fat to absorb and store certain vitamins and to make some of the hormones that control body processes. It is a major component of the membranes that surround each of our cells, and it regulates the flow of nutrients and other substances in and out of the cell body.

There are many different kinds of fat, but for purposes of this section we are going to discuss three: saturated, polyunsaturated, and monounsaturated. You have probably heard a good deal about them, but perhaps don't understand the important differences.

Saturated fats are the lipids we traditionally call "fat." They are solid at room temperature, and are found primarily in animal products. About 50% of the fat in beef, lamb, and pork is saturated, as is 61% of the fat in butter and 40% of the fat in lard. Chicken contains a smaller percentage of saturated fats than other meats, about 30%. The fat in dairy products is butterfat, so a high proportion of the fat in dairy products is saturated, too. However, there are also saturated vegetable fats. In fact, some of the most saturated fat in our diet is found in tropical oils: palm, palm kernel and coconut oil. The oil in coconut oil is a whopping 86% saturated. These tropical oils have been used widely in processed foods such as imitation dairy products, granola and dry mixes, cookies and crackers. However, because many Americans exceed the recommended 10% saturated fats in their diets and because of the growing concern about saturated fats and their link to cholesterol levels, many food manufacturers have removed tropical oils from their products.

Americans get 15% to 20%—too much—of their calories from monounsaturated fats, mostly found in oils. Olive, canola, and peanut oil are high in monounsaturated fats. However, many margarines and hydrogenated vegetable shortenings are also high in monounsaturated fats.

Another 5% to 7% of the calories in the American diet—not enough—comes from polyunsaturated fats, found in the highest proportions in vegetable oils: safflower, sunflower, corn, soybean, and cottonseed mixtures. The fat of some fish also contains a high proportion of polyunsaturated fats.

Cholesterol

Cholesterol is another type of fat essential for many key body functions. It is found in all animal cells and in the human body, it is concentrated in the brain, liver, kidneys and adrenal glands. It is an important component of the fatty sheaths surrounding nerve fibers, and it plays a role in the synthesis of several vital substances, including sex hormones and bile salts. However, cholesterol may also be deposited in arterial walls and cause them to narrow—the process called atherosclerosis.

Most of the cholesterol in our blood, between 70% to 80%, is manufactured by the liver. But your total blood cholesterol (TBC) level is determined by many factors, some of which you have no control over: heredity, sex and age. However, you do have control over your diet which is a significant factor in your cholesterol level.

But, alas, the situation with cholesterol is complicated. Lipids, including cholesterol, cannot mix with water and blood, for the well–known reason that oil and water don't mix. Therefore, the lipids are combined with other substances in the liver, and these *lipoproteins* are the molecules that actually "deliver" cholesterol throughout the body. There are several kinds of lipoproteins, including *low-density lipoproteins* (LDLs), and *high-density lipoproteins* (HDLs).

LDLs are sometimes called "bad cholesterol" because they are associated with excess cholesterol that is deposited in places where it may cause damage—the best example is the inside walls of the arteries.

HDL's are known as "good cholesterol" because they work as scavengers in the blood stream, picking up excess cholesterol and returning it to the liver. Obviously, this helps reduce cholesterol levels.

Thus, your LDL and HDL levels are also important factors. Doctors generally use the total blood cholesterol level to screen patients, then measure lipoprotein levels if the total level is high. The ratio between HDLs and total blood cholesterol has become an important indicator of the risk of coronary heart disease. The TBC/HDL ratio indicates approximately how much more LDL than HDL is present in your blood. The higher the ratio of LDLs to HDLs, the higher the risk of coronary heart disease. The average American male has a ratio of 4.5, the average woman, 4.0.

Dietary Control of Blood Cholesterol Levels

Nutrition can lower cholesterol, improve your TBC/HDL ratio, and therefore lower risk of heart disease. Reducing cholesterol intake directly is one obvious adjustment. But the best way is to reduce your saturated fat intake, because the liver uses saturated fat to *manufacture* cholesterol. An excessive intake of saturated fat can significantly raise your blood cholesterol level.

Therefore, unsaturated fats are the more desirable fats for your diet because they can help lower your cholesterol level. However, the fats should still comprise only 10% of your total fat intake.

Fat, Cholesterol and Food Labeling

In 1991, the Federal Drug Administration (FDA) mandated the most significant changes in food labeling in the last 50 years. The new regulations affect virtually all solid food in grocery stores, many of which are the foods that contain fat and cholesterol. Under the new regulations, food labels must provide nutritional information and meet the FDA's regulations regarding descriptions on the label, serving size and health claims.

The new regulations will restrict food descriptions. Terms such as "lite," "low-calorie" and "fat-free," widely used in the food industry with varying meanings, can now be used only if they fit the FDA's definition of that term. With regard to fats and cholesterol, "lowfat" will mean less than 3 grams of fat per serving. "Reduced fat" will mean at least a 50% reduction from the company's or industry's similar products. In general, "reduced" may be used if the food contains less than one-third the standard amount. "Less" and "fewer" may be used if the reduction is at least 25%.

The new regulations also will set uniform serving sizes for

all foods, stopping manufacturers from manipulating serving sizes to make their products appear low in undesirable products. It will also make it easier for the consumer to compare nutritional information of different brands. Currently, three different brands of yogurt will probably dispense nutritional information based on three different serving sizes. You would need a calculator to make a true comparison.

Under the regulations, health claims will be allowed only in the following areas: fat and heart disease, fat and cancer, sodium and high blood pressure, and calcium and osteoporosis. The rules will also restrict advertising the absence of an undesirable ingredient such as cholesterol if there was never any cholesterol in the product in the first place.

Although some of the manufacturers represented in this book have already made changes in their food labeling, many have not. Most of the changes mandated by these regulations will not appear until 1993.

How to Use This Book

Food Values: Fats and Cholesterol provides important information on thousands of foods: total grams of fat, grams of saturated, monounsaturated, and polyunsaturated fats; milligrams of cholesterol; and calories.

The foods are divided into forty-nine categories. If you don't find a food in the expected category, check the note at the beginning of that category, or refer to the Table of Contents. When products could be classified in more than one category, we have included a "see also" reference.

Each category begins with an alphabetical listing of generic food items, with fresh products listed before processed foods; for instance, fresh peaches come before canned peaches. Brand name products follow generic, alphabetized by the name that is *most easily recognized*, either the manufacturing company or the product itself. For instance, Campbells' soups are listed under Campbell, the manufacturer's name; Ortega sauces are listed under Ortega, the product line, rather than the manufacturer, Nabisco; Kit Kat candy bar is listed under Kit Kat, because it is better known by its product name than by the fact that it is a Hershey product.

Under each brand name, specific products are generally listed alphabetically; Aunt Jemima French toast, for example, precedes Aunt Jemima pancakes. We have found, however, as most alphabetizers do, that some items can be listed in more than one way. Split peas are under "s" in this book but might be under "p" in another. If you don't find a food under the first letter of the first word of its name, try looking for it under the first letter of another word in the name. The cross-references will help here, too.

Be sure to look for foods in the form in which you eat them: the way foods are prepared changes their nutrient values. A soup prepared with whole milk, for example, contains more fat, saturated fat, cholesterol, and calories than the same soup prepared with water.

We've used the portion sizes that Americans use—cups, ounces, or serving units—and when available, we've used two kinds of measures; for example, "3 cookies = 1 oz." Serving units are the easiest portions to measure: it's easier to count cookies than to weigh them. However, you can only compare serving units of the same weight. If a Brand X chocolate chip cookie weighs 1 ounce, and Brand Y chocolate chip cookie weighs 1/4 ounce, the Brand X cookie will contain more fat and cholesterol because it is larger. But the Brand X chocolate chip cookie might actually contain less fat and cholesterol per unit of weight. To compare the two products you would have to multiply the values for the Brand Y cookie by 4 to find out how much fat and cholesterol it contains per ounce. When two similar products of different sizes weigh more than an ounce, divide the values for each product by the number of ounces it contains, and then compare the values per ounce.

Please note the difference between weight measures and volume measures. Measuring cups measure fluid ounces. An ounce of water by weight fills a measuring cup to the 1-ounce line. But volume and weight are very different kinds of measures for solid foods. An ounce of unpopped popcorn, which is dense, wouldn't fill a measuring cup, for example, but an ounce of popped popcorn, which is airy, would fill more than one. In this book, portions for solid food given in ounces refer to weight. Fluid ounces (fl oz), cups (c), tea-spoons (t), and tablespoons (T) refer to volume measure-ments. Since we don't ordinarily weigh our food, we've given volume and weight measurements when both are available and useful. For example, we've indicated how much of a measuring cup would be filled by an ounce of a given cold cereal when this information is available.

All values given in this book are approximations. No two apples, chicken breasts, or rolls are exactly alike. Data repre-sent averages for several samples.

Figures provided by different sources may not be exactly comparable. The U.S. Department of Agriculture (USDA) and various manufacturers may use different analytical procedures to analyze nutrient content, and may round off the data in different ways. In the USDA *Composition of Food* series, the information source for generic and fresh food, values are given to hundredths and thousandths. We rounded off calorie figures to the nearest whole unit. For example, we list 68.4 calories as 68 calories and 68.5 calories as 69 calories. When an item contained less than .5 calories we listed the value as a "trace" (tr).

Many manufacturers use a simpler rounding-off system for calories, approved by the Food and Drug Administration, which regulates food labels. Calories between 0 and 20 may be given in increments of 2; between 20 and 50, in increments of 5; and above 50, in increments of 5 or 10. This means that there's no point in counting single calories when comparing products; a product listed as containing 197 calories, another as 195 calories, and a third as 200 calories may actually contain the same amount of food energy. For most practical purposes, these small differences don't matter. If you need about 2,000 calories a day, it doesn't matter if you get 2,005 one day and 1,991 the next.

This book contains the best and most complete information now available. When information about the content of a particular nutrient in a food is not available or has not been determined, we put a question mark in the appropriate column. Since food manufacturers constantly change recipes and product sizes and develop new products, some of the data contained here may quickly become outdated.

Calculating the Amount of Fat and Cholesterol in Your Diet

To get an idea of how many grams of fat and saturated fat and how many milligrams of cholesterol are in your present diet, keep a complete record of everything you eat and drink for three days, preferably including a weekend day. Right after you finish a meal or snack or cup of coffee, write down what you ate, how it was prepared, and the portion by volume (cups, tablespoons), weight (ounces, pounds), or units (one medium apple, one English muffin), or all three if you can. To get a feeling for different food sizes, measure your food when you are at home. For example, instead of just pouring milk from the carton over your cereal, pour it into a measuring cup first to see how much you use. Use tablespoons to measure the milk you pour into your tea or coffee. Look at the measurements on the side of a bar of butter or margarine and see how much you cut off when you butter your toast (a teaspoon? ½ teaspoon?). You may find that the portion sizes used in the book are smaller than the ones you use. For example, for many American adults, a typical main course portion of spaghetti is 2 cups, not the 1 cup portion listed as a portion here.

At the end of three days, look up the grams of fat, saturated, monounsaturated, and polyunsaturated fats, milligrams of cholesterol, and calorie values for every food on your list.

To calculate the total cholesterol in your diet for these three days, add the cholesterol figures together. To calculate your daily average, divide your total cholesterol figure by three.

As indicated earlier, the information you need about fat is not the average number of grams but the *percentage* of the calories in your diet that come from fats. We'll give you two ways to do this. We'll show you how to calculate the actual percentage of fats in your diet and we will also show you how to calculate the number of grams that equals the recommended percentages.

To calculate the percentage of total fat in your diet, you first need to find your daily average intake of calories and your average daily intake of fat. Simply total each category for the three days you've recorded and divide by three. Then, take your daily average intake of fat, multiply that number by 9, the number of calories in a gram of fat, and divide that total by your average daily intake of calories.

Percentage of Calories Provided by Total Fat =

$$\frac{85 \text{ grams (Ave. daily fat intake)} \times 9 \text{ grams (\# of grams in a cal. of fat)}}{2000 \text{ (Ave. daily caloric intake)}} = .38 \text{ or } 38\%$$

You can use the same formula for calculating the percentages of saturated, polyunsaturated, and monounsaturated fats. Simply multiply the average daily intake of each by 9, and divide by the average total caloric intake.

Percentage of Calories Provided by Individual Fats =

$$\frac{\text{Average daily intake of SFA, PFA or MFA} \times 9}{\text{Average Daily Caloric Intake}} = \begin{array}{l}\text{\% Calories}\\\text{from SFA,}\\\text{PFA or MFA}\end{array}$$

Sometimes it's easier to think in terms of grams of fat you can eat, rather than percentages. To find out how many grams of fat would equal 30% of your total calories you multiply your average total intake of calories by .3 and divide that by 9, the number of calories in each gram of fat.

Allowable Grams of Total Fat =

$$\frac{\begin{array}{c}2000 \text{ (Average total calories)} \times\\.3 \text{ (Allowable \%)}\end{array}}{9 \text{ (calories per gram of fat)}} = 67 \text{ grams}$$

You can also do this calculation in one step:

Average daily caloric × .033 = Grams of fat needed to supply 30% of daily caloric intake

To find the percentage of fats in your diet or the number of allowable grams of each in your diet, use either of the two following formulas.

Allowable Grams of Individual Fats =

$$\frac{\text{Allowable grams of fat}}{3} = \begin{array}{l}\text{Allowable grams of SFA,}\\\text{PFA or MFA}\end{array}$$

or:

Average daily caloric intake × .011 = Grams of fat needed to supply 10% of daily caloric intake

The following chart may be helpful to you.

Daily Calories	# Grams of Fat = 30% Daily Caloric Intake	# Grams of SFA, PFA or MFA = 10% Daily Caloric Intake
1500	50	16–17
1800	60	20
2000	67	22–23
2250	75	25
2500	83	27–28
2700	90	30
3000	100	33–34

Since values are not available for many foods, you may have to estimate these nutrients. To get a rough estimate you can get some idea of the "missing" values of prepared processed foods by checking the ingredient list on the label. By law, the ingredients are listed on the label in order of weight. If a fat or oil is at the beginning of the list, the product is probably high in fat.

If want to be more specific about your estimate you can look up the "missing value fat" in the "Fats, Oils and Shortenings" or "Butter and Margarine Spreads" sections of this book. For example, if hydrogenated soybean–cotton seed oil blends is your "missing value," you'll find that one cup consists of 218 grams of fat, of which 39 grams are saturated. That means that these blends are about 18% saturated fat:

$$\frac{39 \text{ grams of saturated fat}}{218 \text{ grams of total fat}} = .18 \text{ or } 18\%$$

If this book or the product label gives the number of grams of total fat in a product and you know from the ingredient list what kind of fat it contains, you can estimate the number of grams of specific fats in the food. For example, if the label says that one serving of the product contains 14 grams of fat, and the only fat listed as an ingredient is hydrogenated soy–bean cottonseed oil, which is 18% saturated, then the serving contains about 2½ grams of saturated fat (18% of 14 grams).

If you want to calculate the percentage of calories supplied by fat in a product by using information on the label, multiply the number of grams of total fat by 9 and divide by the total calories. The percentage of calories supplied by fat will be *much higher* than the percentage of weight that is fat, because fat has more than twice as many calories per unit weight then either protein or carbohydrate. For example, when milk is labeled 3.3% fat, that means that 3.3% of the weight of the milk is fat, but 49% of milk's calories come from fat. This is important to note: even some products that advertise themselves as less than 5% fat, or less than 2% fat, are actually comparatively fatty.

Nutrition is not a hard science; recommendations about the most healthful diet are made on the basis of the evidence we have now. That evidence is still incomplete—which is why, when it comes to diet, doctors often disagree. The one recommendation about which there is a consensus is the most healthful diet is a moderate, balanced one, which includes a variety of foods and tastes good enough so that people will stick to it. We hope this book will help you find tasty ways to reduce the amount of fat and cholesterol in your diet.

Explanation of table headings:

Portion	Serving size
Chol (mg)	Cholesterol in milligrams
Total Fat (g)	Total fat in grams
Satur'd Fat (g)	Saturated fat in grams
Mono Fat (g)	Monounsaturated fat in grams
Poly Fat (g)	Polyunsaturated fat in grams
Total Calor	Total calories

Sources

1. *Food Values of Portions Commonly Used, 14th Edition,*
   Jean A. T. Pennington and Helen Nichols Church, Harper
   & Row, 1985.
2. *Nutritive Value of Foods,* U.S. Department of Agriculture,
   Nutrition Information Service, Home and Garden Bulletin
   #72, revised 1981.
3. *Composition of Food Series,* U.S. Department of Agriculture, Science and Education Administration:

   8-1   *Dairy and Egg Products,* revised November 1976.
   8-3   *Baby Foods,* revised December 1978.
   8-4   *Fats and Oils,* revised June 1979.
   8-5   *Poultry Products,* revised August 1979.
   8-6   *Soups, Sauces and Gravies,* revised February 1980.
   8-7   *Sausages and Luncheon Meats,* revised September
         1980.
   8-8   *Breakfast Cereals,* revised July 1982.
   8-9   *Fruits and Fruit Juices,* revised August 1982.
   8-10 *Pork Products,* revised August 1983.
   8-11 *Vegetables and Vegetable Products,* revised August
         1984.
   8-12 *Nut and Seed Products,* revised September 1984.
   8-13 *Beef Products,* revised August 1986.
   8-14 *Beverages,* revised May 1986.
   8-15 *Finfish and Shellfish Products,* revised September
         1987.
   8-16 *Legumes and Legume Products,* revised December
         1986.

Information about brand-name products was supplied by the
food processing companies themselves or taken from the
above sources.

Abbreviations

c = cup
cal = calories
chol = cholesterol
diam = diameter
g = grams
lb = pounds
mg = milligrams
oz = ounces
pkg = package
pkt = packet
sat fat = saturated fat
T = tablespoon ≈ 2 t
t = teaspoon
tr = trace
var = varies
w/ = with
w/out = without
? = not available, or not known at this time
< = less than
≤ = less than or equal to

	Portion	Chol (mg)	Total Fat(g)	Satur'd Fat(g)	Mono Fat(g)	Poly Fat(g)	Total Calor

❑ ALCOHOLIC BEVERAGES
See BEVERAGES

❑ BABY FOOD *See* INFANT & TODDLER FOODS

❑ BAKING INGREDIENTS

	Portion	Chol (mg)	Total Fat(g)	Satur'd Fat(g)	Mono Fat(g)	Poly Fat(g)	Total Calor
baking powder, all types	1 t	0	0	0	?	?	5
baking soda	1 t	0	0	0	?	?	0
candied fruit							
apricot	1 medium	0	tr	?	?	?	101
cherry	3 large	0	tr	?	?	?	51
citron	1 oz	0	tr	?	?	?	89
fig	1 piece	0	tr	?	?	?	90
ginger root	1 oz	0	tr	?	?	?	95
peel of grapefruit/ lemon/orange	1 oz	0	tr	?	?	?	89
pineapple	1 slice	0	tr	?	?	?	120
cornmeal *See* FLOURS & CORNMEALS							
cornstarch *See* FLOURS & CORNMEALS							
flour *See* FLOURS & CORNMEALS							
pastry puff dough	1 oz	?	10	?	?	?	129
patty shell	1 shell	?	19	?	?	?	240
piecrust							
from mix w/vegetable shortening	2-crust 9" pie	0	93	23	?	?	1,485
from sticks	1/6 double crust = 2 oz	?	18	?	?	?	290
frozen	1/16 crust = 1 oz	?	8	?	?	?	130
graham cracker	4.8 oz	?	10	?	?	?	159
homemade w/vegetable shortening	for 9" pie	0	60	15	?	?	900
yeast							
baker's, dry, active	1 pkg	0	tr	tr	?	?	20
brewer's dry	1 T	0	tr	tr	?	?	25
torula	1 T	0	tr	tr	?	?	28

▪ BRAND NAME

Baker's
COCONUT

	Portion	Chol (mg)	Total Fat(g)	Satur'd Fat(g)	Mono Fat(g)	Poly Fat(g)	Total Calor
Angel Flake, bag	1/3 c	0	8	?	?	?	120

	Portion	Chol (mg)	Total Fat(g)	Satur'd Fat(g)	Mono Fat(g)	Poly Fat(g)	Total Calor
Angel Flake, can	⅓ c	0	9	?	?	?	110
Angel Flake Toasted	⅓ c	0	17	?	?	?	200

CHOCOLATE

	Portion	Chol (mg)	Total Fat(g)	Satur'd Fat(g)	Mono Fat(g)	Poly Fat(g)	Total Calor
Big Chip milk chocolate chips	¼ c	10	13	?	?	?	240
Big Chip semisweet chocolate chips	¼ c	0	13	?	?	?	220
German's sweet chocolate	1 oz	0	10	?	?	?	140
milk chocolate chips	1 oz	5	8	?	?	?	140
semisweet chocolate	1 oz	0	9	?	?	?	140
semisweet chocolate-flavored chips	¼ c	0	9	?	?	?	200
semisweet real chocolate chips	¼ c	0	11	?	?	?	200
unsweetened chocolate	1 oz	0	15	?	?	?	140
Davis							
baking powder	1 t	?	0	?	?	?	8
Hershey's							
milk chocolate chips	1 oz	10	12	?	?	?	150
milk chocolate chunks	1 oz	?	9	?	?	?	160
premium bakig bar	1 oz	?	8	?	?	?	140
semisweet chocolate chips, regular & miniature	¼ c or 1½ oz	0	12	?	?	?	220
semisweet chunks	1 oz	?	8	?	?	?	140
unsweetened baking chocolate	1 oz	0	16	?	?	?	190
vanilla milk chips	1½ oz	?	14	?	?	?	240
Nestle							
Toll House Premier White Treasures	1 oz	?	10	?	?	?	160
Toll House Merry Morsels	1 oz	?	5	?	?	?	140
Toll House Semisweet Chocolate Mini-Morsels	1 oz	?	8	?	?	?	140
Toll House Semisweet Mini-Morsels	1 oz	?	8	?	?	?	140
Toll House Milk Chocolate Morsels	1 oz	?	7	?	?	?	150
Toll House Butterscotch Flavored Morsels	1 oz	?	8	?	?	?	150
Toll House Milk Chocolate Treasures	1 oz	?	9	?	?	?	150
Semisweet Chocolate Baking Bars	1 oz	?	9	?	?	?	160
Unsweetened Chocolate Baking Bars	1 oz	?	14	?	?	?	180

	Portion	Chol (mg)	Total Fat(g)	Satur'd Fat(g)	Mono Fat(g)	Poly Fat(g)	Total Calor
Choco Bake Unsweetened Pre-melted Baking Chocolate	1 oz	?	16	?	?	?	190
Premier White Baking Bars	½ oz	?	5	?	?	?	80
Reese's							
peanut butter flavored chips	¼ c or 1½ oz	3	13	11	?	?	230

❏ BAKING MIXES

all-purpose biscuit/ pancake mix	½ c	?	8	?	?	?	240

cakes & pastries, prepared from mix *See* DESSERTS: CAKES, PASTRIES, & PIES
pancakes, prepared from mix *See* BREAKFAST FOODS, PREPARED
pie fillings *See* DESSERTS: CUSTARDS, GELATINS, PUDDINGS, & PIE FILLINGS
waffles, prepared from mix *See* BREAKFAST FOODS, PREPARED

▪ BRAND NAME

Arrowhead Mills

	Portion	Chol (mg)	Total Fat(g)	Satur'd Fat(g)	Mono Fat(g)	Poly Fat(g)	Total Calor
biscuit mix	2 oz	tr	1	?	?	?	100
blue corn muffin mix	1 muffin	?	4	?	?	?	110
bran muffin mix	2 muffins	tr	7	?	?	?	270
corn bread mix	1 oz	tr	1	?	?	?	100
wheat free oat bran muffin mix	1 muffin	?	5	?	?	?	100

Aunt Jemima

Easy Mix coffee cake	1.3 oz	1	4	1	2	<1	156
Easy Mix corn bread	1.7 oz	13	6	1	2	1	196

Betty Crocker

SUPER MOIST CAKE MIXES

butter pecan	¹/₁₂ cake	55	11	3	4	4	250
No cholesterol recipe	¹/₁₂ cake	0	4	2	3	2	220
butter yellow	¹/₁₂ cake	75	11	6	4	1	260
carrot	¹/₁₂ cake	55	10	2	4	4	250
No cholesterol recipe	¹/₁₂ cake	0	6	2	2	2	210
chocolate chip	¹/₁₂ cake	55	15	3	6	6	290
No cholesterol recipe	¹/₁₂ cake	0	8	2	4	2	220
chocolate fudge	¹/₁₂ cake	55	12	3	5	4	260
devil's food	¹/₁₂ cake	55	12	3	5	4	260
No cholesterol recipe	¹/₁₂ cake	0	7	2	3	2	220
german chocolate	¹/₁₂ cake	55	12	3	5	4	260
No cholesterol recipe	¹/₁₂ cake	0	7	2	3	2	220
golden vanilla	¹/₁₂ cake	55	14	3	5	6	260
No cholesterol recipe	¹/₁₂ cake	0	7	2	3	2	220
lemon	¹/₁₂ cake	55	11	3	4	4	260
No cholesterol recipe	¹/₁₂ cake	0	7	2	3	2	220

	Portion	Chol (mg)	Total Fat(g)	Satur'd Fat(g)	Mono Fat(g)	Poly Fat(g)	Total Calor
marble	1/12 cake	55	11	3	4	4	260
No cholesterol recipe	1/12 cake	0	7	2	3	2	220
milk chocolate	1/12 cake	55	12	3	5	4	260
No cholesterol recipe	1/12 cake	0	7	2	3	2	210
sour cream chocolate	1/12 cake	55	12	3	5	4	260
No cholesterol recipe	1/12 cake	0	8	2	4	2	220
spice	1/12 cake	55	11	3	4	4	260
No cholesterol recipe	1/12 cake	0	7	2	3	2	220
white	1/12 cake	0	9	2	3	4	240
No cholesterol recipe	1/12 cake	0	7	2	3	2	220
yellow	1/12 cake	55	11	3	4	4	260
No cholesterol recipe	1/12 cake	0	7	2	3	2	220

MICRORAVE CAKE MIXES

	Portion	Chol (mg)	Total Fat(g)	Satur'd Fat(g)	Mono Fat(g)	Poly Fat(g)	Total Calor
apple streusel	1/6 cake	45	11	3	5	3	240
No cholesterol recipe	1/6 cake	0	8	2	3	<1	210
cinnamon pecan streusel	1/6 cake	35	12	3	6	3	280
No cholesterol recipe	1/6 cake	0	7	2	4	1	230
devil's food/chocolate frosting	1/6 cake	35	17	5	6	6	310
No cholesterol recipe	1/6 cake	0	9	3	4	2	240
german chocolate/ coconut pecan frosting	1/6 cake	35	18	5	7	6	320
yellow/chocolate frosting	1/6 cake	35	17	4	7	6	300
No cholesterol recipe	1/6 cake	0	9	3	4	2	230

SUPER MOIST LIGHT CAKE MIXES

	Portion	Chol (mg)	Total Fat(g)	Satur'd Fat(g)	Mono Fat(g)	Poly Fat(g)	Total Calor
devil's food	1/12 cake	55	4	2	1	<1	200
No cholesterol recipe	1/12 cake	0	3	1	1	<1	180
white	1/12 cake	0	3	1	1	<1	180
yellow	1/12 cake	55	4	2	1	<1	200
No cholesterol recipe	1/12 cake	0	3	1	1	<1	190

ANGEL FOOD CAKE MIXES

	Portion	Chol (mg)	Total Fat(g)	Satur'd Fat(g)	Mono Fat(g)	Poly Fat(g)	Total Calor
confetti	1/12 cake	0	0	?	?	?	150
lemon custard	1/12 cake	0	0	?	?	?	150
traditional	1/12 cake	0	0	?	?	?	130

CLASSIC DESSERT MIXES

	Portion	Chol (mg)	Total Fat(g)	Satur'd Fat(g)	Mono Fat(g)	Poly Fat(g)	Total Calor
Boston creme pie	1/8 pie	?	6	?	?	?	270
gingerbread mix	1/9 cake	30	7	2	4	<1	220
No cholesterol recipe	1/9 cake	0	6	2	3	<1	?
golden pound cake	1/12 cake	35	9	3	5	1	200
lemon chiffon cake mix	1/12 cake	?	5	?	?	?	200
pineapple upsidedown cake	1/9 cake	40	10	4	5	4	250
No cholesterol recipe	1/9 cake	0	9	3	5	1	240
chocolate pudding cake	1/6 cake	?	5	?	?	?	230
lemon pudding cake	1/6 cake	?	5	?	?	?	230

	Portion	Chol (mg)	Total Fat(g)	Satur'd Fat(g)	Mono Fat(g)	Poly Fat(g)	Total Calor
MICRORAVE SINGLES							
devil's food cake	1 cake	50	10	3	5	2	250
w/chocolate RTS frosting	1 cake	50	18	6	10	2	440
yellow cake	1 cake	50	11	3	6	2	260
w/chocolate RTS frosting	1 cake	50	19	6	10	3	440
brownie mix	1 brownie	0	9	2	5	2	240
w/hot fudge topping	1 brownie	0	12	3	6	3	350
CREAMY DELUXE READY-TO-SPREAD FROSTING							
butter pecan	1/12 tub	0	7	2	4	<1	170
cherry	1/12 tub	0	6	2	3	<1	160
chocolate	1/12 tub	0	7	2	4	<1	160
chocolate chip	1/12 tub	0	7	3	3	<1	170
coconut pecan	1/12 tub	0	9	3	5	1	160
cream cheese	1/12 tub	0	7	2	4	<1	170
dark dutch fudge	1/12 tub	0	7	2	4	<1	160
lemon	1/12 tub	0	6	2	3	<1	170
milk chocolate	1/12 tub	0	6	2	3	<1	160
sour cream chocolate	1/12 tub	0	7	2	4	<1	160
sour cream white	1/12 tub	0	6	2	3	<1	160
vanilla	1/12 tub	0	6	2	3	<1	160
chocolate w/dinosaurs	1/12 tub	0	7	2	4	<1	160
chocolate w/candy coated choc. chips	1/12 tub	0	7	2	4	<1	160
chocolate w/turbo racers	1/12 tub	0	7	2	4	<1	160
vanilla w/teddy bears	1/12 tub	0	6	2	3	<1	160
CREAMY DELUXE LIGHT READY-TO-SPREAD FROSTING							
chocolate	1/12 tub	0	2	1	1	0	130
milk chocolate	1/12 tub	0	2	1	1	0	140
vanilla	1/12 tub	0	2	1	1	0	140
CREAMY FROSTING MIX							
chocolate fudge	1/2 frosting	0	6	2	3	1	180
coconut pecan	1/2 frosting	0	8	3	3	2	150
creamy milk chocolate	1/2 frosting	0	5	1	3	1	170
creamy vanilla	1/2 frosting	0	5	1	3	1	170
FLUFFY FROSTING MIX							
white	1/2 frosting	0	0	?	?	?	70
MUFFIN MIXES							
apple cinnamon	1 muffin	25	4	1	2	1	120
No cholesterol recipe	1 muffin	0	3	1	1	1	110
banana nut	1 muffin	25	5	1	3	1	120
No cholesterol recipe	1 muffin	0	4	1	2	1	110
oat bran	1 muffin	35	8	2	4	2	190
No cholesterol recipe	1 muffin	0	7	2	3	2	180
wild blueberry	1 muffin	25	4	1	2	1	120
No cholesterol recipe	1 muffin	0	3	<1	2	<1	110

	Portion	Chol (mg)	Total Fat(g)	Satur'd Fat(g)	Mono Fat(g)	Poly Fat(g)	Total Calor
twice the bluberries	1 muffin	20	4	1	2	1	120
No cholesterol recipe	1 muffin	0	3	1	1	1	110
light muffins							
wild strawberry	1 muffin	20	<1	?	?	?	70
No cholesterol recipe	1 muffin	0	<1	?	?	?	70
BROWNIE MIXES							
supreme caramel	1 brownie	10	4	1	2	1	120
supreme chocolate chip	1 brownie	10	6	2	2	2	140
supreme frosted	1 brownie	10	6	2	2	2	160
fudge-regular size	1 brownie	15	6	1	3	2	150
supreme German chocolate	1 brownie	10	7	2	3	2	160
supreme original	1 brownie	10	6	1	3	2	140
supreme walnut	1 brownie	10	7	1	3	3	140
LIGHT BROWNIES							
fudge	1 brownie	0	1	?	?	?	100
MICRORAVE BROWNIES							
frosted	1 brownie	0	7	2	4	1	180
fudge	1 brownie	0	6	2	3	1	150
walnut	1 brownie	0	7	2	3	2	160
BIG BATCH COOKIE MIX							
chocolate chip	2 cookies	?	6	?	?	?	120
PIE CRUST							
mix	1/16 package	0	8	2	5	<1	120
sticks	1/8 stick	0	8	2	5	<1	120
Dromedary							
corn bread, prepared	2" times 2" piece	?	3	?	?	?	130
corn muffin, prepared	1 muffin	?	4	?	?	?	120
gingerbread, prepared	2" times 2" piece	?	2	?	?	?	100
pound cake, prepared	1/2" slice	?	6	?	?	?	150
Flako							
corn muffin mix	1 oz	?	3	1	1	<1	196
pie crust mix	1.7 oz	9	15	5	5	2	116
Hain							
apple/cinnamon oat bran muffin mix	1 muffin	0	3	?	?	?	140
banana nut oat bran muffin mix	1 muffin	0	4	?	?	?	140
walnut wheat baking mix	1 1/2 oz	?	1	?	?	?	150
Royal							
chocolate mousse pie mix	1/8 pie	0	4	0	?	?	130
lemon meringue pie mix	1/8 pie	?	5	?	?	?	210

	Portion	Chol (mg)	Total Fat(g)	Satur'd Fat(g)	Mono Fat(g)	Poly Fat(g)	Total Calor
lite cheese cake mix	⅛ pie	5	3	0	?	?	130
real cheese cake mix	⅛ pie	?	3	?	?	?	160

❏ BEANS *See* LEGUMES & LEGUME PRODUCTS

❏ BEEF, FRESH & CURED
See also PROCESSED MEAT & POULTRY PRODUCTS

Beef, Fresh

BRISKET

Lean & Fat

	Portion	Chol (mg)	Total Fat(g)	Satur'd Fat(g)	Mono Fat(g)	Poly Fat(g)	Total Calor
whole, all grades, braised	3 oz cooked	79	28	11	?	?	332
flat half, all grades, braised	3 oz cooked	78	30	12	?	?	347
point half, all grades, braised	3 oz cooked	81	25	10	?	?	311

Lean Only

whole, all grades, braised	3 oz cooked	79	11	4	?	?	205
flat half, all grades, braised	3 oz cooked	77	13	5	?	?	223
point half, all grades, braised	3 oz cooked	81	7	3	?	?	181

CHUCK, ARM ROAST

Lean & Fat

all grades, braised	3 oz cooked	84	22	9	?	?	297
choice, braised	3 oz cooked	84	23	9	?	?	301
good, braised	3 oz cooked	84	21	9	?	?	287
prime, braised	3 oz cooked	84	26	11	?	?	332

Lean Only

all grades, braised	3 oz cooked	85	8	3	?	?	196
choice, braised	3 oz cooked	85	7	3	?	?	199
good, braised	3 oz cooked	85	8	3	?	?	189
prime, braised	3 oz cooked	85	11	4	?	?	222

	Portion	Chol (mg)	Total Fat(g)	Satur'd Fat(g)	Mono Fat(g)	Poly Fat(g)	Total Calor
CHUCK, BLADE ROAST							
Lean & Fat							
all grades, braised	3 oz cooked	87	26	11	?	?	325
choice, braised	3 oz cooked	87	26	11	?	?	330
good, braised	3 oz cooked	88	24	10	?	?	311
prime, braised	3 oz cooked	87	29	12	?	?	354
Lean Only							
all grades, braised	3 oz cooked	90	13	5	?	?	230
choice, braised	3 oz cooked	90	13	5	?	?	234
good, braised	3 oz cooked	90	12	5	?	?	218
prime, braised	3 oz cooked	90	17	7	?	?	270
FLANK							
Lean & Fat							
choice							
braised	3 oz cooked	61	13	6	?	?	218
broiled	3 oz cooked	60	14	6	?	?	216
Lean Only							
choice							
braised	3 oz cooked	60	12	5	?	?	208
broiled	3 oz cooked	60	13	5	?	?	207
GROUND BEEF							
Extra Lean							
baked							
medium	3 oz cooked	70	14	5	?	?	213
well done	3 oz cooked	91	14	5	?	?	232
broiled							
medium	3 oz cooked	71	14	5	?	?	217
well done	3 oz cooked	84	13	5	?	?	225
pan-fried							
medium	3 oz cooked	69	14	5	?	?	216

	Portion	Chol (mg)	Total Fat(g)	Satur'd Fat(g)	Mono Fat(g)	Poly Fat(g)	Total Calor
well done	3 oz cooked	79	14	5	?	?	224
Lean							
baked							
medium	3 oz cooked	66	16	6	?	?	227
well done	3 oz cooked	84	16	6	?	?	248
broiled							
medium	3 oz cooked	74	16	6	?	?	231
well done	3 oz cooked	86	15	6	?	?	238
pan-fried							
medium	3 oz cooked	71	16	6	?	?	234
well done	3 oz cooked	81	15	6	?	?	235
Regular							
baked							
medium	3 oz cooked	74	18	7	?	?	244
well done	3 oz cooked	92	18	7	?	?	269
broiled							
medium	3 oz cooked	76	18	7	?	?	246
well done	3 oz cooked	86	17	7	?	?	248
pan-fried							
medium	3 oz cooked	75	19	8	?	?	260
well done	3 oz cooked	83	16	6	?	?	243
GROUND, FROZEN PATTIES							
broiled, medium	3 oz cooked	80	17	7	?	?	240
RIB, WHOLE (RIBS 6–12)							
Lean & Fat							
all grades							
broiled	3 oz cooked	73	25	11	?	?	308
roasted	3 oz cooked	72	27	11	?	?	324
choice							
broiled	3 oz cooked	73	26	11	?	?	313
roasted	3 oz cooked	72	27	12	?	?	328

	Portion	Chol (mg)	Total Fat(g)	Satur'd Fat(g)	Mono Fat(g)	Poly Fat(g)	Total Calor
good							
broiled	3 oz cooked	72	23	10	?	?	289
roasted	3 oz cooked	72	25	11	?	?	306
prime							
broiled	3 oz cooked	73	30	13	?	?	347
roasted	3 oz cooked	73	31	13	?	?	361
Lean Only							
all grades							
broiled	3 oz cooked	69	11	5	?	?	194
roasted	3 oz cooked	68	12	5	?	?	204
choice							
broiled	3 oz cooked	69	12	5	?	?	198
roasted	3 oz cooked	68	12	5	?	?	209
good							
broiled	3 oz cooked	69	10	4	?	?	181
roasted	3 oz cooked	68	10	4	?	?	191
prime							
broiled	3 oz cooked	69	16	7	?	?	238
roasted	3 oz cooked	68	17	7	?	?	248

RIB, EYE, SMALL END (RIBS 10–12)

Lean & Fat

	Portion	Chol (mg)	Total Fat(g)	Satur'd Fat(g)	Mono Fat(g)	Poly Fat(g)	Total Calor
choice, broiled	3 oz cooked	70	18	7	?	?	250

Lean Only

	Portion	Chol (mg)	Total Fat(g)	Satur'd Fat(g)	Mono Fat(g)	Poly Fat(g)	Total Calor
choice, broiled	3 oz cooked	68	10	4	?	?	191

RIB, LARGE END (RIBS 6–9)

Lean & Fat

	Portion	Chol (mg)	Total Fat(g)	Satur'd Fat(g)	Mono Fat(g)	Poly Fat(g)	Total Calor
all grades							
broiled	3 oz cooked	74	27	12	?	?	321
roasted	3 oz cooked	72	26	11	?	?	313
choice							
broiled	3 oz cooked	74	28	12	?	?	327

	Portion	Chol (mg)	Total Fat(g)	Satur'd Fat(g)	Mono Fat(g)	Poly Fat(g)	Total Calor
roasted	3 oz cooked	72	26	11	?	?	316
good							
broiled	3 oz cooked	73	25	11	?	?	301
roasted	3 oz cooked	72	24	10	?	?	304
prime							
broiled	3 oz cooked	74	32	14	?	?	361
roasted	3 oz cooked	72	29	13	?	?	346

Lean Only

	Portion	Chol (mg)	Total Fat(g)	Satur'd Fat(g)	Mono Fat(g)	Poly Fat(g)	Total Calor
all grades							
broiled	3 oz cooked	70	12	5	?	?	198
roasted	3 oz cooked	68	12	5	?	?	207
choice							
broiled	3 oz cooked	70	13	5	?	?	203
roasted	3 oz cooked	68	12	7	?	?	210
good							
broiled	3 oz cooked	70	10	4	?	?	183
roasted	3 oz cooked	68	11	5	?	?	197
prime							
broiled	3 oz cooked	70	18	8	?	?	250
roasted	3 oz cooked	68	16	7	?	?	241

RIB, SMALL END (RIBS 10–12)

Lean & Fat

	Portion	Chol (mg)	Total Fat(g)	Satur'd Fat(g)	Mono Fat(g)	Poly Fat(g)	Total Calor
all grades							
broiled	3 oz cooked	71	21	9	?	?	277
roasted	3 oz cooked	72	25	11	?	?	305
choice							
broiled	3 oz cooked	71	22	9	?	?	282
roasted	3 oz cooked	72	26	11	?	?	312
good							
broiled	3 oz cooked	71	19	8	?	?	263
roasted	3 oz cooked	72	22	9	?	?	283

	Portion	Chol (mg)	Total Fat(g)	Satur'd Fat(g)	Mono Fat(g)	Poly Fat(g)	Total Calor
prime							
broiled	3 oz cooked	71	25	10	?	?	309
roasted	3 oz cooked	72	31	13	?	?	357
Lean Only							
all grades							
broiled	3 oz cooked	68	10	4	?	?	188
roasted	3 oz cooked	68	11	5	?	?	201
choice							
broiled	3 oz cooked	68	10	4	?	?	191
roasted	3 oz cooked	68	12	5	?	?	206
good							
broiled	3 oz cooked	68	8	4	?	?	178
roasted	3 oz cooked	68	10	4	?	?	183
prime							
broiled	3 oz cooked	68	13	6	?	?	221
roasted	3 oz cooked	68	18	8	?	?	259
RIB, SHORT							
Lean & Fat							
choice, braised	3 oz cooked	80	36	15	?	?	400
Lean Only							
choice, braised	3 oz cooked	79	15	7	?	?	251
ROUND, FULL CUT							
Lean & Fat							
choice, broiled	3 oz cooked	71	16	6	?	?	233
good, broiled	3 oz cooked	71	14	6	?	?	222
Lean Only							
choice, broiled	3 oz cooked	70	7	2	?	?	165
good, broiled	3 oz cooked	70	6	2	?	?	157

	Portion	Chol (mg)	Total Fat(g)	Satur'd Fat(g)	Mono Fat(g)	Poly Fat(g)	Total Calor
ROUND, BOTTOM							
Lean & Fat							
all grades, braised	3 oz cooked	81	13	5	?	?	222
choice, braised	3 oz cooked	81	13	5	?	?	224
good, braised	3 oz cooked	81	12	5	?	?	215
prime, braised	3 oz cooked	81	16	6	?	?	253
Lean Only							
all grades, braised	3 oz cooked	81	8	3	?	?	189
choice, braised	3 oz cooked	81	8	3	?	?	191
good, braised	3 oz cooked	81	7	3	?	?	182
prime, braised	3 oz cooked	81	11	4	?	?	212
ROUND, EYE OF							
Lean & Fat							
all grades, roasted	3 oz cooked	62	12	5	?	?	206
choice, roasted	3 oz cooked	62	12	5	?	?	207
good, roasted	3 oz cooked	62	12	5	?	?	201
prime, roasted	3 oz cooked	61	13	5	?	?	213
Lean Only							
all grades, roasted	3 oz cooked	59	6	2	?	?	155
choice, roasted	3 oz cooked	59	6	2	?	?	156
good, roasted	3 oz cooked	59	5	2	?	?	151
prime, roasted	3 oz cooked	59	7	3	?	?	168
ROUND, TIP							
Lean & Fat							
all grades, roasted	3 oz cooked	70	13	5	?	?	213
choice, roasted	3 oz cooked	70	13	5	?	?	216
good, roasted	3 oz cooked	70	12	5	?	?	205

	Portion	Chol (mg)	Total Fat (g)	Satur'd Fat (g)	Mono Fat (g)	Poly Fat (g)	Total Calor
prime, roasted	3 oz cooked	71	16	7	?	?	242
Lean Only							
all grades, roasted	3 oz cooked	69	6	2	?	?	162
choice, roasted	3 oz cooked	69	7	2	?	?	164
good, roasted	3 oz cooked	69	6	2	?	?	156
prime, roasted	3 oz cooked	69	9	3	?	?	181
ROUND, TOP							
Lean & Fat							
all grades, broiled	3 oz cooked	72	7	3	?	?	179
choice							
broiled	3 oz cooked	72	8	3	?	?	181
pan-fried	3 oz cooked	82	15	6	?	?	246
good, broiled	3 oz cooked	72	7	3	?	?	176
prime, broiled	3 oz cooked	72	10	4	?	?	201
Lean Only							
all grades, broiled	3 oz cooked	72	5	2	?	?	162
choice							
broiled	3 oz cooked	72	5	2	?	?	165
pan-fried	3 oz cooked	83	7	2	?	?	193
good, broiled	3 oz cooked	72	5	2	?	?	156
prime, broiled	3 oz cooked	72	8	3	?	?	183
SHANK CROSSCUTS							
Lean & Fat							
choice, simmered	3 oz cooked	67	10	4	?	?	208
Lean Only							
choice, simmered	3 oz cooked	66	5	2	?	?	171

	Portion	Chol (mg)	Total Fat(g)	Satur'd Fat(g)	Mono Fat(g)	Poly Fat(g)	Total Calor
SHORT LOIN, PORTERHOUSE							
Lean & Fat							
choice, broiled	3 oz cooked	70	18	7	?	?	254
Lean Only							
choice, broiled	3 oz cooked	68	9	4	?	?	185
SHORT LOIN, T-BONE STEAK							
Lean & Fat							
choice, broiled	3 oz cooked	71	21	9	?	?	276
Lean Only							
choice, broiled	3 oz cooked	68	9	4	?	?	182
SHORT LOIN, TENDERLOIN							
Lean & Fat							
all grades							
broiled	3 oz cooked	73	15	6	?	?	226
roasted	3 oz cooked	74	19	8	?	?	258
choice							
broiled	3 oz cooked	73	15	6	?	?	230
roasted	3 oz cooked	74	19	8	?	?	262
good							
broiled	3 oz cooked	73	13	5	?	?	216
roasted	3 oz cooked	74	17	7	?	?	245
prime							
broiled	3 oz cooked	73	20	8	?	?	270
roasted	3 oz cooked	75	24	10	?	?	305
Lean Only							
all grades							
broiled	3 oz cooked	72	8	3	?	?	174
roasted	3 oz cooked	73	10	4	?	?	186
choice							
broiled	3 oz cooked	72	8	3	?	?	176

	Portion	Chol (mg)	Total Fat(g)	Satur'd Fat(g)	Mono Fat(g)	Poly Fat(g)	Total Calor
roasted	3 oz cooked	73	10	4	?	?	189
good							
broiled	3 oz cooked	72	7	3	?	?	167
roasted	3 oz cooked	73	9	3	?	?	177
prime							
broiled	3 oz cooked	72	11	4	?	?	197
roasted	3 oz cooked	73	13	5	?	?	217
SHORT LOIN, TOP							
Lean & Fat							
all grades, broiled	3 oz cooked	67	16	7	?	?	238
choice, broiled	3 oz cooked	68	17	7	?	?	243
good, broiled	3 oz cooked	67	14	6	?	?	223
prime, broiled	3 oz cooked	68	22	9	?	?	288
Lean Only							
all grades, broiled	3 oz cooked	65	8	3	?	?	172
choice, broiled	3 oz cooked	65	8	3	?	?	176
good, broiled	3 oz cooked	65	6	3	?	?	162
prime, broiled	3 oz cooked	65	12	5	?	?	208
WEDGE-BONE SIRLOIN							
Lean & Fat							
all grades, broiled	3 oz cooked	77	15	6	?	?	238
choice							
broiled	3 oz cooked	77	16	7	?	?	240
pan-fried	3 oz cooked	84	21	9	?	?	288
good, broiled	3 oz cooked	77	15	6	?	?	232
prime, broiled	3 oz cooked	77	19	8	?	?	271
Lean Only							
all grades, broiled	3 oz cooked	76	7	3	?	?	177

	Portion	Chol (mg)	Total Fat(g)	Satur'd Fat(g)	Mono Fat(g)	Poly Fat(g)	Total Calor
choice							
broiled	3 oz cooked	76	8	3	?	?	180
pan-fried	3 oz cooked	85	9	4	?	?	202
good, broiled	3 oz cooked	76	7	3	?	?	170
prime, broiled	3 oz cooked	76	10	4	?	?	201

Beef, Variety Meats

	Portion	Chol (mg)	Total Fat(g)	Satur'd Fat(g)	Mono Fat(g)	Poly Fat(g)	Total Calor
brains							
pan-fried	3 oz cooked	1696	13	3	?	?	167
simmered	3 oz cooked	1746	11	2	?	?	136
heart, simmered	3 oz cooked	164	5	1	?	?	148
kidneys, simmered	3 oz cooked	329	3	1	?	?	122
liver							
braised	3 oz cooked	331	4	2	?	?	137
pan-fried	3 oz cooked	410	7	2	?	?	184
lungs, braised	3 oz cooked	236	3	1	?	?	102
suet, raw	1 oz	19	27	15	?	?	242
tongue, simmered	3 oz cooked	91	18	8	?	?	241
tripe, raw	1 oz	27	1	1	?	?	28

Beef, Cured

	Portion	Chol (mg)	Total Fat(g)	Satur'd Fat(g)	Mono Fat(g)	Poly Fat(g)	Total Calor
breakfast strips, cooked	3 slices or 1/5 of 12 oz pkg	40	12	5	?	?	153
breakfast strips, cooked	6 oz	202	58	24	?	?	764
corned beef brisket, cooked	3 oz cooked	83	16	5	?	?	213
pastrami	1 oz	26	8	3	?	?	99

	Portion	Chol (mg)	Total Fat(g)	Satur'd Fat(g)	Mono Fat(g)	Poly Fat(g)	Total Calor

❑ BEVERAGES

See also MILK, MILK SUBSTITUTES, & MILK PRODUCTS
See also FAST FOODS

Beverages, Alcoholic

BEER & ALE

all types	1	0	0	0	?	?	?

COCKTAILS & MIXED DRINKS

Bloody Mary, daiquiri, gin & tonic, manhattan, martini, screwdriver, tequila sunrise, Tom Collins, whiskey sour	1	0	0 or tr	0 or tr	?	?	?
eggnog *See* FLAVORED MILK BEVERAGES, below							
piña colada, canned	6–8 fl oz	?	17	15	?	?	525
piña colada cocktail	4½ fl oz	0	3	1	?	?	262

CORDIALS & LIQUEURS

54 proof (22.1% alcohol by weight)	1 fl oz	0	0	0	?	?	97
coffee liqueur (53 proof)	1½ fl oz	0	tr	tr	?	?	174
coffee w/cream liqueur (34 proof)	1½ fl oz	?	7	5	?	?	154
crème de menthe liqueur (72 proof)	1½ fl oz	0	tr	tr	?	?	186

DISTILLED SPIRITS

gin, rum, vodka, whiskey 100 proof	1 fl oz	0	0	0	?	?	82
94 proof	1 fl oz	0	0	0	?	?	76
gin, 90 proof	1½ fl oz	0	0	0	?	?	110
rum, 80 proof	1½ fl oz	0	0	0	?	?	97
vodka, 80 proof	1½ fl oz	0	0	0	?	?	97
whiskey, 86 proof	1½ fl oz	0	0	0	?	?	105

WINES

dessert wine, sweet, 18.8% alcohol by volume	1 fl oz	0	0	0	?	?	46
table wine, 11½% alcohol by volume							
red	1 fl oz	0	0	0	?	?	21
rosé	1 fl oz	0	0	0	?	?	21
white	1 fl oz	0	0	0	?	?	20

	Portion	Chol (mg)	Total Fat(g)	Satur'd Fat(g)	Mono Fat(g)	Poly Fat(g)	Total Calor

Beverages, Carbonated

	Portion	Chol (mg)	Total Fat(g)	Satur'd Fat(g)	Mono Fat(g)	Poly Fat(g)	Total Calor
sodas, all flavors	12 oz	0	0	0	?	?	?

Coffees & Coffee Substitutes

	Portion	Chol (mg)	Total Fat(g)	Satur'd Fat(g)	Mono Fat(g)	Poly Fat(g)	Total Calor
coffee, brewed	6 fl oz	0	0	tr	?	?	4
coffee, instant, regular & decaffeinated, powder prepared w/water	6 fl oz water + 1 rounded t powder	0	0	tr	?	?	4
coffee substitute, cereal grain beverage, powder							
prepared w/water	6 fl oz water + 1 t powder	0	tr	tr	?	?	9
prepared w/whole milk	6 fl oz milk + 1 t powder	25	6	4	?	?	121

Fruit & Vegetable Juices

	Portion	Chol (mg)	Total Fat(g)	Satur'd Fat(g)	Mono Fat(g)	Poly Fat(g)	Total Calor
all types	1	0	0 or tr	0 or tr	?	?	?

Fruit Juice Drinks (10–50% Fruit Juice), Juice Ades, Juice-flavored Drinks & Powders

	Portion	Chol (mg)	Total Fat(g)	Satur'd Fat(g)	Mono Fat(g)	Poly Fat(g)	Total Calor
all types	1	0	0 or tr	0 or tr	?	?	?

Flavored Milk Beverages

	Portion	Chol (mg)	Total Fat(g)	Satur'd Fat(g)	Mono Fat(g)	Poly Fat(g)	Total Calor
carob flavor mix powder	3 t	0	0	tr	?	?	45
powder, prepared w/whole milk	1 c milk + 3 t powder	33	8	5	?	?	195
chocolate dairy drink mix, reduced cal, aspartame sweetened, powder prepared w/water	1/2 c water + 3 ice cubes + 1 3/4 oz pkt	?	1	tr	?	?	64
chocolate flavor mix powder	2–3 heaping t	0	1	tr	?	?	75
powder, prepared w/whole milk	1 c milk + 2–3 heaping t powder	33	9	5	?	?	226
chocolate milk							
low-fat, 1%	1 c	7	3	2	?	?	158
low-fat, 2%	1 c	17	5	4	?	?	179

	Portion	Chol (mg)	Total Fat(g)	Satur'd Fat(g)	Mono Fat(g)	Poly Fat(g)	Total Calor
whole	1 c	30	8	5	?	?	208
chocolate syrup							
w/added nutrients	1 T	0	tr	tr	?	?	46
prepared w/whole milk	1 c milk + 1 T syrup	33	8	5	?	?	196
w/out added nutrients	1 fl oz	0	tr	tr	?	?	82
prepared w/whole milk	1 c whole milk + 2 T syrup	33	9	5	?	?	232
cocoa, homemade w/whole milk	6 fl oz	24	7	4	?	?	164
cocoa, homemade w/whole milk	1 c	33	9	6	?	?	218
cocoa mix, powder, prepared w/water							
reduced-calorie, aspartame- sweetened,	6 fl oz water + 1/23 oz pkt	?	tr	tr	?	?	48
w/added nutrients	6 fl oz water + 1 pkt	?	3	2	?	?	120
w/out added nutrients	6 fl oz water + 3–4 heaping t powder	?	1	1	?	?	103
eggnog, dairy	1 c	149	19	11	?	?	342
eggnog flavor mix, powder, prepared w/whole milk	1 c whole milk + 2 heaping t powder	33	8	5	?	?	260

Malt & Chocolate Malt-flavored Beverages

	Portion	Chol (mg)	Total Fat(g)	Satur'd Fat(g)	Mono Fat(g)	Poly Fat(g)	Total Calor
gelatin, drinking, orange flavor, powder	1 pkt	?	tr	tr	?	?	67
malt beverage	12 fl oz	0	0	0	?	?	32
malted milk flavor mix, chocolate							
w/added nutrients							
powder	3/4 oz or 4–5 heaping t	?	1	tr	?	?	75
powder prepared w/whole milk	1 c whole milk + 4 or 5 heaping t powder	33	9	5	?	?	225
w/out added nutrients							
powder	3 heaping t or 3/4 oz	1	1	tr	?	?	79

	Portion	Chol (mg)	Total Fat(g)	Satur'd Fat(g)	Mono Fat(g)	Poly Fat(g)	Total Calor
powder prepared w/whole milk	1 c whole milk + 3 heaping t powder	34	9	6	?	?	229
malted milk flavor mix, natural w/added nutrients							
powder	¾ oz or 4–5 heaping t	?	1	tr	?	?	80
powder prepared w/whole milk	1 c whole milk + 4–5 heaping t powder	33	9	5	?	?	230
w/out added nutrients							
powder	¾ oz or 3 heaping t	4	2	1	?	?	87
powder prepared w/whole milk	1 c whole milk + 3 heaping t powder	37	10	6	?	?	237
shake, thick							
chocolate	10 oz	30	8	5	?	?	335
vanilla	10 oz	33	9	5	?	?	315
strawberry flavor mix, powder, prepared w/whole milk	1 c milk + 2–3 heaping t powder	33	8	5	?	?	234

Tea

	Portion	Chol (mg)	Total Fat(g)	Satur'd Fat(g)	Mono Fat(g)	Poly Fat(g)	Total Calor
brewed	6 fl oz	0	0	0	?	?	2
herb, brewed	6 fl oz	0	0	0	?	?	0
iced							
lemon flavored, from instant	1.3 g powder in 8 fl oz water	0	0	0	?	?	2
sugar sweetened	12 fl oz	0	0	0	?	?	146
instant, powder							
low cal, sodium saccharin sweetened, lemon flavored	2 t	0	0	0	?	?	5
sugar sweetened, lemon flavored	3 rounded t	0	tr	tr	?	?	87
sweetened	3 t in 8 fl oz water	0	tr	tr	?	?	86
unsweetened,	1 t	0	0	0	?	?	2
unsweetened, lemon flavored	1 rounded t	0	0	0	?	?	4

	Portion	Chol (mg)	Total Fat(g)	Satur'd Fat(g)	Mono Fat(g)	Poly Fat(g)	Total Calor
water							
municipal	1 c	0	0	0	?	?	0

▪ BRAND NAME

Carnation's
hot cocoa mix
rich chocolate	1 envelope	<1	1	<1	<1	<1	110
with marshmallows	1 envelope	<1	1	<1	<1	<1	110
with chocolate marshmallows	1 envelope	2	1	<1	<1	<1	110
milk chocolate	1 envelope	1	1	<1	<1	<1	110
70–calorie	1 envelope	1	<1	<1	<1	<1	70
sugar free diet	1 envelope	1	<1	<1	<1	<1	25
sugar free rich chocolate	1 envelope	3	<1	<1	<1	<1	50
sugar free mocha	1 envelope	2	<1	<1	<1	<1	50

malted milk
original flavor	3 heaping t	0	2	1	<1	<1	90
chocolate	3 heaping t	0	1	<1	<1	<1	80

Hershey's
cocoa	⅓ c	0	4	?	?	?	120
european cocoa	⅓ c	0	3	?	?	?	90

General Foods International Coffee
SWEETENED W/SUGAR
cafe Amaretto	6 fl oz	0	2	?	?	?	50
cafe Francais	6 fl oz	0	3	?	?	?	60
cafe Irish creme	6 fl oz	0	2	?	?	?	50
cafe Vienna	6 fl oz	0	2	?	?	?	60
Irish mocha mint	6 fl oz	0	2	?	?	?	50
suisse mocha	6 fl oz	0	3	?	?	?	50

SUGAR-FREE
cafe Francais	6 fl oz	0	2	?	?	?	35
cafe Vienna	6 fl oz	0	2	?	?	?	30
orange cappuccino	6 fl oz	0	2	?	?	?	30
suisse mocha	6 fl oz	0	2	?	?	?	30

Nestle
QUIK
chocolate flavor	approx. 2½ heaping t with 8 oz whole milk	?	9	?	?	?	230

	Portion	Chol (mg)	Total Fat(g)	Satur'd Fat(g)	Mono Fat(g)	Poly Fat(g)	Total Calor
chocolate flavor	approx. 2½ heaping t with 8 oz low fat 2% milk	?	5	?	?	?	210
chocolate flavor	approx. 2½ heaping t with 8 oz skim milk	?	1	?	?	?	170
sugar free chocolate flavor	approx. 2½ heaping t with 8 oz low fat 2% milk	?	5	?	?	?	140
strawberry flavor	approx. 2½ heaping t with 8 oz whole milk	?	8	?	?	?	220
strawberry flavor	approx. 2½ heaping t with 8 oz low fat 2% milk	?	5	?	?	?	200
strawberry flavor	approx. 2½ heaping t with 8 oz skim milk	?	0	?	?	?	160
ready to drink							
chocolate milk	8 oz	?	9	?	?	?	230
strawberry milk	8 oz	?	8	?	?	?	230
lite ready to drink							
chocolate low fat milk	8 oz	?	5	?	?	?	130
lowfat milk							
strawberry	8 oz	?	4	?	?	?	200
vanilla	8 oz	?	4	?	?	?	200
chocolate	8 oz	?	5	?	?	?	200
banana	8 oz	?	4	?	?	?	190

HOT COCOA MIX

	Portion	Chol (mg)	Total Fat(g)	Satur'd Fat(g)	Mono Fat(g)	Poly Fat(g)	Total Calor
rich chocolate flavor	1 oz with 6 oz whole milk	?	8	?	?	?	230
rich chocolate flavor	1 oz with 6 oz low fat 2% milk	?	5	?	?	?	210

	Portion	Chol (mg)	Total Fat(g)	Satur'd Fat(g)	Mono Fat(g)	Poly Fat(g)	Total Calor
rich chocolate flavor	1 oz with 6 oz skim milk	?	1	?	?	?	180
Ovaltine							
chocolate & malt	¾ oz dry mix	tr	tr	?	?	?	80
chocolate & malt	¾ oz dry mix w/8 oz 2% milk	20	5	?	?	?	200
cocoa							
hot 'n rich	1 oz or 5 t	?	3	?	?	?	120
50 cal	0.45 oz or about 2½ t	?	2	?	?	?	50
lactose free	1 oz	?	4	?	?	?	130
sugar free	0.41 oz or about 2½ t	?	1	?	?	?	40
Perrier							
water, bottled	1 c	0	0	0	?	?	0
Postum							
instant hot beverage	6 fl oz	0	0	0	?	?	12
coffee flavor instant hot beverage	6 fl oz	0	0	0	?	?	12
Swiss Miss							
HOT COCOA							
milk chocolate	6 oz mixed	5	1	?	?	?	110
bavarian chocolate	6 oz mixed	2	3	2	?	<1	110
double rich	6 oz mixed	0	1	?	?	?	110
COCOA MIX							
with mini marshmallows	6 oz mixed	5	1	?	?	<1	110
diet	6 oz mixed	2	<1	?	?	?	20
sugar free	6 oz mixed	2	<1	?	?	?	50
with sugar free marshmallows	6 oz mixed	1	<1	?	?	?	70
lite	6 oz mixed	1	<1	?	?	?	70

❑ BISCUITS *See* BREADS, ROLLS, BISCUITS, & MUFFINS

❑ BREADCRUMBS, CROUTONS, STUFFINGS, & SEASONED COATINGS

breadcrumbs							
enriched, dry, grated	1 c		5	5	2	?	?	390

	Portion	Chol (mg)	Total Fat(g)	Satur'd Fat(g)	Mono Fat(g)	Poly Fat(g)	Total Calor
white bread, enriched soft	1 c	0	2	1	?	?	120
bread cubes, white, enriched	1 c	0	1	tr	?	?	80
cornflake crumbs	1 oz	0	0	0	?	?	110
croutons, herb seasoned	7/10 oz	?	0	0	?	?	70
stuffing, from mix							
bread	1/2 c	?	12	?	?	?	198
cornbread	1/2 c	?	23	?	?	?	117
enriched bread							
dry type	1 c	0	31	6	?	?	500
moist type	1 c	67	26	5	?	?	420

▪ BRAND NAME

Betty Crocker
STUFFING MIX

	Portion	Chol (mg)	Total Fat(g)	Satur'd Fat(g)	Mono Fat(g)	Poly Fat(g)	Total Calor
chicken + 6 of added ingred.	1/6 package (1/2 c)	?	9	?	?	?	180
traditional herb + 6 of added ingred.	1/6 package (1/2 c)	?	8	?	?	?	180

Pepperidge Farm
CROUTONS

	Portion	Chol (mg)	Total Fat(g)	Satur'd Fat(g)	Mono Fat(g)	Poly Fat(g)	Total Calor
onion & garlic	1/2 oz	0	?	?	?	?	70
seasoned	1/2 oz	0	?	?	?	?	70
sour cream & chive	1/2 oz	0	?	?	?	?	70
cheese & garlic	1/2 oz	0	?	?	?	?	70

STUFFING

	Portion	Chol (mg)	Total Fat(g)	Satur'd Fat(g)	Mono Fat(g)	Poly Fat(g)	Total Calor
herb seasoned	1 oz	?	1	?	?	?	110
corn bread	1 oz	?	1	?	?	?	110
cubes	1 oz	?	1	?	?	?	110
country style	1 oz	?	1	?	?	?	100

DISTINCTIVE STUFFING

	Portion	Chol (mg)	Total Fat(g)	Satur'd Fat(g)	Mono Fat(g)	Poly Fat(g)	Total Calor
apple & raisin	1 oz	?	1	?	?	?	110
harvest vegetable & almond	1 oz	?	3	?	?	?	110
wild rice & mushroom	1 oz	?	5	?	?	?	130
classic chicken	1 oz	?	1	?	?	?	110

Progresso

	Portion	Chol (mg)	Total Fat(g)	Satur'd Fat(g)	Mono Fat(g)	Poly Fat(g)	Total Calor
plain	2 T	0	<1	?	?	?	60
italian style	2 T	0	<1	?	?	?	60

Rice-A-Roni Stuffing Mixes

	Portion	Chol (mg)	Total Fat(g)	Satur'd Fat(g)	Mono Fat(g)	Poly Fat(g)	Total Calor
chicken flavor	1 oz dry mix	<1	1	<1	<1	<1	106

	Portion	Chol (mg)	Total Fat(g)	Satur'd Fat(g)	Mono Fat(g)	Poly Fat(g)	Total Calor
corn bread	1 oz dry mix	<1	1	<1	<1	<1	105
herb & butter	1 oz dry mix	<1	1	<1	<1	<1	104
w/wild rice	1 oz dry mix	<1	1	<1	<1	<1	108
Shake 'n Bake oven fry coatings							
Italian herb recipe	¼ pouch	0	1	?	?	?	80
original recipe							
for chicken	¼ pouch	0	2	?	?	?	80
for fish	¼ pouch	0	1	?	?	?	70
for pork	¼ pouch	0	1	?	?	?	80
for pork barbeque	¼ pouch	0	2	?	?	?	80
country milk recipe	¼ pouch	0	4	?	?	?	80
extra crispy							
for chicken	¼ pouch	0	2	?	?	?	110
for pork	¼ pouch	0	3	?	?	?	120
homestyle for chicken	¼ pouch	0	2	?	?	?	80
Stove Top							
FLEXIBLE SERVING STUFFING MIX							
chicken flavor w/salted butter	½ c	15	9	?	?	?	170
cornbread flavor w/salted butter	½ c	15	9	?	?	?	180
homestyle herb w/salted butter	½ c	15	9	?	?	?	170
pork flavor	½ c	15	9	?	?	?	170
MICROWAVE STUFFING MIX							
broccoli & cheese w/salted butter	½ c	15	8	?	?	?	170
chicken flavor w/salted butter	½ c	10	7	?	?	?	160
homestyle cornbread w/salted butter	½ c	10	7	?	?	?	160
mushroom & onion flavor w/salted butter	½ c	10	7	?	?	?	170
STUFFING MIX							
Americana San Francisco w/salted butter	½ c	20	9	?	?	?	170
beef w/salted butter	½ c	20	9	?	?	?	180
chicken flavor w/salted butter	½ c	20	9	?	?	?	180
cornbread w/salted butter	½ c	20	9	?	?	?	170
long grain & wild rice w/salted butter	½ c	20	9	?	?	?	180

	Portion	Chol (mg)	Total Fat(g)	Satur'd Fat(g)	Mono Fat(g)	Poly Fat(g)	Total Calor
mushroom & onion w/salted butter	½ c	20	9	?	?	?	180
pork w/salted butter	½ c	20	9	?	?	?	170

❏ BREADS, ROLLS, BISCUITS, & MUFFINS

Biscuits

	Portion	Chol (mg)	Total Fat(g)	Satur'd Fat(g)	Mono Fat(g)	Poly Fat(g)	Total Calor
baking powder, prepared w/enriched flour & vegetable shortening							
from mix	1 (2″ diam)	tr	3	1	?	?	95
from refrigerator dough	1 (2″ diam)	1	2	1	?	?	65
homemade	1 (2″ diam)	tr	5	1	?	?	100
buttermilk, from refrigerator dough	2	?	6	?	?	?	130
flaky, from refrigerator dough	2	?	9	?	?	?	180

Bread & Bread Sticks

	Portion	Chol (mg)	Total Fat(g)	Satur'd Fat(g)	Mono Fat(g)	Poly Fat(g)	Total Calor
Boston brown bread, canned	1.6 oz slice	3	1	tr	?	?	95
bread sticks							
regular	1	?	tr	?	?	?	23
garlic	1	?	tr	?	?	?	26
sesame	1	?	4	?	?	?	56
coffee cakes *See* DESSERTS: CAKES, PASTRIES, & PIES							
cornbread							
from mix	2 oz	?	4	?	?	?	160
homemade							
w/enriched cornmeal	2.9 oz	?	7	?	?	?	198
w/whole-ground cornmeal	2.7 oz	?	7	?	?	?	172
cracked-wheat bread	1 lb loaf	0	16	3	?	?	1,190
cracked-wheat bread	0.9 oz slice	1	0	1	tr	?	65
danishes *See* DESSERTS: CAKES, PASTRIES, & PIES							
French bread	1 lb loaf	0	18	4	?	?	1,270
French bread	1.2 oz slice	0	1	tr	?	?	100
Vienna bread	0.9 oz slice	0	1	tr	?	?	70
fruit & nut quick bread, from mix	1.4 oz slice	?	2	?	?	?	118

	Portion	Chol (mg)	Total Fat(g)	Satur'd Fat(g)	Mono Fat(g)	Poly Fat(g)	Total Calor
honey wheatberry bread	1 oz slice	?	1	?	?	?	70
Italian bread, enriched	1 lb loaf	0	4	1	?	?	1,255
Italian bread, enriched	1 oz slice	0	tr	tr	?	?	85
matzo *See* CRACKERS							
mixed grain bread	1 lb loaf	0	17	3	?	?	1,165
mixed grain bread	0.9 oz slice	1	0	1	tr	?	65
oatmeal bread	1 lb loaf	0	20	4	?	?	1,145
oatmeal bread	0.9 oz slice	0	1	tr	?	?	65
pita bread, enriched, white	1 piece (6½″ diam)	0	1	tr	?	?	165
pumpernickel bread	1 lb loaf	0	16	3	?	?	1,160
pumpernickel bread	1.1 oz slice	0	1	tr	?	?	80
raisin bread, enriched	1 lb loaf	0	18	4	?	?	1,260
raisin bread, enriched	0.9 oz slice	0	1	tr	?	?	65
roman meal bread	1 slice	?	1	?	?	?	68
rye bread, light	1 lb loaf	0	17	3	?	?	1,190
rye bread, light	0.9 oz slice	0	1	tr	?	?	65
sourdough bread	1 oz slice	?	1	?	?	?	68
wheat bread, enriched	1 lb loaf	0	19	4	?	?	1,160
wheat bread, enriched	0.9 oz slice (18/ loaf)	0	1	tr	?	?	65
wheatberry bread	1 oz slice	?	1	?	?	?	70
white bread, enriched	1 lb loaf	0	18	6	?	?	1,210
white bread, enriched	0.9 oz slice	0	1	tr	?	?	65
white bread, enriched	0.7 oz slice	0	1	tr	?	?	55
whole-wheat bread	1 lb loaf	0	20	6	?	?	1,110
whole-wheat bread	1 slice (16/ loaf)	0	1	tr	?	?	70

Muffins

	Portion	Chol (mg)	Total Fat(g)	Satur'd Fat(g)	Mono Fat(g)	Poly Fat(g)	Total Calor
blueberry							
from mix	1.6 oz	45	5	1	?	?	140
homemade	1.6 oz	19	5	2	?	?	135
bran							
from mix	1.6 oz	28	4	1	?	?	140
homemade	1.6 oz	24	6	1	?	?	125
corn							
from mix	1.6 oz	42	6	2	?	?	145
homemade	1.6 oz	23	5	2	?	?	145
English	202	0	1	tr	?	?	140
English, sourdough	202	0	1	?	?	?	129

	Portion	Chol (mg)	Total Fat(g)	Satur'd Fat(g)	Mono Fat(g)	Poly Fat(g)	Total Calor
Rolls & Bagels							
bagel, plain or water enriched	1 (3½" diam)	0	2	tr	?	?	200
bagel, egg	1 (3½" diam)	44	2	tr	?	?	200
brown & serve roll	1	?	2	?	?	?	92
butterflake roll, from refrigerator dough	1	?	3	?	?	?	110
buttermilk roll, from mix	1	?	5	?	?	?	113
crescent roll, from refrigerator dough	2	?	10	?	?	?	200
croissant	2 oz	13	12	4	?	?	235
dinner rolls							
commercial	1 oz	tr	2	1	?	?	85
homemade	1.2 oz	12	3	1	?	?	120
frankfurter or hamburger roll	1 (8 per 11½ oz pkg)	1	tr	2	1	?	115
French bread roll, enriched	1	?	tr	?	?	?	137
hard roll, commercial	1.2 oz	tr	2	tr	?	?	155
hoagie or submarine roll	4.8 oz	tr	8	2	?	?	400
parkerhouse roll	0.6 oz	?	2	?	?	?	59
popover							
from mix	1	?	5	?	?	?	170
homemade	1.8 oz	?	5	?	?	?	112
raisin roll	2.1 oz	?	2	?	?	?	165
rye roll	0.6 oz	?	2	?	?	?	55
dark, hard	1 oz	?	1	?	?	?	80
light, hard	1 oz	?	1	?	?	?	79
sandwich roll	1.8 oz	?	3	?	?	?	162
sesame seed roll	0.6 oz	?	2	?	?	?	59
sweet roll See DESSERTS: CAKES, PASTRIES, & PIES							
wheat roll	0.6 oz	?	2	?	?	?	52
white rolls							
from mix	2	?	4	?	?	?	190
from refrigerator dough	1	?	1	?	?	?	90
homemade	1.2 oz	?	3	?	?	?	119
whole-wheat roll, homemade	1	?	1	?	?	?	90
Tortillas							
taco/tostada shell, corn	0.4 oz	?	2	?	?	?	50
tortilla, corn	1.1 oz	0	1	tr	?	?	65
canned	1.2 oz	?	1	?	?	?	75
tortilla, flour	1.1 oz	?	2	?	?	?	95

	Portion	Chol (mg)	Total Fat(g)	Satur'd Fat(g)	Mono Fat(g)	Poly Fat(g)	Total Calor

■ **BRAND NAME**

Health Valley
FAT-FREE MUFFINS

	Portion	Chol (mg)	Total Fat(g)	Satur'd Fat(g)	Mono Fat(g)	Poly Fat(g)	Total Calor
apple spice	1 muffin	0	<1	?	?	?	130
banana muffin	1 muffin	0	<1	?	?	?	130
raisin spice	1 muffin	0	<1	?	?	?	140
oat bran fancy fruit							
almond & dates	1 muffin	0	<1	?	?	?	140
raisin	1 muffin	0	<1	?	?	?	140
blueberry	1 muffin	0	<1	?	?	?	140
Old El Paso							
taco shells	1	?	3	?	?	?	55
super taco shells	1	0	6	?	?	?	100
tostada shells	1	0	5	?	?	?	100
mini taco shells	3	0	4	?	?	?	70
flour tortillas	1	?	3	?	?	?	150
Pepperidge Farm							
WHITE BREADS							
white thin sliced enriched	1 slice	0	2	0	0	0	80
toasting white sliced enriched	1 slice	0	1	0	0	0	70
sandwich white enriched	2 slices	0	2	0	0	0	130
1½ POUND BREADS							
hearty slice-seven grain	2 slices	0	2	0	0	1	180
oatmeal	1 slice	0	1	?	?	?	90
crunchy oat	2 slices	0	4	1	2	1	190
sesame wheat	2 slices	0	3	1	1	1	190
country white	2 slices	0	2	1	0	1	190
honey bran	1 slice	0	1	?	?	?	90
wheat	1 slice	0	2	?	?	?	90
HEARTH BREADS							
twin French enriched	1 oz	0	1	?	?	?	80
sliced soft rye	1 slice	0	1	0	0	0	70
sliced Italian	1 slice	0	1	0	0	0	70
brown & serve Italian enriched	1 oz	0	1	1	1	0	80
vienna thick sliced enriched	1 slice	0	1	0	0	0	70
fully baked French style enriched	1 oz	0	1	0	1	0	80
RYE/PUMPERNICKEL BREADS							
dijon rye	1 slice	0	1	0	0	0	50
thick sliced dijon rye	1 slice	0	1	0	0	0	70

	Portion	Chol (mg)	Total Fat(g)	Satur'd Fat(g)	Mono Fat(g)	Poly Fat(g)	Total Calor
family pumpernickel	1 slice	0	1	0	0	0	80
family rye	1 slice	0	1	0	0	0	80
seedless family rye	1 slice	0	1	0	0	0	80
party rye slices	4 slices	0	1	0	0	0	60
party pumpernickel slices	4 slices	0	1	0	0	0	60

VERY THIN SLICED BREADS

	Portion	Chol (mg)	Total Fat(g)	Satur'd Fat(g)	Mono Fat(g)	Poly Fat(g)	Total Calor
oatmeal	1 slice	0	1	?	?	?	40
white enriched	1 slice	0	1	?	?	?	40
wheat	1 slice	0	1	0	0	0	35

LIGHT STYLE BREADS

	Portion	Chol (mg)	Total Fat(g)	Satur'd Fat(g)	Mono Fat(g)	Poly Fat(g)	Total Calor
light vienna	1 slice	0	0	0	0	0	45
light oatmeal	1 slice	0	0	0	0	0	45
light wheat	1 slice	0	0	0	0	0	45

HEARTY SLICES

	Portion	Chol (mg)	Total Fat(g)	Satur'd Fat(g)	Mono Fat(g)	Poly Fat(g)	Total Calor
country white	2 slices	0	2	1	?	1	190
seven grain	2 slices	0	2	0	?	1	180
sesame wheat	2 slices	0	3	1	?	1	190
crunchy oat	2 slices	0	4	1	?	1	190

SWIRL BREADS

	Portion	Chol (mg)	Total Fat(g)	Satur'd Fat(g)	Mono Fat(g)	Poly Fat(g)	Total Calor
cinnamon	1 slice	0	3	0	?	0	90
raisin w/cinnamon	1 slice	0	2	0	?	0	90
date walnut	1 slice	0	3	0	?	2	90

VARIETY BREADS

	Portion	Chol (mg)	Total Fat(g)	Satur'd Fat(g)	Mono Fat(g)	Poly Fat(g)	Total Calor
oatmeal	1 slice	0	1	?	?	?	70
sprouted wheat sliced	1 slice	0	2	?	?	?	70

QUARTET ROLLS

	Portion	Chol (mg)	Total Fat(g)	Satur'd Fat(g)	Mono Fat(g)	Poly Fat(g)	Total Calor
croissant sandwich quartets	1 roll	?	7	?	?	?	170

DINNER ROLLS

	Portion	Chol (mg)	Total Fat(g)	Satur'd Fat(g)	Mono Fat(g)	Poly Fat(g)	Total Calor
country style classic	1 roll	0	1	0	1	0	50
12 dinner enriched	1 roll	<5	2	0	1	0	60
10 soft family enriched	1 roll	0	2	1	1	0	100
12 old fashioned enriched	1 roll	5	2	1	1	0	50
party 20 enriched	1 roll	0	1	0	0	0	30
finger poppy seed 12 enriched	1 roll	<5	2	0	1	0	50
parker house 12 enriched	1 roll	5	1	0	1	0	60

FRANKFURTER/HAMBURGER ROLLS

	Portion	Chol (mg)	Total Fat(g)	Satur'd Fat(g)	Mono Fat(g)	Poly Fat(g)	Total Calor
8 frankfurter rolls enriched (top sliced)	1 roll	0	3	1	1	0	140

	Portion	Chol (mg)	Total Fat(g)	Satur'd Fat(g)	Mono Fat(g)	Poly Fat(g)	Total Calor
8 frankfurter rolls enriched (side sliced)	1 roll	0	3	1	1	0	140
dijon frankfurter rolls	1 roll	0	5	1	1	1	160
8 frankfurter rolls with poppy seeds	1 roll	0	2	1	1	0	130
potato sandwich buns	1 roll	0	4	1	0	2	160
8 sliced hamburger enriched	1 roll	0	2	1	1	0	130

SANDWICH ROLLS

	Portion	Chol (mg)	Total Fat(g)	Satur'd Fat(g)	Mono Fat(g)	Poly Fat(g)	Total Calor
onion 8 sliced sandwich buns with poppy seeds	1 roll	0	3	1	1	1	150
sandwich 8 sliced sandwich buns with sesame seeds	1 roll	0	3	1	1	1	150

DELI CLASSIC ROLLS

	Portion	Chol (mg)	Total Fat(g)	Satur'd Fat(g)	Mono Fat(g)	Poly Fat(g)	Total Calor
salad sandwich rolls	1 roll	10	4	?	?	?	110
soft hoagie rolls	1 roll	0	5	1	2	1	210
brown 'n serve 2 french enriched	½ roll	0	2	1	1	0	180
brown 'n serve 3 french enriched	½ roll	0	1	0	1	0	120
brown 'n serve 6 club enriched	1 roll	0	1	0	0	0	100
brown 'n serve 12 hearth enriched	1 roll	0	1	0	0	0	50
heat 'n serve 6 golden twist enriched	1 roll	5	5	2	2	0	110
heat 'n serve 6 butter crescent enriched	1 roll	15	6	3	1	0	110
9 French style enriched	1 roll	0	1	0	0	0	100
9 sourdough style French enriched	1 roll	0	1	0	0	0	100
4 French style enriched	½ roll	?	2	?	?	?	120

CROISSANTS

	Portion	Chol (mg)	Total Fat(g)	Satur'd Fat(g)	Mono Fat(g)	Poly Fat(g)	Total Calor
petite all butter	1 croissant	?	6	?	?	?	120

CROISSANT TOASTER TARTS

	Portion	Chol (mg)	Total Fat(g)	Satur'd Fat(g)	Mono Fat(g)	Poly Fat(g)	Total Calor
cheese	1 tart	10	10	3	5	1	190
apple cinnamon	1 tart	0	7	2	4	0	170
strawberry	1 tart	0	7	2	4	0	190

ENGLISH MUFFINS

	Portion	Chol (mg)	Total Fat(g)	Satur'd Fat(g)	Mono Fat(g)	Poly Fat(g)	Total Calor
regular	1 muffin	0	1	0	0	0	140
cinnamon chip	1 muffin	0	3	0	0	0	160
cinnamon raisin	1 muffin	0	2	0	0	0	150
sourdough	1 muffin	0	1	0	0	0	135

	Portion	Chol (mg)	Total Fat(g)	Satur'd Fat(g)	Mono Fat(g)	Poly Fat(g)	Total Calor
cinnamon apple	1 muffin	0	1	0	0	0	140

OLD FASHIONED MUFFINS, FROZEN

banana nut	1 muffin	30	6	1	2	2	170
cholesterol free multi-grain muesli	1 muffin	0	8	1	3	2	200
cholesterol free oatbran with apple	1 muffin	0	7	1	3	2	190
corn	1 muffin	30	7	1	3	2	180
blueberry	1 muffin	25	7	1	3	2	170
cholesterol free raisin bran	1 muffin	0	6	1	2	2	170
cinnamon swirl	1 muffin	35	6	1	2	2	190

DANISH, FROZEN

apple	1 danish	?	8	?	?	?	220
cheese	1 danish	?	14	?	?	?	240
cinnamon raisin	1 danish	?	11	?	?	?	250

CINNAMON ROLLS

2-pack	2¼ oz	?	14	?	?	?	280

Pillsbury

BISCUITS

country	1 biscuit	0	1	0	?	0	50
buttermilk	1 biscuit	0	1	0	?	0	50
butter	1 biscuit	0	1	0	?	0	50
big country butter tastin'	1 biscuit	0	4	<1	?	0	100
big country buttermilk	1 biscuit	0	4	<1	?	0	100
ballard oven ready	1 biscuit	0	1	0	?	0	50
ballard oven ready buttermilk	1 biscuit	0	1	0	?	0	50
1869 brand baking powder	1 biscuit	0	5	1	?	0	100
1869 brand buttermilk	1 biscuit	0	5	1	?	0	100
1869 brand butter tastin'	1 biscuit	0	5	1	?	0	100
hungry jack extra rich buttermilk	1 biscuit	0	1	0	?	0	50
hungry jack flaky	1 biscuit	0	4	<1	?	0	80
hungry jack buttermilk fluffy	1 biscuit	0	4	1	?	0	90
good 'n buttery fluffly	1 biscuit	0	5	1	?	0	90
tender layer buttermilk	1 biscuit	0	1	0	?	0	50
hungry jack honey tastin' flaky	1 biscuit	0	4	<1	0	?	90
heat 'n eat buttermilk	2 biscuits	0	5	1	?	0	170
big premium heat 'n eat	2 biscuits	0	15	3	?	<1	280

BREADS

pipin' hot white loaf	1 inch slice	0	2	0	?	0	70

	Portion	Chol (mg)	Total Fat(g)	Satur'd Fat(g)	Mono Fat(g)	Poly Fat(g)	Total Calor
pipin' hot wheat loaf	1 inch slice	0	2	0	?	0	70
soft bread sticks	1 stick	0	2	<1	?	<1	100
crusty French loaf	1 inch slice	0	<1	0	?	0	60
cornbread twists	1 twist	0	<1	<1	?	0	70
DINNER ROLLS							
butter flavored butterflake	1 roll	0	5	1	?	0	140
crescent	1 roll	0	6	1	?	0	100
Sara Lee							
BAGELS							
plain	1	0	1	?	?	?	190
cinnamon & raisin	1	0	2	?	?	?	200
onion	1	0	1	?	?	?	190
poppy seed	1	0	1	?	?	?	190
sesame	1	0	1	?	?	?	190
oat bran	1	0	1	?	?	?	180
CINNAMON ROLLS							
all butter	1	?	11	?	?	?	230
L'ORIGINAL CROISSANTS							
all butter	1	?	9	?	?	?	170
petite size	1	?	6	?	?	?	120
free & light blueberry	1	0	3	?	?	?	150
ham & swiss cheese	1	20	16	?	?	?	310
cheese & broccoli	1	15	17	?	?	?	310
MUFFINS							
apple spice	1	0	8	?	?	?	220
blueberry	1	25	12	?	?	?	220
golden corn	1	40	14	?	?	?	260
raisin bran	1	0	7	?	?	?	220
oat bran	1	0	8	?	?	?	210
chocolate chunk	1	?	8	?	?	?	220
Weight Watchers							
MUFFINS							
banana nut	2½ oz	5	4	1	3	1	170
blueberry	2½ oz	10	5	1	3	1	170
BREAD							
white	1 slice	?	<1	?	?	?	40
wheat	1 slice	?	<1	?	?	?	40
rye	1 slice	?	<1	?	?	?	40
multi-grain	1 slice	?	<1	?	?	?	40
oatbran	1 slice	?	<1	?	?	?	40

	Portion	Chol (mg)	Total Fat(g)	Satur'd Fat(g)	Mono Fat(g)	Poly Fat(g)	Total Calor

❏ BREAKFAST CEREALS, COLD & HOT

Cold Cereal

	Portion	Chol (mg)	Total Fat(g)	Satur'd Fat(g)	Mono Fat(g)	Poly Fat(g)	Total Calor
corn flakes, low sodium	1 oz or about 1 c	?	tr	?	?	?	113
crisp rice, low sodium	1 oz or about 1 c	?	tr	?	?	?	114
granola, homemade	1 oz or about ¼ c	?	8	1	?	?	138
granola, homemade	1 c	?	33	6	?	?	595
oat flakes, fortified	1 oz or about ⅔ c	?	tr	?	?	?	105
oat flakes, fortified	1 c	?	1	?	?	?	177
rice, puffed	½ oz or about 1 c	?	tr	?	?	?	57
wheat, puffed, plain	½ oz or about 1 c (heaping)	?	tr	?	?	?	52
wheat, shredded large biscuit	2 round biscuits	?	1	?	?	?	133
small biscuit	1 oz or about ⅔ c	?	1	?	?	?	102
small biscuit	⅞ oz box	?	1	?	?	?	89
wheat germ, toasted, plain	1 oz or about ¼ c	?	3	1	?	?	108
wheat germ, toasted, plain	1 c	?	12	2	?	?	431
wheat germ, toasted, w/brown sugar & honey	1 oz or about ¼ c	?	2	tr	?	?	107
wheat germ, toasted, w/brown sugar & honey	1 c	?	9	2	?	?	426

Hot Cereal

	Portion	Chol (mg)	Total Fat(g)	Satur'd Fat(g)	Mono Fat(g)	Poly Fat(g)	Total Calor
corn grits, regular & quick							
dry	1 c	?	2	?	?	?	579
dry	1 T	?	tr	?	?	?	36
cooked	1 c	?	1	?	?	?	146
cooked	¾ c	?	tr	?	?	?	110
corn grits, instant, prepared							
plain	1 pkt	?	tr	?	?	?	82

	Portion	Chol (mg)	Total Fat(g)	Satur'd Fat(g)	Mono Fat(g)	Poly Fat(g)	Total Calor
w/artificial cheese flavor	1 pkt	?	1	?	?	?	107
w/imitation bacon bits	1 pkt	?	1	?	?	?	104
w/imitation ham bits	1 pkt	?	tr	?	?	?	103
oats, regular, quick, & instant (nonfortified)							
dry	1/3 c	?	2	tr	?	?	104
cooked	1 c	?	2	tr	?	?	145
cooked	3/4 c	?	2	tr	?	?	108
whole-wheat hot natural cereal							
dry	1/3 c	?	1	?	?	?	106
cooked	1 c	?	1	?	?	?	151
cooked	3/4 c	?	1	?	?	?	113

▪ BRAND NAME

Arrowhead Mills
COLD CEREAL

	Portion	Chol (mg)	Total Fat(g)	Satur'd Fat(g)	Mono Fat(g)	Poly Fat(g)	Total Calor
Arrowhead Crunch	1 oz	0	3	?	?	?	120
Bran Flakes	1 oz	0	1	?	?	?	100
Corn, Puffed	1/2 oz	0	0	?	?	?	50
Corn Flakes	1 oz	0	1	?	?	?	110
Granola							
Apple Amaranth	2 oz	0	6	?	?	?	225
Maple Nut	2 oz	0	9	?	?	?	260
Millet, Puffed	1/2 oz	0	0	?	?	?	50
Nature O's	1 oz	0	1	?	?	?	110
Oat Bran Flakes	1 oz	?	2	?	?	?	110
Rice, Puffed	1/2 c	0	0	?	?	?	50
Wheat Bran	2 oz	0	2	?	?	?	200
Wheat Flakes	1 oz	?	1	?	?	?	110
Wheat Germ, Raw	2 oz	0	6	?	?	?	210

HOT CEREAL

	Portion	Chol (mg)	Total Fat(g)	Satur'd Fat(g)	Mono Fat(g)	Poly Fat(g)	Total Calor
Bear Mush	1 oz	0	0	?	?	?	100
Corn Grits							
white	2 oz	0	1	?	?	?	200
yellow	2 oz	0	1	?	?	?	200
4 Grain & Flax	2 oz	0	1	?	?	?	94
Oat Bran	1 oz	0	2	?	?	?	110
Oatmeal, instant	1 oz	0	2	?	?	?	100
Oats, steel cut	2 oz	0	4	?	?	?	220
Rice & Shine	1/4 c	0	1	?	?	?	160
Seven Grain	1 oz	0	1	?	?	?	100

Erewhon
COLD CEREAL

	Portion	Chol (mg)	Total Fat(g)	Satur'd Fat(g)	Mono Fat(g)	Poly Fat(g)	Total Calor
Aztec	1 oz	0	0	?	?	?	100
Crispy Brown Rice, regular or low-sodium	1 oz	0	1	?	?	?	110

	Portion	Chol (mg)	Total Fat(g)	Satur'd Fat(g)	Mono Fat(g)	Poly Fat(g)	Total Calor
Fruit 'n Wheat	1 oz	0	1	?	?	?	100
Granola							
Date Nut	1 oz	0	6	?	?	?	130
Honey Almond	1 oz	0	6	?	?	?	130
Maple	1 oz	0	5	?	?	?	130
#9 w/Bran	1 oz	0	6	?	?	?	130
Spiced Apple	1 oz	0	6	?	?	?	130
Sunflower Crunch	1 oz	0	4	?	?	?	130
Right Start	1 oz	0	0	?	?	?	90
Right Start w/raisins	1 oz	0	0	?	?	?	90
Super O's	1 oz	0	0	?	?	?	110
Uncle Sam Laxative Cereal	1 oz	0	2	?	?	?	110

HOT CEREAL

	Portion	Chol (mg)	Total Fat(g)	Satur'd Fat(g)	Mono Fat(g)	Poly Fat(g)	Total Calor
Barley Plus	1 oz dry	0	1	?	?	?	110
Brown Rice Cream	1 oz dry	0	1	?	?	?	110
Instant Oatmeal							
apple cinnamon	1.25 oz	?	3	?	?	?	145
apple raisin	1.25 oz	?	3	?	?	?	150
maple spice	1.25 oz	?	3	?	?	?	140
raisins, dates & walnuts	1.25 oz	?	3	?	?	?	130
w/added oat bran	1.25 oz	?	3	?	?	?	125

Familia

	Portion	Chol (mg)	Total Fat(g)	Satur'd Fat(g)	Mono Fat(g)	Poly Fat(g)	Total Calor
Original	1.45 oz w/¹/₂ c milk	0	2	?	?	?	190
No sugar added	1.45 oz w/¹/₂ c milk	0	3	?	?	?	190
Crunchy Muesli	1.45 oz w/¹/₂ c milk	0	4	?	?	?	200
25% Bran	1.45 oz w/¹/₂ c milk	0	3	?	?	?	180

General Mills

COLD CEREAL

	Portion	Chol (mg)	Total Fat(g)	Satur'd Fat(g)	Mono Fat(g)	Poly Fat(g)	Total Calor
Basic 4	1.3 oz (³/₄ c)	0	2	?	?	?	130
Cheerios	1 oz (1¹/₄ c)	0	2	tr	?	?	110
regular							
apple-cinnamon	1 oz (³/₄ c)	0	2	?	?	?	110
honey nut	1 oz (³/₄ c)	0	1	tr	?	?	110
Cinnamon Toast Crunch	1 oz (³/₄ c)	0	3	?	?	?	120
Clusters	1 oz (¹/₂ c)	0	2	?	?	?	110
Cocoa Puffs	1 oz (1 c)	0	1	?	?	?	110
Country Corn Flakes	1 oz (1 c)	0	1	?	?	?	110
Crispy Wheats 'n Raisins	1 oz (³/₄ c)	0	1	?	?	?	100
Fiber One	1 oz (¹/₂ c)	0	1	?	?	?	60

	Portion	Chol (mg)	Total Fat(g)	Satur'd Fat(g)	Mono Fat(g)	Poly Fat(g)	Total Calor
Fruity Yummy Mummy	1 oz (1 c)	0	1	?	?	?	110
Golden Grahams	1 oz (¾) c	0	1	1	?	?	110
Kix	1 oz (1½ c)	0	1	tr	?	?	110
Lucky Charms	1 oz (1 c)	0	1	tr	?	?	110
Oatmeal Crisp	1 oz (½ c)	0	2	?	?	?	110
Oatmeal Raisin Crisp	1.2 oz (½ c)	0	2	?	?	?	130
Raisin Nut Bran	1 oz (½ c)	0	3	?	?	?	110
S'mores Grahams	1 oz (¾ c)	0	2	?	?	?	120
Total	1 oz (1 c)	0	1	tr	?	?	100
Total Corn Flakes	1 oz (1 c)	0	<1	?	?	?	110
Total Raisin Bran	1.5 oz (1 c)	0	1	?	?	?	140
Triples	1 oz (¾ c)	0	1	?	?	?	110
Trix	1 oz (1 c)	0	1	?	?	?	110
Wheaties	1 oz (1 c)	0	1	tr	?	?	100
Health Valley							
Amaranth w/Banana	1 oz (¼ c)	0	2	?	?	?	100
Amaranth Crunch w/Raisins	1 oz (¼ c)	0	3	?	?	?	110
Fat-Free granola							
almond/date	1 oz	0	<1	?	?	?	90
raisin/cinnamon	1 oz	0	<1	?	?	?	90
tropical	1 oz	0	<1	?	?	?	90
sprouts							
banana	1 oz	0	<1	?	?	?	90
raisin	1 oz	0	<1	?	?	?	90
Fruit Lites							
Corn	½ oz (½ c)	0	0	?	?	?	43
Rice	½ oz (½ c)	0	0	?	?	?	45
Wheat	½ oz (½ c)	0	0	?	?	?	43
Lites							
corn, rice or wheat, puffed	½ oz (½ c)	0	0	?	?	?	50
No Fat Added healthy crunch							
almond/date	1 oz	0	1	?	?	?	90
apple/cinnamon	1 oz	0	1	?	?	?	90
real oat bran							
almond/date	1 oz	0	1	?	?	?	90
hawaiian fruit	1.2 oz	0	1	?	?	?	100
raisin	1.2 oz	0	1	?	?	?	100
swiss breakfast							
raisin	1 oz	0	1	?	?	?	80
tropical fruit	1 oz	0	1	?	?	?	80

	Portion	Chol (mg)	Total Fat(g)	Satur'd Fat(g)	Mono Fat(g)	Poly Fat(g)	Total Calor
Oat Bran Flakes							
plain or w/almonds & dates	1 oz (1/2 c)	0	2	?	?	?	110
Sprouts 7, w/bananas & Hawaiian fruit or w/raisins	1 oz (1/4 c)	0	1	?	?	?	100
Heartland							
Natural Cereal, plain	1 oz	0	4	?	?	?	130
Natural Cereal w/Raisins	1 oz	?	4	?	?	?	130
Kellogg's							
COLD CEREAL							
All-Bran	1 oz (1/3 c)	0	1	?	?	?	70
Apple Jacks	1 oz (1 c)	0	0	?	?	?	110
Bigg Mixx	1 oz (1/2 c)	0	2	?	?	?	110
w/raisins	1 oz + .3 oz raisins (1/2 c)	0	2	?	?	?	140
Bran Buds	1 oz (1/3 c)	0	1	?	?	?	70
Bran Flakes	1 oz (2/3 c)	0	0	?	?	?	90
Cocoa Krispies	1 oz (3/4 c)	0	0	?	?	?	110
Common Sense Oat Bran	1 oz (1/2 c)	0	1	?	?	?	100
w/raisins	1 oz + .3 oz raisins (1/2 c)	0	1	?	?	?	120
Corn Flakes	1 oz (1 c)	0	0	?	?	?	100
Corn Pops	1 oz (1 c)	0	0	?	?	?	110
Cracklin' Oat Bran	1 oz (1/2 c)	0	4	?	?	?	110
Crispix	1 oz (1 c)	0	0	?	?	?	110
Froot Loops	1 oz (1 c)	0	1	?	?	?	110
Frosted Flakes	1 oz (3/4 c)	0	0	?	?	?.	110
Frosted Krispies	1 oz (3/4 c)	0	0	?	?	?	110
Fruitful Bran	1.3 oz (2/3 c)	0	0	?	?	?	110
Fruity Marshmallow Krispies	1.3 oz (1 1/4 c)	0	0	?	?	?	140
Heartwise	1 oz (2/3 c)	0	1	?	?	?	90
Honey Smacks	1 oz (3/4 c)	0	1	?	?	?	110
Just Right							
w/fiber	1 oz (2/3 c)	0	1	?	?	?	100
w/fruit & nuts	1.3 oz (3/4 c)	0	1	?	?	?	140
Müeslix Crispy Blend	1.5 oz (2/3 c)	0	2	?	?	?	160
Müeslix Golden Crunch	1.2 oz (1/2 c)	0	2	?	?	?	120
Nut & Honey Crunch	1 oz (2/3 c)	0	1	?	?	?	110
Nut & Honey Crunch O's	1 oz (2/3 c)	0	2	?	?	?	110

	Portion	Chol (mg)	Total Fat(g)	Satur'd Fat(g)	Mono Fat(g)	Poly Fat(g)	Total Calor
Nutri-Grain							
Almond Raisin	1.4 oz (2/3 c)	0	1	?	?	?	130
Wheat	1 oz (2/3 c)	0	0	?	?	?	100
Oatbake Honey Bran	1 oz (1/3 c)	0	3	?	?	?	110
Oatbake Raisin Nut	1 oz (1/3 c)	0	3	?	?	?	110
Product 19	1 oz (1 c)	0	0	?	?	?	100
Raisin Bran	1.4 oz (3/4 c)	0	1	?	?	?	120
Rice Krispies	1 oz (1 c)	0	0	?	?	?	110
Shredded Wheat Squares							
apple cinnamon	1 oz (1/2 c)	0	0	?	?	?	90
blueberry	1 oz (1/2 c)	0	0	?	?	?	90
raisin	1 oz (1/2 c)	0	0	?	?	?	90
strawberry	1 oz (1/2 c)	0	0	?	?	?	90
Special K	1 oz (1 c)	0	0	?	?	?	110
Malt-o-Meal							
Malt-o-Meal, plain or chocolate							
cooked	3/4 c	0	tr	?	?	?	92
Nabisco							
COLD CEREAL							
Fruit Wheats							
Apple	1 oz	?	0	?	?	?	90
100% Bran	1 oz (1/2 c)	0	1	1	?	?	70
Shredded Wheat							
regular	1 biscuit	0	1	0	?	0	80
w/oat bran	1 oz	0	1	0	?	0	100
spoon size	1 oz	0	1	0	?	0	90
Shredded Wheat 'n bran	1 oz	0	0	?	?	?	90
Team	1 oz	0	1	?	?	?	110
HOT CEREAL							
Cream of Rice	1 oz dry	0	0	0	?	?	100
Cream of Wheat							
regular	1 oz	0	0	0	?	0	100
instant & quick	1 oz	<5	<1	<1	0	<1	100
Mix 'n Eat							
Original	1 oz dry	0	0	0	?	?	100
w/apple & cinnamon, w/brown sugar cinnamon, or w/maple brown sugar)	1¼ oz dry						
Nature Valley							
cinnamon & raisin	1 oz (1/3 c)	0	4	?	?	?	120

	Portion	Chol (mg)	Total Fat(g)	Satur'd Fat(g)	Mono Fat(g)	Poly Fat(g)	Total Calor
fruit & nut	1 oz (⅓ c)	0	4	?	?	?	130
toasted oat	1 oz (⅓ c)	0	4	?	?	?	130
Post							
Alpha-Bits	1 oz	0	1	?	?	?	110
Cocoa Pebbles	1 oz	0	1	?	?	?	110
C.W. Post Hearty Granola	1 oz	0	4	?	?	?	130
Fruit & Fibre							
Dates, Raisins, Walnuts w/oat clusters	1.25 oz	0	2	?	?	?	120
Peaches, Raisins, Almonds w/oat clusters	1.25 oz	0	2	?	?	?	120
Tropical Fruit w/oat clusters	1.25 oz	0	3	?	?	?	120
Fruity Pebbles	1 oz	0	1	?	?	?	110
Grape-Nuts							
regular	1 oz	0	0	0	?	?	110
raisin	1 oz	0	0	0	?	?	100
Grape-Nuts Flakes	1 oz	0	1	?	?	?	100
Honey Bunches of Oats							
w/almonds	1 oz	0	3	?	?	?	120
honey roasted	1 oz	0	2	?	?	?	110
Honeycomb	1 oz	0	0	0	?	?	110
Natural Bran Flakes	1 oz	0	0	0	?	?	90
Natural Raisin Bran	1.4 oz	0	0	0	?	?	120
oat flakes	1 oz	0	1	?	?	?	110
Post Toasties	1 oz	0	0	0	?	?	110
Smurf-Magic Berries	1 oz	0	1	?	?	?	120
Quaker Oats							
COLD CEREAL							
Cap'n Crunch	1 oz (¾ c)	?	2	1	<1	<1	113
Cap'n Crunch w/Crunchberries	1 oz (¾ c)	?	2	1	<1	<1	113
Cap'n Crunch Peanut Butter Cereal	1 oz (¾ c)	?	3	1	0	1	119
Crunchy Nut Oh!s	1 oz (1 c)	?	4	2	<1	<1	127
Honey Graham Oh!s	1 oz (1 c)	?	3	2	<1	<1	122
Kretschmer Wheat Germ							
regular	1 oz (¼ c)	0	3	1	?	2	103
honey crunch	1 oz (¼ c)	0	3	<1	?	2	105
toasted wheat bran	1 oz (⅓ c)	0	2	<1	?	1	57
Life							
regular	1 oz (⅔ c)	?	2	?	?	?	101
cinnamon	1 oz (⅔ c)	?	2	?	?	?	101

	Portion	Chol (mg)	Total Fat(g)	Satur'd Fat(g)	Mono Fat(g)	Poly Fat(g)	Total Calor
Crunchy Bran	1 oz (²/₃ c)	?	1	<1	?	<1	89
Oat Bran	1 oz (²/₃ c)	0	2	<1	?	<1	100
Oat Squares	1 oz (¹/₂ c)	?	2	?	?	?	105
100% Natural Cereal							
Plain	1 oz (¹/₄ c)	?	6	3	?	1	127
w/apples & cinnamon	1 oz (¹/₄ c)	?	5	3	?	1	126
w/raisins & dates	1 oz (¹/₄ c)	?	5	3	?	1	123
Puffed Rice	1 oz (1 c)	0	<1	0	?	0	54
Puffed Wheat	1 oz (1 c)	0	<1	0	<1	0	50
Shredded Wheat	1.4 oz (2 biscuits)	?	1	?	?	?	132
Sun Country Granola							
w/Almonds	1 oz (¹/₄ c)	0	5	1	1	0	130
w/Raisins	1 oz (¹/₄ c)	0	5	<1	1	0	125
HOT CEREAL							
Oats, quick and old-fashioned	¹/₃ c un-cooked (²/₃ c cooked)	0	2	<1	1	1	99
Oatmeal, Instant							
regular	1 packet	0	2	<1	1	1	94
w/apples & cinnamon	1 packet	0	2	<1	1	1	118
w/cinnamon & spice	1 packet	0	2	<1	1	1	164
w/peaches & cream flavor	1 packet	0	2	1	<1	1	129
w/raisins, dates, & walnuts	1 packet	0	4	<1	1	2	141
w/raisins & spice	1 packet	0	2	<1	1	1	149
w/strawberries & cream flavor	1 packet	0	2	1	1	1	129
Extra Fortified Instant Oatmeal							
regular	1 packet	0	2	<1	<1	1	95
apples & spice	1 packet	0	2	<1	1	1	133
raisins & cinnamon	1 packet	0	2	<1	<1	1	129
Quaker & Mother's							
oat bran	¹/₃ c un-cooked (²/₃ c cooked)	0	2	<1	1	1	92
whole wheat hot natural cereal	¹/₃ c un-cooked (²/₃ c cooked)	0	1	<1	<1	<1	92
Ralston Purina							
COLD CEREAL							
Almond Delight	1 oz (³/₄ c)	0	2	?	?	?	110
Bran News	1 oz (³/₄ c)	0	0	?	?	?	100
Cookie Crisp	1 oz (1 c)	?	1	?	?	?	110

	Portion	Chol (mg)	Total Fat(g)	Satur'd Fat(g)	Mono Fat(g)	Poly Fat(g)	Total Calor
Corn Chex	1 oz (1 c)	?	0	?	?	?	110
Double Chex	1 oz (2/3 c)	0	0	?	?	?	110
Honey Graham Chex	1 oz (2/3 c)	0	1	?	?	?	110
Honey Nut Oat Chex	1 oz (1/2 c)	0	1	?	?	?	100
Muesli							
apple almond	1.45 oz (1/2 c)	0	2	?	?	?	150
cranberry walnut	1.45 oz (1/2 c)	0	3	?	?	?	150
date almond	1.45 oz (1/2 c)	0	2	?	?	?	140
peach pecan	1.45 oz (1/2 c)	0	3	?	?	?	150
Multi-Bran Chex	1 oz (2/3 c)	0	0	?	?	?	90
Wheat Chex	1 oz (2/3 c)	0	0	?	?	?	100
HOT CEREAL							
High Fiber	1 oz (1/3 c un-cooked)	0	1	?	?	?	90
Wheatena							
Wheatena							
dry	1/4 c	?	1	?	?	?	125
cooked	1 c	?	1	?	?	?	135
cooked	3/4 c	?	1	?	?	?	101

❏ BREAKFAST FOODS, PREPARED
See also EGGS & EGG SUBSTITUTES; FAST FOODS

	Portion	Chol (mg)	Total Fat(g)	Satur'd Fat(g)	Mono Fat(g)	Poly Fat(g)	Total Calor
French toast, homemade	1 slice	112	7	2	?	?	155
pancakes							
from mix							
plain	1 pancake (4" diam)	16	2	1	?	?	60
buckwheat	1 (4" diam)	20	2	1	?	?	55
extra light	3 pancakes (4" diam)	?	7	?	?	?	200
homemade							
plain	1 pancake (4" diam)	16	2	1	?	?	60
cornmeal	1 pancake (4" diam)	?	1	?	?	?	68
soy	1 (4" diam)	?	2	?	?	?	68
waffles							
from mix, egg & milk added	1 (7" diam)	59	8	3	?	?	205
frozen	1	?	3	?	?	?	95

	Portion	Chol (mg)	Total Fat(g)	Satur'd Fat(g)	Mono Fat(g)	Poly Fat(g)	Total Calor
homemade	1 (7″ diam)	102	13	4	?	?	245

■ BRAND NAME

Arrowhead Mills
blue corn	½ c	?	5	?	?	?	330
buckwheat	½ c	tr	2	?	?	?	270
griddle lite	½ c	tr	3	?	?	?	260
multigrain	½ c	tr	2	?	?	?	350
oat bran	½ c	?	2	?	?	?	200

Aunt Jemima
French Toast, Frozen
plain	2 slices	46	4	1	1	1	166
cinnamon swirl	2 slices	41	4	1	1	1	171
raisin	2 slices	46	4	1	1	1	172

Pancake & Waffle Mixes
original flavor	1.23 oz dry mix	0	1	<1	<1	<1	116
buttermilk	1.3 oz dry mix	1	1	<1	<1	<1	122
whole wheat	1.8 oz dry mix	0	1	<1	<1	<1	161
complete	2.5 oz dry mix	16	4	1	1	1	253
buttermilk complete	2.3 oz dry mix	8	3	1	1	1	231

Pancake Batter, Frozen
plain	3 (4″ diam) pancakes	19	2	1	1	1	183
blueberry	3 (4″ diam) pancakes	27	4	1	1	1	204
buttermilk	3 (4″ diam) pancakes	27	2	1	1	1	180

Pancakes, Frozen
original flavor	3 (4″ diam) pancakes	19	2	1	1	1	183
blueberry	3 (4″ diam) pancakes	27	4	1	1	1	204
buttermilk	3 (4″ diam) pancakes	27	2	1	1	1	180

Waffles, Frozen
original flavor	2 waffles	6	6	1	2	1	173
apple & cinnamon	2 waffles	6	6	1	1	1	176
blueberry	2 waffles	5	5	1	2	<1	175
buttermilk	2 waffles	7	6	1	2	1	179
whole grain	2 waffles	?	3	?	?	?	154

	Portion	Chol (mg)	Total Fat(g)	Satur'd Fat(g)	Mono Fat(g)	Poly Fat(g)	Total Calor
Bisquick							
Shake & Pour pancake and waffle mixes							
apple cinnamon	3 (4" diam) pancakes	0	3	?	?	?	240
blueberry	3 (4" diam) pancakes	0	3	?	?	?	270
buttermilk	3 (4" diam) pancakes	0	3	?	?	?	250
original	3 (4" diam) pancakes	0	3	?	?	?	250
Carnation							
Instant Breakfast							
coffee	1 envl. mixed w/8 oz Vit D milk	3	0	0	0	0	130
chocolate	1 envl. mixed w/8 oz Vit D milk	2	1	<1	<1	<1	130
vanilla	1 envl. mixed w/8 oz Vit D milk	3	0	0	0	0	130
chocolate malt	1 envl. mixed w/8 oz Vit D milk	3	2	1	<1	<1	130
strawberry	1 envl. mixed w/8 oz Vit D milk	3	0	0	0	0	130
diet							
chocolate	1 envl. mixed w/8 oz lowfat milk	2	1	1	<1	<1	70
chocolate malt	1 envl. mixed w/8 oz lowfat milk	2	2	1	<1	<1	70
strawberry	1 envl. mixed w/8 oz lowfat milk	3	0	0	0	0	70

	Portion	Chol (mg)	Total Fat(g)	Satur'd Fat(g)	Mono Fat(g)	Poly Fat(g)	Total Calor
vanilla	1 envl. mixed w/8 oz lowfat milk	3	0	0	0	0	70
Breakfast Bars							
peanut butter & chocolate chips	1 bar	<1	11	3	5	2	200
peanut butter crunch	1 bar	0	10	3	5	2	190
chocolate crunch	1 bar	0	10	4	4	2	190
chocolate chip	1 bar	0	11	4	5	1	200

Kellog's

FROZEN WAFFLES

	Portion	Chol (mg)	Total Fat(g)	Satur'd Fat(g)	Mono Fat(g)	Poly Fat(g)	Total Calor
Common Sense							
oatbran	1	?	4	?	?	?	110
oatbran w/nut & fruit	1	?	5	?	?	?	120
Eggo							
apple cinnamon	1	?	5	?	?	?	130
blueberry	1	?	5	?	?	?	130
buttermilk	1	?	5	?	?	?	120
Homestyle	1	?	5	?	?	?	120
strawberry	1	?	5	?	?	?	130
Nutri-Grain							
original	1	?	5	?	?	?	130
raisin & bran	1	?	5	?	?	?	130

POP-TARTS

See DESSERTS: CAKES, PASTRIES, & PIES

Nabisco

Toastettes *See* DESSERTS: CAKES, PASTRIES, & PIES

Pillsbury

HUNGRY JACK PANCAKE MIXES

	Portion	Chol (mg)	Total Fat(g)	Satur'd Fat(g)	Mono Fat(g)	Poly Fat(g)	Total Calor
blueberry, regular recipe	3 4" pancakes	45	14	3	?	7	320
buttermilk							
regular recipe	3 4" pancakes	55	9	2	?	4	210
no-cholesterol recipe	3 4" pancakes	0	7	1	?	4	200
buttermilk complete, regular recipe	3 4" pancakes	5	1	<1	?	0	180
complete pancakes, regular recipe	3 4" pancakes	0	3	<1	?	0	180
extra lights							
regular recipe	3 4" pancakes	55	6	1	?	2	190
no-cholesterol recipe	3 4" pancakes	0	4	<1	?	2	170
extra lights complete, regular recipe	3 4" pancakes	0	2	<1	?	0	190

	Portion	Chol (mg)	Total Fat(g)	Satur'd Fat(g)	Mono Fat(g)	Poly Fat(g)	Total Calor
Swanson							
GREAT STARTS BREAKFASTS							
Belgian waffles & sausage	2.85 oz	?	19	?	?	?	280
Belgian waffles & sausage w/strawberries	3½ oz	?	8	?	?	?	210
French toast (cinnamon swirl)	5½ oz	?	21	?	?	?	390
French toast w/sausage	5½ oz	?	21	?	?	?	380
ham & cheese on a bagel	3 oz	?	8	?	?	?	240
mini french toast w/sausage	2½ oz	?	9	?	?	?	190
oatmeal french toast w/light links	4.65 oz	?	13	?	?	?	310
omelets w/cheese sauce & ham	7 oz	?	29	?	?	?	390
pancakes & bacon	4½ oz	?	20	?	?	?	400
pancakes & sausage	6 oz	?	22	?	?	?	460
reduced cholesterol eggs w/mini oatmeal muffins	4¾ oz	?	12	?	?	?	250
scrambled eggs w/home fries	4.6 oz	?	19	?	?	?	260
scrambled eggs & bacon w/home fries	5.6 oz	?	26	?	?	?	340
scrambled eggs & sausage w/hashed brown potatoes	6½ oz	?	34	?	?	?	430
silver dollar pancakes & sausage	3¾ oz	?	14	?	?	?	310
waffle w/bacon	2.2 oz	?	14	?	?	?	230
whole wheat pancakes w/lite links	5½ oz	?	16	?	?	?	350
GREAT STARTS BREAKFAST ON A BISCUIT							
egg, Canadian bacon & cheese	5.2 oz	?	22	?	?	?	420
egg, sausage & cheese	5½ oz	?	28	?	?	?	460
sausage	4.7 oz	?	22	?	?	?	410
GREAT STARTS BREAKFAST ON A MUFFIN							
egg, beefsteak & cheese	4.9 oz	?	20	?	?	?	360
egg, canadian bacon & cheese	4.1 oz	?	15	?	?	?	290
Weight Watchers							
English muffin sandwich	4 oz	160	8	3	4	1	230
sausage biscuit	3 oz	70	11	2	8	1	220
buttermilk pancakes	2½ oz	10	3	1	2	<1	140

	Portion	Chol (mg)	Total Fat(g)	Satur'd Fat(g)	Mono Fat(g)	Poly Fat(g)	Total Calor
French toast w/cinnamon	3 oz	5	4	<1	2	<1	160
French toast w/links	4 ½ oz	15	11	3	6	2	270
pancakes w/links	4 oz	15	10	4	3	3	220
pancakes w/blueberry topping	4 ¾ oz	10	3	1	1	1	200
pancakes w/strawberry topping	4 ¾ oz	10	3	1	1	1	200

❑ BROWNIES *See* COOKIES, BARS, & BROWNIES

❑ BUTTER & MARGARINE SPREADS

Butter

See also NUTS & NUT-BASED BUTTERS, FLOURS, MEALS, MILKS, PASTES, POWDERS, SEEDS & SEED-BASED BUTTERS, FLOURS, & MEALS

	Portion	Chol (mg)	Total Fat(g)	Satur'd Fat(g)	Mono Fat(g)	Poly Fat(g)	Total Calor
salted or unsalted	1 t	11	4	2½	?	?	36
salted or unsalted	1 stick (4 oz or about ½ c)	247	92	57	?	?	813
whipped, salted	1 t	8	3	2	?	?	27
whipped, salted	1 stick (4 oz or about ½ c)	165	61	38	?	?	542

Margarine

REGULAR

Hard, Stick or Brick

	Portion	Chol (mg)	Total Fat(g)	Satur'd Fat(g)	Mono Fat(g)	Poly Fat(g)	Total Calor
coconut, safflower, coconut (hydrogenated) & palm (hydrogenated)	1 stick	0	91	65	?	?	815
coconut, safflower, coconut (hydrogenated) & palm (hydrogenated)	1 t	0	4	3	?	?	34
corn (hydrogenated)	1 stick	0	91	15	?	?	815
corn (hydrogenated)	1 t	0	4	1	?	?	34
corn & corn (hydrogenated)	1 stick	0	91	16	?	?	815
corn & corn (hydrogenated)	1 t	0	4	1	?	?	34

	Portion	Chol (mg)	Total Fat (g)	Satur'd Fat (g)	Mono Fat (g)	Poly Fat (g)	Total Calor
corn, soybean (hydrogenated), & cottonseed (hydrogenated)							
salted	1 stick	0	91	17	?	?	815
salted	1 t	0	4	1	?	?	34
unsalted	1 stick	0	91	17	?	?	810
unsalted	1 t	0	4	1	?	?	34
lard (hydrogenated)	1 stick	57	91	36	?	?	831
lard (hydrogenated)	1 t	2	4	2	?	?	35
safflower & soybean (hydrogenated)	1 stick	0	91	16	?	?	815
safflower & soybean (hydrogenated)	1 t	0	4	1	?	?	34
safflower, soybean (hydrogenated), & cottonseed (hydrogenated)	1 stick	0	91	15	?	?	815
safflower, soybean (hydrogenated), & cottonseed (hydrogenated)	1 t	0	4	1	?	?	34
safflower, soybean, soybean (hydrogenated), & cottonseed (hydrogenated)	1 stick	0	91	16	?	?	815
safflower, soybean, soybean (hydrogenated), & cottonseed (hydrogenated)	1 t	0	4	1	?	?	34
soybean (hydrogenated)	1 stick	0	91	19	?	?	815
soybean (hydrogenated)	1 t	0	4	1	?	?	34
soybean & soybean (hydrogenated)	1 stick	0	91	15	?	?	815
soybean & soybean (hydrogenated)	1 t	0	4	1	?	?	34
soybean (hydrogenated) & cottonseed	1 stick	0	91	19	?	?	815
soybean (hydrogenated) & cottonseed	1 t	0	4	1	?	?	34
soybean (hydrogenated) & cottonseed (hydrogenated)	1 stick	0	91	17	?	?	815
soybean (hydrogenated) & cottonseed (hydrogenated)	1 t	0	4	1	?	?	34
soybean (hydrogenated) & palm (hydrogenated)	1 stick	0	91	17	?	?	815
soybean (hydrogenated) & palm (hydrogenated)	1 t	0	4	1	?	?	34

	Portion	Chol (mg)	Total Fat(g)	Satur'd Fat(g)	Mono Fat(g)	Poly Fat(g)	Total Calor
soybean (hydrogenated), corn, & cottonseed (hydrogenated)	1 stick	0	91	23	?	?	815
soybean (hydrogenated), corn, & cottonseed (hydrogenated)	1 t	0	4	1	?	?	34
soybean (hydrogenated), cottonseed (hydrogenated), & soybean	1 stick	0	91	18	?	?	815
soybean (hydrogenated), cottonseed (hydrogenated), & soybean	1 t	0	4	1	?	?	34
soybean (hydrogenated), palm (hydrogenated), & palm	1 stick	0	91	20	?	?	815
soybean (hydrogenated), palm (hydrogenated), & palm	1 t	0	4	1	?	?	34
sunflower, soybean (hydrogenated), & cottonseed (hydrogenated)	1 stick	0	91	14	?	?	815
sunflower, soybean (hydrogenated), & cottonseed (hydrogenated)	1 t	0	4	1	?	?	34
Liquid, Bottle							
soybean (hydrogenated), soybean, & cottonseed	1 c	0	183	30	?	?	1637
soybean (hydrogenated), soybean, & cottonseed	1 t	0	4	1	?	?	34
Soft, Tub							
corn & corn (hydrogenated)	1 c	0	183	32	?	?	1,626
corn & corn (hydrogenated)	1 t	0	4	1	?	?	34
safflower, cottonseed (hydrogenated), & peanut (hydrogenated)	1 c	0	183	30	?	?	1,626
safflower, cottonseed (hydrogenated), & peanut (hydrogenated)	1 t	0	4	1	?	?	34

	Portion	Chol (mg)	Total Fat(g)	Satur'd Fat(g)	Mono Fat(g)	Poly Fat(g)	Total Calor
safflower & safflower (hydrogenated)	1 c	0	183	21	?	?	1,626
safflower & safflower (hydrogenated)	1 t	0	4	tr	?	?	34
soybean (hydrogenated)							
salted	1 c	0	183	31	?	?	1,626
salted	1 t	0	4	1	?	?	34
unsalted	1 c	0	182	31	?	?	1,626
unsalted	1 t	0	4	1	?	?	34
soybean (hydrogenated) & cottonseed	1 c	0	183	37	?	?	1,626
soybean (hydrogenated) & cottonseed	1 t	0	4	1	?	?	34
soybean (hydrogenated) & cottonseed (hydrogenated)							
salted	1 c	0	183	32	?	?	1,626
salted	1 t	0	4	1	?	?	34
unsalted	1 c	0	182	32	?	?	1,626
unsalted	1 t	0	4	1	?	?	34
soybean (hydrogenated), & safflower	1 c	0	183	24	?	?	1,626
soybean (hydrogenated), & safflower	1 t	0	4	1	?	?	34
soybean (hydrogenated), cottonseed (hydrogenated), & soybean	1 c	0	183	35	?	?	1,626
soybean (hydrogenated), cottonseed (hydrogenated), & soybean	1 t	0	4	1	?	?	34
soybean (hydrogenated), palm (hydrogenated), & palm	1 c	0	183	39	?	?	1,626
soybean (hydrogenated), palm (hydrogenated), & palm	1 t	0	4	1	?	?	34
soybean, soybean (hydrogenated), & cottonseed (hydrogenated)	1 c	0	183	37	?	?	1,626
soybean, soybean (hydrogenated), & cottonseed (hydrogenated)	1 t	0	4	1	?	?	34
sunflower, cottonseed (hydrogenated), & peanut (hydrogenated)	1 c	0	183	29	?	?	1,626

	Portion	Chol (mg)	Total Fat(g)	Satur'd Fat(g)	Mono Fat(g)	Poly Fat(g)	Total Calor
sunflower, cottonseed (hydrogenated), & peanut (hydrogenated)	1 t	0	4	1	?	?	34

IMITATION (ABOUT 40% FAT)

	Portion	Chol (mg)	Total Fat(g)	Satur'd Fat(g)	Mono Fat(g)	Poly Fat(g)	Total Calor
corn & corn (hydrogenated)	1 c	0	90	15	?	?	801
corn & corn (hydrogenated)	1 t	0	2	tr	?	?	17
soybean (hydrogenated)	1 c	0	90	15	?	?	801
soybean (hydrogenated)	1 t	0	2	tr	?	?	17
soybean (hydrogenated) & cottonseed	1 c	0	90	19	?	?	801
soybean (hydrogenated) & cottonseed	1 t	0	2	tr	?	?	17
soybean (hydrogenated) & cottonseed (hydrogenated)	1 c	0	90	17	?	?	801
soybean (hydrogenated) & cottonseed (hydrogenated)	1 t	0	2	tr	?	?	17
soybean (hydrogenated), palm (hydrogenated), & palm	1 c	0	90	24	?	?	801
soybean (hydrogenated), palm (hydrogenated), & palm	1 t	0	2	1	?	?	17
unspecified ingredient oils	1 c	0	90	18	?	?	801
unspecified ingredient oils	1 t	0	2	tr	?	?	17

SPREAD, MARGARINE (ABOUT 60% FAT)

stick

	Portion	Chol (mg)	Total Fat(g)	Satur'd Fat(g)	Mono Fat(g)	Poly Fat(g)	Total Calor
soybean (hydrogenated) & palm (hydrogenated)	1 c	0	139	32	?	?	1,236
soybean (hydrogenated) & palm (hydrogenated)	1 t	0	3	1	?	?	26

tub

	Portion	Chol (mg)	Total Fat(g)	Satur'd Fat(g)	Mono Fat(g)	Poly Fat(g)	Total Calor
soybean (hydrogenated), & cottonseed (hydrogenated)	1 c	0	139	28	?	?	1,236
soybean (hydrogenated), & cottonseed (hydrogenated)	1 t	0	3	1	?	?	26

	Portion	Chol (mg)	Total Fat(g)	Satur'd Fat(g)	Mono Fat(g)	Poly Fat(g)	Total Calor
soybean (hydrogenated), palm (hydrogenated), & palm	1 c	0	139	31	?	?	1,236
soybean (hydrogenated), palm (hydrogenated), & palm	1 t	0	3	1	?	?	26
unspecified ingredient oils	1 c	0	139	29	?	?	1,236
unspecified ingredient oils	1 t	0	3	1	?	?	26

■ BRAND NAME

Blue Bonnet
better blend

	Portion	Chol (mg)	Total Fat(g)	Satur'd Fat(g)	Mono Fat(g)	Poly Fat(g)	Total Calor
stick	1 T	<2	11	2	?	2	90
soft	1 T	<2	11	2	?	3	90
margarine, stick	1 T	0	11	2	?	3	100
spread, 48% fat	1 T	0	7	1	?	2	60
spread stick, 75% fat	1 T	0	11	2	?	3	90
soft margarine	1 T	0	11	2	?	4	100
whipped margarine stick	1 T	0	7	1	?	2	70

Fleischmann's
margarine

	Portion	Chol (mg)	Total Fat(g)	Satur'd Fat(g)	Mono Fat(g)	Poly Fat(g)	Total Calor
diet or diet w/lite salt	1 T	0	6	1	?	2	50
light corn oil spread, soft or stick	1 T	0	8	1	?	3	80
stick	1 T	0	11	2	?	4	100
squeeze	1 T	0	10	1	?	5	90
whipped, lightly salted or unsalted	1 T	0	7	2	?	3	70
soft	1 T	0	11	2	?	5	100
sweet unsalted, soft	1 T	0	11	2	?	5	100
sweet unsalted, stick	1 T	0	11	2	?	4	100
extra light corn oil, spread or stick	1 T	0	6	1	?	2	50

Hain
margarine

	Portion	Chol (mg)	Total Fat(g)	Satur'd Fat(g)	Mono Fat(g)	Poly Fat(g)	Total Calor
safflower	1 T	0	11	2	?	5	100
soft safflower	1 T	0	11	2	?	6	100
unsalted safflower	1 T	0	11	2	?	5	100

Hollywood
margarine

	Portion	Chol (mg)	Total Fat(g)	Satur'd Fat(g)	Mono Fat(g)	Poly Fat(g)	Total Calor
soft spread	1 T	0	10	1	?	3	90
safflower	1 T	0	11	2	?	5	100
sweet unsalted safflower	1 T	0	11	2	?	5	100

	Portion	Chol (mg)	Total Fat(g)	Satur'd Fat(g)	Mono Fat(g)	Poly Fat(g)	Total Calor
Kraft							
margarine							
touch of butter							
bowl (40% fat)	1 T	0	6	1	?	2	50
stick (70% fat)	1 T	0	10	2	?	1	90
chiffon							
soft cup	1 T	0	10	1	?	4	90
soft stick	1 T	0	11	2	?	3	100
soft unsalted	1 T	0	10	2	?	4	90
whipped	1 T	0	8	1	?	3	70
parkay							
regular	1 T	0	11	2	?	2	100
soft	1 T	0	11	2	?	4	100
soft diet reduced calorie	1 T	0	6	1	?	2	50
spread (50% vegetable oil)	1 T	0	7	1	?	2	60
squeeze spread	1 T	0	10	2	?	6	90
whipped (cup)	1 T	0	7	1	?	2	70
whipped (stick)	1 T	0	7	1	?	1	70
miracle brand							
whipped (cup)	1 T	0	7	1	?	2	60
whipped (stick)	1 T	0	7	1	?	1	70
Land O'Lakes							
butter							
stick, lightly salted or unsalted	1 t	10	4	2	1	<1	35
whipped ,lightly salted or unsalted	1 t	5	3	2	1	<1	25
Country Morning Blend							
stick, lightly salted or unsalted	1 t	4	4	1	1	1	35
lightly salted soft (tub)	1 t	4	3	1	1	1	30
Country Morning Blend Light							
stick or tub, lightly salted	1 t	2-½	2	1	1	<1	20
Spread with Sweet Cream							
stick, lightly salted or unsalted	1 t	0	4	1	2	1	30
lightly salted soft (tub)	1 t	0	3	<1	1	1	25
margarine							
regular (soy oil), stick or soft tub	1 t	0	4	1	2	1	35
Mazola							
margarine							
diet-reduced calorie	1 T	0	6	1	?	?	50
light corn oil spread	1 T	0	6	1	?	?	50

	Portion	Chol (mg)	Total Fat(g)	Satur'd Fat(g)	Mono Fat(g)	Poly Fat(g)	Total Calor
Weight Watchers							
margarine							
reduced calorie tub	1 T	?	6	1	?	2	50
sweet unsalted tub	1 T	?	6	1	?	2	50
reduced calorie sticks	1 T	?	7	1	?	2	60

❑ CAKES *See* DESSERTS: CAKES, PASTRIES, & PIES

❑ CANDIED FRUIT *See* BAKING INGREDIENTS

❑ CANDY

	Portion	Chol (mg)	Total Fat(g)	Satur'd Fat(g)	Mono Fat(g)	Poly Fat(g)	Total Calor
butterscotch	6 pieces	?	3	?	?	?	116
butterscotch chips	1 oz	tr	7	?	?	?	150
caramels							
plain or chocolate	3	?	3	?	?	?	112
chocolate							
chocolate fudge center	1	?	5	?	?	?	129
chocolate fudge w/nuts center	1	?	6	?	?	?	127
coconut center	1	?	5	?	?	?	123
cream center	1	?	4	?	?	?	102
vanilla cream center	1	?	4	?	?	?	114
chocolate chips							
chocolate-flavored	¼ c	tr	8	2	?	?	195
dark	1 oz	?	8	?	?	?	148
milk chocolate	¼ c	7	11	?	?	?	218
semisweet	1 c or 6 oz	0	61	36	?	?	860
chocolate-covered almonds	1 oz	?	12	?	?	?	159
chocolate-covered peanuts	1 oz	?	9	?	?	?	153
chocolate-covered raisins	1 oz	?	4	?	?	?	115
chocolate kisses	6	?	9	?	?	?	154
English toffee	1 oz	?	17	?	?	?	193
fondant, uncoated (mints, candy corn, other)	1 oz	0	0	0	?	?	105
fudge							
chocolate, plain	1 oz	1	3	2	?	?	115
chocolate w/nuts	1 oz	?	5	?	?	?	119
vanilla	1 oz	?	3	?	?	?	111
vanilla w/nuts	1 oz	?	5	?	?	?	119

granola bars *See* COOKIES, BARS, & BROWNIES

	Portion	Chol (mg)	Total Fat(g)	Satur'd Fat(g)	Mono Fat(g)	Poly Fat(g)	Total Calor
gum drops	1 oz	0	tr	tr	?	?	100
jelly beans	10	0	0	0	?	?	66
malted milk balls	14	?	7	?	?	?	135
marshmallows	1 oz	0	0	0	?	?	90
marshmallows	1 large	0	0	0	?	?	25
mints	14	?	1	?	?	?	104
peanut brittle	1 oz	?	4	?	?	?	123
sugar-coated almonds	7	?	5	?	?	?	128

■ BRAND NAME

NOTE: Candies may be listed under product name (such as Milky Way) or company name (such as Cadbury or Hershey).

	Portion	Chol (mg)	Total Fat(g)	Satur'd Fat(g)	Mono Fat(g)	Poly Fat(g)	Total Calor
Almond Joy	1.76 oz	0	14	?	?	?	250
Baby Ruth	2.2 oz	0	13	6	?	2	300
Baker's chocolate See BAKING INGREDIENTS							
Bar None	1.5 oz	10	14	?	?	?	240
Beechies candy-coated gum, all flavors	1 piece	?	0	?	?	?	6
Beech-Nut							
cough drops, all flavors	1	?	0	?	?	?	10
gums, all flavors	1 piece	?	0	?	?	?	10
Bit-O-Honey	1.7 oz	?	4	?	?	?	200
Bonkers!, all flavors	1 piece	?	0	?	?	?	20
Breath Savers Mints, sugar-free, all flavors	1	?	0	?	?	?	8
Bubble Yum bubble gum, all flavors							
sugarless	1 piece	?	0	?	?	?	20
Butterfinger	2.1 oz	0	12	5	?	2	280
Cadbury							
chocolate almond	1 oz	6	9	?	?	?	153
chocolate Brazil nut	1 oz	?	9	?	?	?	156
chocolate hazelnut	1 oz	4	9	?	?	?	153
chocolate Krisp	1 oz	?	7	?	?	?	146
creme eggs	1 oz	?	6	?	?	?	136
fruit & nut	1 oz	6	8	?	?	?	148
Caramello	1.6 oz	10	11	?	?	?	220
Care-Free							
sugarless bubble gum, all flavors	1 piece	?	0	?	?	?	10
sugarless gum, all flavors	1 piece	?	0	?	?	?	8
Charlestown Chew	1 oz	?	3	?	?	?	120
Chunky							
original	1.4 oz	?	12	?	?	?	210
Fifth Avenue	2 oz	5	13	?	?	?	290
Golden Almond Chocolate Bar	1.6 oz (½ bar)	5	17	?	?	?	260
Golden III Chocolate Bar	1.6 oz (½ bar)	10	15	?	?	?	250

	Portion	Chol (mg)	Total Fat(g)	Satur'd Fat(g)	Mono Fat(g)	Poly Fat(g)	Total Calor
Goobers Milk Chocolate-covered Peanuts	1-3/8 oz	?	13	?	?	?	220
Hershey							
chocolate chips & unsweetened chocolate *See* BAKING INGREDIENTS							
chocolate Kisses	9 (1.46 oz)	10	13	?	?	?	220
Krackel	1.6 oz	10	13	?	?	?	230
milk chocolate	1.55 oz	10	14	?	?	?	240
milk chocolate w/almonds	1.45 oz	15	14	?	?	?	230
Special Dark sweet chocolate	1.45 oz	0	12	?	?	?	220
Junior Mints	12	?	3	?	?	?	120
Kit Kat	1.6 oz	10	13	?	?	?	250
Life Savers							
roll candy, all flavors, regular or sugar-free	1 piece	?	0	?	?	?	10
M&M's							
regular	1 oz	?	6	?	?	?	140
peanut	1 oz	?	7	?	?	?	140
peanut butter	1 oz	?	7	?	?	?	140
Milky Way	1 bar	?	11	?	?	?	280
Mounds	1.9 oz	0	14	?	?	?	260
Mr. Goodbar	1.75 oz	15	19	?	?	?	290
Nestlé							
Alpine White Bar w/almonds	1.25 oz	?	13	?	?	?	200
Alpine White Holiday Singles	5 pieces	?	10	?	?	?	160
Alpine White Nesteggs	5 pieces	?	10	?	?	?	160
Crunch	1.4 oz	?	10	?	?	?	210
milk chocolate	1.45 oz	?	13	?	?	?	220
milk chocolate w/almonds	1.45 oz	?	14	?	?	?	230
Crunch Holiday Singles	5 pieces	?	7	?	?	?	150
Crunch Nesteggs	5 pieces	?	7	?	?	?	150
Oh Henry!	2 oz	?	14	?	?	?	280
Pom Poms	1/2 box	?	3	?	?	?	100
Raisinet Milk Chocolate-covered Raisins	1 3/8 oz	?	6	?	?	?	180
Reese's							
Peanut Butter Cup	1.8 oz	10	17	?	?	?	280
Peanut Butter-flavored Chips	1/4 c	5	13	?	?	?	230
Pieces	1.85 oz	5	11	?	?	?	260
Rolo	8 pieces (1.93 oz)	15	12	?	?	?	270
Skor	1.4 oz	25	14	?	?	?	220
Snickers	1 bar	?	13	?	?	?	280
Sugar Babies	1 pkg	?	2	?	?	?	180
Sugar Daddy	1 bar	?	1	?	?	?	150
Symphony Almond Toffee Chips	1.4 oz	?	14	?	?	?	220

	Portion	Chol (mg)	Total Fat(g)	Satur'd Fat(g)	Mono Fat(g)	Poly Fat(g)	Total Calor
Symphony Chocolate	1.4 oz	10	13	?	?	?	200
Whatchamacallit	1.8 oz	10	13	?	?	?	260
Y&S							
Bites	1 oz	0	1	?	?	?	100
Nibs Cherry Candy	1 oz	0	1	?	?	?	100
Twizzlers	1 oz	0	1	?	?	?	100
York Peppermint Pattie	1.5 oz	0	4	?	?	?	180

❏ CANNED MEATS *See* PROCESSED MEAT & POULTRY PRODUCTS

❏ CEREAL, BREAKFAST *See* BREAKFAST CEREALS, COLD & HOT

❏ CHEESE & CHEESE FOODS

Natural Cheese

	Portion	Chol (mg)	Total Fat(g)	Satur'd Fat(g)	Mono Fat(g)	Poly Fat(g)	Total Calor
bleu	1 oz	21	8	5	?	?	100
bleu	1 c, crumbled, not packed	102	39	25	?	?	477
brick	1" cube	16	5	3	?	?	64
brick	1 oz	27	8	5	?	?	105
Brie	1 oz	28	8	?	?	?	95
Brie	4½ oz	128	35	?	?	?	427
Camembert	1 oz	20	7	4	?	?	85
Camembert	3⅓ oz	27	9	6	?	?	114
caraway	1 oz	?	8	?	?	?	107
cheddar	1 oz	30	9	6	?	?	114
cheddar	1 c, shredded, not packed	119	37	24	?	?	455
Cheshire	1 oz	29	9	?	?	?	110
Colby	1" cube	16	6	3	?	?	68
Colby	1 oz	27	9	6	?	?	112
cottage							
creamed, small curd	4 oz	17	5	3	?	?	117
creamed, small curd	1 c, not packed	31	9	6	?	?	217
fruit added	4 oz	13	4	2	?	?	140
fruit added	1 c, not packed	25	8	5	?	?	279
dry curd	4 oz	8	tr	tr	?	?	96
dry curd	1 c, not packed	10	tr	tr	?	?	123

	Portion	Chol (mg)	Total Fat(g)	Satur'd Fat(g)	Mono Fat(g)	Poly Fat(g)	Total Calor
low-fat							
2%	4 oz	9	2	1	?	?	101
2%	1 c, not packed	19	4	3	?	?	203
1%	4 oz	5	1	tr	?	?	82
1%	1 c, not packed	10	2	1.46	?	?	164
cream	1 oz	31	10	6	?	?	99
cream	3 oz	93	30	19	?	?	297
Edam	1 oz	25	8	5	?	?	101
Edam	7 oz	177	55	35	?	?	706
feta, from sheep's milk	1 oz	25	6	4	?	?	75
fontina	1 oz	33	9	5	?	?	110
fontina	8 oz	263	71	44	?	?	883
gjetost, from goat's & cow's milk	1 oz	?	8	5	?	?	132
gjetost, from goat's & cow's milk	8 oz	?	67	43	?	?	1,057
Gouda	1 oz	32	8	5	?	?	101
Gouda	7 oz	226	54	35	?	?	705
Gruyère	1 oz	31	9	5	?	?	117
Gruyère	6 oz	187	55	32	?	?	702
Limburger	1 oz	26	8	5	?	?	93
Limburger	1 pkg, 8 oz	204	62	38	?	?	742
Monterey Jack	1 oz	?	9	?	?	?	106
Monterey Jack	6 oz	?	51	?	?	?	635
mozzarella	1 oz	22	6	4	?	?	80
low moisture	1" cube	16	4	3	?	?	56
low moisture	1 oz	25	7	4	?	?	90
part skim	1" cube	10	3	2	?	?	49
part skim	1 oz	15	5	3	?	?	79
part skim	1 oz	16	5	3	?	?	72
Muenster	1 oz	27	9	5	?	?	104
Muenster	6 oz	163	51	32	?	?	626
Neufâchatel	1 oz	22	7	4	?	?	74
Neufâchatel	3 oz	65	20	13	?	?	221
Parmesan							
grated	1 T	4	2	1	?	?	23
grated	1 oz	22	9	5	?	?	129
hard	1 oz	19	7	5	?	?	111
hard	5 oz	96	37	23	?	?	557
Port du Salut	1 oz	35	8	5	?	?	100
Port du Salut	6 oz	209	48	28	?	?	598
provolone	1 oz	20	8	5	?	?	100
provolone	6 oz	117	45	29	?	?	598
ricotta							
whole milk	½ c	63	16	10	?	?	216
part skim milk	½ c	38	10	6	?	?	171
Romano, hard	1 oz	29	8	?	?	?	110
Romano, hard	5 oz	148	38	?	?	?	549

	Portion	Chol (mg)	Total Fat(g)	Satur'd Fat(g)	Mono Fat(g)	Poly Fat(g)	Total Calor
Roquefort, from sheep's milk	1 oz	26	9	5	?	?	105
Roquefort, from sheep's milk	1 pkg net wt 3 oz	76	26	16	?	?	314
Swiss	1" cube	14	4	3	?	?	56
Swiss	1 oz	20	8	5	?	?	107
Tilsit	1 oz	29	7	5	?	?	96
Tilsit	6 oz	173	44	29	?	?	578

whey *See* MILK, MILK SUBSTITUTES, & MILK PRODUCTS

Processed Cheese & Cheese Food

CHEESE FOOD

	Portion	Chol (mg)	Total Fat(g)	Satur'd Fat(g)	Mono Fat(g)	Poly Fat(g)	Total Calor
American							
cold pack	1 oz	18	7	4	?	?	94
cold pack	8 oz	144	56	35	?	?	752
pasteurized process	1 oz	18	7	4	?	?	93
pasteurized process	8 oz	145	56	35	?	?	745
Swiss, pasteurized process	1 oz	23	7	?	?	?	92
Swiss, pasteurized process	8 oz	186	55	?	?	?	734

CHEESE SPREAD

	Portion	Chol (mg)	Total Fat(g)	Satur'd Fat(g)	Mono Fat(g)	Poly Fat(g)	Total Calor
American, pasteurized process	1 oz	16	6	4	?	?	82
American, pasteurized process	5 oz	78	30	19	?	?	412
American	1" cube	17	5	3	?	?	66
American	1 oz	27	9	6	?	?	106
pimiento	1" cube	16	5	3	?	?	66
pimiento	1 oz	27	9	6	?	?	106
Swiss	1" cube	15	4	3	?	?	60
Swiss	1 oz	24	7	5	?	?	95

■ BRAND NAME

Bonbel
See FROMAGERIES BEL, below

Friendship

	Portion	Chol (mg)	Total Fat(g)	Satur'd Fat(g)	Mono Fat(g)	Poly Fat(g)	Total Calor
cottage cheese							
California style, 4% milk fat	½ c	17	5	?	?	?	120
Friendship n' Fruit low-fat	6 oz	6	1	?	?	?	100
regular & lactose reduced, both 1% milk fat	½ c	5	1	?	?	?	90
large curd pot style, 2% milk fat	½ c	9	2	?	?	?	100

	Portion	Chol (mg)	Total Fat(g)	Satur'd Fat(g)	Mono Fat(g)	Poly Fat(g)	Total Calor
no salt added, 1% milk fat	½ c	5	1	?	?	?	90
w/pineapple, 1% milk fat	½ c	5	1	?	?	?	110
w/pineapple, 4% milk fat	½ c	17	4	?	?	?	140
cream cheese	1 oz	31	<10	?	?	?	103
farmer cheese, regular & no salt added	½ c	40	12	?	?	?	160
natural hoop cheese ½% milk fat, no salt added	4 oz	8	<1	?	?	?	84
Fromageries Bel							
Babybel	1 oz	10	7	5	?	?	90
Bonbel	1 oz	25	8	5	?	?	100
Edam	1 oz	25	8	?	?	?	100
Gouda	1 oz	30	9	6	?	?	110
Mini Babybel	¾ oz	15	6	4	?	?	70
Mini Bonbel	¾ oz	15	6	4	?	?	70
Mini Gouda	¾ oz	20	6	4	?	?	80
Reduced Mini	¾ oz	10	3	2	?	?	45
Kraft							
NATURAL CHEESE							
blue	1 oz	30	9	5	?	0	100
brick	1 oz	30	9	5	?	0	110
cheddar	1 oz	30	9	5	?	0	110
Colby	1 oz	30	9	5	?	0	110
Gouda	1 oz	30	9	5	?	0	110
Edam	1 oz	20	7	4	?	0	90
Mohawk Valley Little Gem Size Limburger	1 oz	25	8	5	?	0	90
Monterey Jack	1 oz	30	9	5	?	0	110
low-moisture mozzarella	1 oz	20	7	4	?	0	90
low-moisture part-skim mozzarella	1 oz	15	5	3	?	0	80
string cheese low-moisture part-skim mozzarella w/jalepeño pepper	1 oz	20	5	3	?	0	80
grated Parmesan	1 oz	30	9	5	?	0	130
Parmesan	1 oz	20	7	4	?	0	100
provolone	1 oz	25	7	4	?	0	100
grated Romano	1 oz	30	9	6	?	0	130
Natural Romano	1 oz	20	7	4	?	0	100
Swiss	1 oz	25	8	5	?	0	110
Casino Swiss	1 oz	30	8	5	?	0	110
Cracker Barrel Baby Swiss	1 oz	25	9	5	?	0	110
Very Low Sodium (75% less sodium)	1 oz	25	8	5	?	0	110

	Portion	Chol (mg)	Total Fat(g)	Satur'd Fat(g)	Mono Fat(g)	Poly Fat(g)	Total Calor
Taco Shredded Cheese	1 oz	30	9	5	?	0	110

NATURAL REDUCED FAT CHEESE

	Portion	Chol (mg)	Total Fat(g)	Satur'd Fat(g)	Mono Fat(g)	Poly Fat(g)	Total Calor
Cracker Barrel Light Cheddar Sharp-white	1 oz	20	5	3	?	0	80
Light Cheddar	1 oz	20	5	3	?	0	80
Light Mild Cheddar	1 oz	20	5	3	?	0	80
Light Shredded Colby & Monterey Jack	1 oz	20	5	3	?	0	80
Light Mozzerella	1 oz	15	4	3	?	0	80
Light Swiss	1 oz	20	5	3	?	0	90

PHILADELPHIA BRAND CREAM CHEESE

	Portion	Chol (mg)	Total Fat(g)	Satur'd Fat(g)	Mono Fat(g)	Poly Fat(g)	Total Calor
plain	1 oz	30	10	6	?	0	100
plain w/chives	1 oz	30	9	5	?	0	90
plain w/pimiento	1 oz	30	9	5	?	0	90
light-Neufâchatel	1 oz	25	7	4	?	0	90
light pasteurized process product	1 oz	10	5	3	?	0	60
soft	1 oz	30	10	5	?	0	100
soft w/chives & onion	1 oz	30	9	5	?	0	100
soft w/herb & garlic	1 oz	25	9	5	?	0	90
soft w/olives & pimiento	1 oz	25	8	5	?	0	90
soft w/pineapple	1 oz	25	8	5	?	0	90
soft w/smoked salmon	1 oz	25	9	5	?	0	90
soft w/strawberries	1 oz	20	8	5	?	0	90
whipped	1 oz	30	10	6	?	0	100

PROCESSED CHEESES

Process Cheese

	Portion	Chol (mg)	Total Fat(g)	Satur'd Fat(g)	Mono Fat(g)	Poly Fat(g)	Total Calor
deluxe pasteurized American (slices)	1 oz	25	9	5	?	0	110
deluxe pasteurized pimiento (slices)	1 oz	25	8	5	?	0	100
deluxe pasteurized Swiss (slices)	1 oz	25	7	4	?	0	90
Old English sharp pasteurized American (loaf)	1 oz	30	9	5	?	0	110
Old English sharp pasteurized American (slices)	1 oz	30	9	5	?	0	110

Process Cheese Food

	Portion	Chol (mg)	Total Fat(g)	Satur'd Fat(g)	Mono Fat(g)	Poly Fat(g)	Total Calor
Cracker Barrel extra sharp cheddar cold pack	1 oz	20	7	4	?	0	90
Cracker Barrel port wine cheddar cold pack	1 oz	20	7	4	?	0	100
Cracker Barrel sharp cheddar cold pack	1 oz	20	7	4	?	0	100

	Portion	Chol (mg)	Total Fat(g)	Satur'd Fat(g)	Mono Fat(g)	Poly Fat(g)	Total Calor
Golden Image American flavored imitation pasteurized	1 oz	5	6	2	?	2	90
American singles pasteurized	1 oz	25	7	4	?	0	90
American singles pasteurized (white)	1 oz	20	7	4	?	0	90
Cheez 'N Bacon singles pasteurized	1 oz	25	7	4	?	0	90
jalapeño singles pasteurized	1 oz	25	7	4	?	0	90
Monterey Jack singles pasteurized	1 oz	25	7	4	?	0	90
sharp singles pasteurized	1 oz	25	8	5	?	0	100
Swiss singles pasteurized	1 oz	25	7	4	?	0	90
grated American	1 oz	25	7	4	?	0	130
pasteurized w/garlic	1 oz	20	7	4	?	0	90
pasteurized w/jalapeño peppers	1 oz	20	7	4	?	0	90
Nippy pasteurized	1 oz	20	7	4	?	0	90
Velveeta shredded	1 oz	20	7	4	?	0	100
Velveeta hot Mexican shredded pasteurized w/jalapeño pepper	1 oz	25	7	4	?	0	100
Velveeta mild Mexican shredded w/jalapeño pepper	1 oz	25	7	4	?	0	100

Process Cheese Product

	Portion	Chol (mg)	Total Fat(g)	Satur'd Fat(g)	Mono Fat(g)	Poly Fat(g)	Total Calor
Harvest Moon pasteurized American flavor	1 oz	15	4	2	?	0	70
free singles nonfat pasteurized	1 oz	5	0	0	?	0	45
light singles American flavor pasteurized	1 oz	15	4	3	?	0	70
light singles American flavor pasteurized (white)	1 oz	15	4	2	?	0	70
light singles sharp cheddar pasteurized	1 oz	15	4	2	?	0	70
light singles Swiss flavor pasteurized	1 oz	15	3	2	?	0	70
Light 'N Lively singles American flavored pasteurized	1 oz	15	4	3	?	0	70

	Portion	Chol (mg)	Total Fat(g)	Satur'd Fat(g)	Mono Fat(g)	Poly Fat(g)	Total Calor
Light 'N Lively singles American flavored pasteurized (white)	1 oz	15	4	2	?	0	70
Light 'N Lively singles sharp cheddar flavored	1 oz	15	4	2	?	0	70
Light 'N Lively singles Swiss flavored	1 oz	15	3	2	?	0	70
Spreadery Cheese Snack medium cheddar cold pack	1 oz	15	4	2	?	0	70
Spreadery Cheese Snack Vermont white cheddar cold pack	1 oz	15	4	2	?	0	70
Spreadery Cheese Snack mild Mexican cold pack w/jalapeño peppers	1 oz	15	4	3	?	0	70
Spreadery Cheese Snack nacho cold pack	1 oz	15	4	2	?	0	70
Spreadery Cheese Snack Neufâchatel w/Classic Ranch flavor	1 oz	20	7	4	?	0	70
Spreadery Cheese Snack Neufâchatel w/French Onion	1 oz	20	6	4	?	0	70
Spreadery Cheese Snack Neufâchatel w/garden vegetables	1 oz	20	6	3	?	0	70
Spreadery Cheese Snack Neufâchatel w/garlic & herb	1 oz	20	6	4	?	0	70
Spreadery Cheese Snack port wine cold pack	1 oz	15	4	2	?	0	70
Velveeta light singles	1 oz	15	4	2	?	0	70
Process Cheese Spread							
Cheeze Whiz	1 oz	20	6	3	?	0	80
Cheeze Whiz mild Mexican	1 oz	20	6	4	?	0	80
Cheeze Whiz w/jalapeño peppers	1 oz	20	6	4	?	0	80
American	1 oz	15	6	3	?	0	80
w/jalapeño (loaf)	1 oz	20	2	4	?	0	80
w/bacon	1 oz	20	1	4	?	0	80
Mohawk Valley Limburger	1 oz	20	0	3	?	0	70
Old English sharp	1 oz	20	1	4	?	0	80
Squeeze-A-Snack garlic flavor	1 oz	20	7	4	?	0	80

	Portion	Chol (mg)	Total Fat(g)	Satur'd Fat(g)	Mono Fat(g)	Poly Fat(g)	Total Calor
Squeeze-A-Snack hickory smoke flavor	1 oz	20	7	4	?	0	80
Squeeze-A-Snack w/bacon	1 oz	20	7	2	?	0	80
Squeeze-A-Snack w/jalapeño pepper	1 oz	20	6	4	?	0	80
Squeeze-A-Snack sharp	1 oz	20	7	4	?	0	80
Velveeta	1 oz	20	6	4	?	0	80
Velveeta Mexican (hot)	1 oz	20	6	3	?	0	80
Velveeta Mexican (mild)	1 oz	20	6	3	?	0	80
Velveeta pimiento	1 oz	20	6	3	?	0	80

Miscellaneous Cheese Items

	Portion	Chol (mg)	Total Fat(g)	Satur'd Fat(g)	Mono Fat(g)	Poly Fat(g)	Total Calor
Cracker Barrel cheese ball sharp cheddar w/almonds	1 oz	20	4	3	?	0	100
Cracker Barrel cheese log port wine cheddar w/almonds	1 oz	15	4	3	?	0	90
Cracker Barrel cheese log sharp cheddar w/almonds	1 oz	15	6	3	?	0	90
Cracker Barrel cheese log smokey cheddar w/almonds	1 oz	15	6	3	?	0	90
Golden Image mild imitation cheddar	1 oz	5	9	3	?	0	110
Golden Image imitation Colby	1 oz	5	9	3	?	0	110
jalapeño pepper spread	1 oz	15	5	4	?	0	70
olives & pimiento	1 oz	15	5	4	?	3	60
pimiento spread	1 oz	15	5	3	?	0	70
pineapple spread	1 oz	15	5	3	?	0	70
Roka Blue spread	1 oz	20	6	3	?	0	70

Land O'Lakes

CULTURED CHEESE

	Portion	Chol (mg)	Total Fat(g)	Satur'd Fat(g)	Mono Fat(g)	Poly Fat(g)	Total Calor
cottage cheese	4 oz	15	5	3	120		
cottage cheese, 2% milk fat	4 oz	10	2	1	100		

NATURAL CHEESE

	Portion	Chol (mg)	Total Fat(g)	Satur'd Fat(g)	Mono Fat(g)	Poly Fat(g)	Total Calor
brick	1 oz	25	8	5	2	<1	110
cheddar	1 oz	30	9	6	3	<1	110
Colby	1 oz	25	9	6	3	<1	110
Edam	1 oz	25	8	5	2	<1	100
Gouda	1 oz	30	8	5	2	<1	100
Monterey Jack	1 oz	20	9	5	3	<1	110
mozzarella, low-moisture, part skim	1 oz	15	5	3	1	<1	80
Muenster	1 oz	25	9	5	2	<1	100
provolone	1 oz	20	8	5	2	<1	100
Swiss	1 oz	25	8	5	2	<1	110

	Portion	Chol (mg)	Total Fat(g)	Satur'd Fat(g)	Mono Fat(g)	Poly Fat(g)	Total Calor
Chedarella	1 oz	25	8	5	2	<1	100
hot pepper Monterey Jack	1 oz	20	9	5	3	<1	110

PROCESS CHEESE

	Portion	Chol (mg)	Total Fat(g)	Satur'd Fat(g)	Mono Fat(g)	Poly Fat(g)	Total Calor
American	1 oz	30	9	6	3	<1	110
American (sharp)	1 oz	30	9	6	3	<1	100
American & Swiss	1 oz	25	8	5	2	<1	100
cheddar & bacon	1 oz	25	9	5	3	<1	110
cheddar extra sharp	1 oz	30	9	6	2	<1	100
jalapeño jack	1 oz	20	8	5	2	<1	90
cheese food	1 oz	20	6	4	2	<1	90
individually wrapped slices	¾ oz	15	5	3	1	<1	70
individually wrapped slices	⅔ oz	15	4	3	1	<1	60
Italian herb cheese food	1 oz	20	7	4	2	<1	90
jalapeño cheese food	1 oz	20	7	4	2	<1	90
onion cheese food	1 oz	20	7	4	2	<1	90
pepperoni cheese food	1 oz	20	7	4	2	<1	90
salami cheese food	1 oz	20	7	4	2	<1	90
Golden Velvet cheese spread	1 oz	20	6	4	2	<1	80

COTTAGE CHEESE

	Portion	Chol (mg)	Total Fat(g)	Satur'd Fat(g)	Mono Fat(g)	Poly Fat(g)	Total Calor
regular	4 oz	15	5	3	2	<1	120
2%	4 oz	10	2	1	1	<1	100
1%	4 oz	5	1	1	<1	<1	90

Laughing Cow

WEDGES

	Portion	Chol (mg)	Total Fat(g)	Satur'd Fat(g)	Mono Fat(g)	Poly Fat(g)	Total Calor
regular	1 oz	20	6	4	?	?	70
cheddar	1 oz	20	6	4	?	?	70
reduced calorie	1 oz	10	3	2	?	?	50

CUPS

	Portion	Chol (mg)	Total Fat(g)	Satur'd Fat(g)	Mono Fat(g)	Poly Fat(g)	Total Calor
lite	1 oz	5	2	1	?	?	45
regular	1 oz	10	6	4	?	?	70

CUBES

	Portion	Chol (mg)	Total Fat(g)	Satur'd Fat(g)	Mono Fat(g)	Poly Fat(g)	Total Calor
reduced calorie	1 oz	10	2	1	/	?	45
regular	1 oz	20	6	4	?	?	70

Progresso

	Portion	Chol (mg)	Total Fat(g)	Satur'd Fat(g)	Mono Fat(g)	Poly Fat(g)	Total Calor
grated Romano	1 T	6	2	1	?	<1	23
grated Parmesan	1 T	4	2	1	?	<1	23

Weight Watchers

	Portion	Chol (mg)	Total Fat(g)	Satur'd Fat(g)	Mono Fat(g)	Poly Fat(g)	Total Calor
Swiss slices	1 oz	15	2	1	?	?	50
sharp cheddar slices	1 oz	5	2	1	?	?	50
natural mild cheddar (colored/white), regular & low sodium	1 oz	15	5	3	?	?	80

	Portion	Chol (mg)	Total Fat(g)	Satur'd Fat(g)	Mono Fat(g)	Poly Fat(g)	Total Calor
natural mild cheddar (shredded)	1 oz	15	5	3	?	?	80
natural sharp cheddar (colored/white)	1 oz	15	5	3	?	?	80
natural Colby	1 oz	15	5	2	?	?	80
natural Monterey Jack	1 oz	15	5	2	?	?	80
natural mozzerella	1 oz	15	4	2	?	?	70
natural mozzerella (shredded)	1 oz	15	4	2	?	?	80
natural Swiss	1 oz	15	5	3	?	?	90
port wine cup	1 oz	10	3	2	?	?	70
sharp cheddar cup	1 oz	10	3	2	?	?	70
American slices (white), regular & low sodium	1 oz	5	2	1	?	?	50
American slices (colored), regular & low sodium	1 oz	5	2	1	?	?	50
cottage cheese, 1%	½ c	?	1	?	?	?	90
cottage cheese, 2%	½ c	?	2	?	?	?	100
creamed cheese	1 oz	?	2	?	?	?	35

❏ **CHICKEN** *See* **POULTRY, FRESH & PROCESSED**

❏ **CHUTNEYS** *See* **PICKLES, OLIVES, RELISHES, & CHUTNEYS**

❏ **COATINGS, SEASONED** *See* **BREADCRUMBS, CROUTONS, STUFFINGS, & SEASONED COATINGS**

❏ **CONDIMENTS** *See* **SAUCES, GRAVIES, & CONDIMENTS**

❏ **COOKIES, BARS, & BROWNIES**

animal cookies	15		?	3	?	?	120
arrowroot cookies	2		?	2	?	?	47
brownies							
butterscotch	1 oz		?	5	?	?	115
chocolate, from mix	1.1 oz		?	5	?	?	130
chocolate, w/nuts							
commercial, frosted	0.9 oz	14	?	4	2	?	100

	Portion	Chol (mg)	Total Fat(g)	Satur'd Fat(g)	Mono Fat(g)	Poly Fat(g)	Total Calor
homemade	0.7 oz	18	6	1	?	?	95
chocolate cookies	1	?	3	?	?	?	93
chocolate chip cookies							
commercial	4 (2¼" diam)	5	9	3	?	?	180
from refrigerator dough	4 (2¼" diam)	22	11	4	?	?	225
homemade w/vegetable shortening	4 (2⅓" diam)	18	11	4	?	?	185
w/coconut cookies	1	?	4	?	?	?	82
chocolate sandwich cookies	1	?	2	?	?	?	49
chocolate snaps	4	?	2	?	?	?	53
coconut bars	1	?	5	?	?	?	109
fig bars	4 = 2 oz	27	4	1	?	?	210
gingersnaps	3 small	?	1	?	?	?	50
homemade	1	?	2	?	?	?	34
graham crackers	2	0	1	tr	?	?	60
chocolate-covered	1	?	3	?	?	?	62
granola bars	1	?	4	?	?	?	109
macaroons	1	?	3	?	?	?	67
molasses cookies	1	?	3	?	?	?	71
oatmeal cookies	1	?	3	?	?	?	80
from mix	2	?	6	?	?	?	130
homemade	1	?	3	?	?	?	62
oatmeal chocolate chip cookies	1	?	3	?	?	?	57
oatmeal raisin cookies							
from refrigerator dough	1	?	3	?	?	?	61
homemade	4 (2⅝" diam)	2	10	3	?	?	245
peanut butter bars	1	?	10	?	?	?	198
peanut butter cookies							
from refrigerator dough	1	?	3	?	?	?	50
homemade	4 = 1.7 oz	28	14	4	?	?	245
sandwich type cookies, chocolate or vanilla	4 = 1.4 oz	0	8	2	?	?	195
shortbread cookies							
commercial	4 small	27	8	3	?	?	155
homemade w/margarine	2 large	0	8	1	?	?	145
sugar cookies							
from mix	2	?	5	?	?	?	120
from refrigerator dough	4 = 1.7 oz	29	12	2	?	?	235
homemade	1	?	3	?	?	?	89
sugar wafers	2	?	2	?	?	?	53
vanilla cream sandwich cookies	1	?	3	?	?	?	69
vanilla wafers	10 = 1.4 oz	25	7	2	?	?	185

	Portion	Chol (mg)	Total Fat(g)	Satur'd Fat(g)	Mono Fat(g)	Poly Fat(g)	Total Calor
■ BRAND NAME							
Grandma's							
Grab cookie bits							
chocolate	8	0	7	?	?	?	145
peanut butter	8	0	7	?	?	?	145
artificially flavored vanilla	8	5	7	?	?	?	145
Sandwich cremes							
chocolate	6	0	13	?	?	?	260
peanut butter	6	0	12	?	?	?	260
artificially flavored vanilla	6	5	12	?	?	?	260
Big cookies							
chocolate chip	2	5	17	?	?	?	370
fudge chocolate chip	2	5	13	?	?	?	350
oatmeal apple spice	2	10	12	?	?	?	330
Old Time molasses	2	5	9	?	?	?	320
peanut butter	2	10	30	?	?	?	410
soft raisin	2	10	10	?	?	?	320
Candied animal cookies	2	5	9	?	?	?	140
Rich 'N Chewey chocolate chip	3	5	6	?	?	?	140
Health Valley							
Fat-free cookies							
apple spice	2	0	<1	?	?	?	75
apricot delight	3	0	<1	?	?	?	75
date delight	3	0	<1	?	?	?	75
Hawaiian fruit	2	0	<1	?	?	?	75
raisin oatmeal	3	0	<1	?	?	?	75
apple raisin	1	0	<1	?	?	?	70
raspberry	1	0	<1	?	?	?	70
Fat-free bars							
almond/date	1	0	<1	?	?	?	140
apple	1	0	<1	?	?	?	140
banana	1	0	<1	?	?	?	140
raisin	1	0	<1	?	?	?	140
Fruit Jumbos							
almonds & dates	1	0	3	?	?	?	85
raisins & nuts	1	0	3	?	?	?	85
tropical fruit	1	0	3	?	?	?	85
graham crackers							
oat bran	3	0	2	?	?	?	54
Jumbo (cookies) cinnamon	1	0	2	?	?	?	70
peanut butter	1	0	2	?	?	?	70
No fat added							
oat bran almond/date	1	0	2	?	?	?	140
oat bran blueberry	1	0	2	?	?	?	140
oat bran raisin	1	0	2	?	?	?	140

	Portion	Chol (mg)	Total Fat(g)	Satur'd Fat(g)	Mono Fat(g)	Poly Fat(g)	Total Calor
tofu cookies	4	0	3	?	?	?	52
wheat-free cookies	4	0	3	?	?	?	52
Hershey's Granola Snack Bars							
chocolate chip	1	?	8	?	?	?	170
chocolate-covered cocoa creme	1	5	9	?	?	?	180
chocolate-covered cookies & creme	1	?	8	?	?	?	170
chocolate-covered peanut butter	1	5	10	?	?	?	180
Kellogg's							
Smart Start Cereal Bars							
Common Sense oat bran (raspberry filling)	1	0	6	?	?	?	170
Corn Flakes (mixed berry filling)	1	0	7	?	?	?	170
Nutri-Grain blueberry	1	0	8	?	?	?	170
Nutri-Grain strawberry	1	0	8	?	?	?	180
Rice Krispies (w/ almonds)	1	0	6	?	?	?	130
Raisin Bran	1	0	5	?	?	?	160
Nabisco							
Almost Home							
fudge chocolate chip	1	<2	3	<1	?	<1	70
oatmeal raisin	1	<2	3	<1	?	<1	70
real chocolate chip	1	<2	3	1	?	?	60
old fashioned sugar	1	<2	3	<1	?	<1	70
Baker's Bonus Oatmeal	1	<5	3	1	?	<1	80
Baker's Own							
apple-filled	1		2	<1	?	<1	70
blueberry-filled	1	0	2	<1	?	<1	70
raspberry-filled	1	0	2	<1	?	<1	70
Barnum's Animal Crackers	5	<2	2	<1	?	<1	60
Bugs Bunny Graham Crackers	5	0	2	<1	?	<1	60
Cameo Cream Sandwich	1	0	3	1	?	<1	70
Chips Ahoy!							
chewy	1	<2	3	1	?	<1	60
pure chocolate chip	1	0	2	<1	?	<1	50
striped	1	0	5	2	?	<1	90
chocolate chocolate chunk	1	10	5	2	?	<1	90
chocolate chunk pecan	1	10	6	2	?	<1	100
Cookie Break	1	<2	2	<1	?	<1	50
Cookies 'N Fudge							
party grahams	1	<2	3	2	?	<1	70
striped shortbread	1½	0	3	1	?	<1	60
striped wafers	1	0	4	2	?	<1	70

	Portion	Chol (mg)	Total Fat(g)	Satur'd Fat(g)	Mono Fat(g)	Poly Fat(g)	Total Calor
Giggles	1	<2	3	<1	?	<1	60
Grahams & Honey Maid Graham Crackers							
cinnamon	2	<2	1	<1	?	<1	60
honey grahams	2	<2	1	<1	?	<1	60
Heyday Bars (fudge, caramel, peanut)	1	0	6	2	?	1	110
Lorna Doone Shortbread	3	<5	4	<1	?	<1	70
Mallomars	1	0	3	1	?	<1	60
Mystic Mint Sandwich	1	<2	5	3	?	<1	90
Brown Edge Wafers	2½	<2	3	<1	?	<1	70
Chocolate Chip Snaps	3	<2	2	1	?	<1	70
Chocolate Grahams	1	<2	3	2	?	<1	60
Chocolate Snaps	4	<2	2	1	?	<1	70
Famous Chocolate Wafers	2½	<2	2	<1	?	<1	70
Marshmallow Puffs Fudge Cakes	1	0	4	3	?	<1	90
Marshmallow Twirls Fudge Cake	1	0	6	4	?	<1	140
Old Fashioned Ginger Snaps	1	<2	1	<1	?	<1	30
Pure Chocolate Middles	1	<5	5	2	?	<1	80
National Arrowroot Biscuit	1	<2	1	<1	?	<1	20
Apple Newtons	1	<2	2	<1	?	<1	80
Fig Newtons	1	<2	1	<1	?	<1	60
Raspberry Newtons	1	<2	2	<1	?	<1	80
Strawberry Newtons	1	<2	2	<1	?	<1	80
Nilla Wafers	3½	5	2	<1	?	<1	60
Nutter Butter							
peanut butter sandwich	1	<2	3	<1	?	<1	70
peanut creme patties	2	0	4	<1	?	<1	80
Oreo							
chocolate sandwich	1	<2	2	<1	?	<1	50
fudge-covered chocolate sandwich	1	<2	6	4	?	<1	110
Big Stuf	1	<5	12	4	?	<1	250
Double Stuf	1	<2	4	1	?	<1	70
Pantry Molasses Cookies	1	0	3	<1	?	<1	80
Pecan Shortbread	1	<2	5	1	?	<1	80
Pinwheels	1	0	5	?	?	?	130
Social Tea Biscuits	1	<2	1	?	?	?	20
Suddenly S'mores	1	0	4	?	?	?	100
Teddy Grahams							
chocolate	11	0	2	?	?	?	60
cinnamon	11	0	2	?	?	?	60
honey	11	0	2	?	?	?	60
Pepperidge Farm							
DISTINCTIVE ASSORTMENTS							
Original Pirouettes	2	<5	4	1	2	0	70

	Portion	Chol (mg)	Total Fat(g)	Satur'd Fat(g)	Mono Fat(g)	Poly Fat(g)	Total Calor
Chocolate-laced Pirouettes	2	<5	4	1	2	0	70

DISTINCTIVE COOKIES

Bordeaux	2	0	3	1	1	0	70
Brussels	2	0	5	2	2	0	110
Brussels Mint	2	0	7	2	2	1	130
Capri	1	0	5	1	2	0	80
Cappucino	1	<5	3	1	1	0	50
Chantilly	1	<5	2	1	0	0	80
Chessman	2	10	4	2	1	0	90
Geneva	2	0	6	2	2	1	130
Lido	1	<5	5	1	3	1	90
Linzer	1	<5	4	1	2	0	120
Milano	2	5	6	2	3	0	120
Mint Milano	2	5	7	2	4	0	150
Nassau	1	<5	5	1	1	1	80
Orange Milano	2	5	7	2	4	0	150
Orleans	3	0	6	2	2	0	90
Orleans Sandwich	2	0	8	2	4	0	120
Tahiti	1	5	6	2	2	1	90
Zurich	1	0	2	1	1	0	60

SPECIAL SELECTION

chocolate chunk pecan	1	10	4	1	2	0	70
milk chocolate macadamia	1	<5	4	1	2	0	70

BROWNIES

Westport Fudgey Brownies w/walnuts	1	25	11	4	4	2	220
Tahoe Milk Chocolate Pecan	1	25	10	3	5	1	210
Charlotte Fudgey Brownie	1	25	11	4	4	2	220

OLD FASHIONED COOKIES

brownie chocolate nut	2	<5	7	2	2	1	110
chocolate chip	2	5	5	2	2	0	100
chocolate toffee chip	2	5	5	2	0	1	100
Gingerman	2	5	3	0	2	0	70
hazelnut	2	0	6	2	1	1	110
Irish oatmeal	2	5	5	1	2	0	90
lemon nut crunch	2	<5	7	2	3	0	110
molasses crisps	2	0	3	0	2	0	70
oatmeal raisin	2	10	5	2	2	0	110
pecan shortbread	2	0	5	2	0	1	70
shortbread	2	<5	8	2	4	0	150
sugar	2	10	5	2	2	0	100

	Portion	Chol (mg)	Total Fat(g)	Satur'd Fat(g)	Mono Fat(g)	Poly Fat(g)	Total Calor
FRUIT FILLED							
apricot-raspberry	2	10	4	2	2	0	100
strawberry	2	10	5	2	2	0	100
AMERICAN COLLECTION							
Beacon Hill Chocolate Chocolate Walnut	1	5	7	2	2	1	120
Chesapeake Chocolate Chunk Pecan	1	5	7	2	4	1	120
Cheyenne Peanut Butter Milk Chocolate Chunk	1	5	6	2	3	0	110
Dakota Milk Chocolate Oatmeal	1	5	6	2	2	1	110
Nantucket Chocolate Chunk	1	5	6	2	3	0	120
Santa Fe Oatmeal Raisin	1	<5	4	1	2	0	100
Sausalito Milk Chocolate Macadamia	1	5	7	2	3	0	120
OLD FASHIONED LARGE COOKIES							
brownie nut	1	5	8	3	3	0	140
chocolate chip	1	5	6	2	3	1	130
oatmeal	1	5	6	1	3	1	120
KITCHEN HEARTH COOKIES							
date pecan	2	10	5	2	2	0	110
raisin bran	2	<5	5	2	2	0	110
Quaker Oats							
CHEWY GRANOLA BARS							
chocolate chip	1	<1	5	2	1	<1	128
chocolate, graham & marshmallow	1	<1	4	1	1	<1	126
chunky nut & raisin	1	<1	6	1	1	<1	131
honey & oats	1	<1	4	1	1	1	125
peanut butter	1	<1	5	1	1	1	128
peanut butter & chocolate chip	1	<1	6	2	2	1	131
raisin & cinnamon	1	<1	5	1	1	1	128
GRANOLA DIPS							
caramel nut	1	2	6	3	2	<1	148
chocolate chip	1	1	6	3	2	<1	139
chocolate fudge	1	?	8	?	?	?	160
peanut butter	1	2	9	3	3	1	170
peanut butter chocolate chip	1	?	10	?	?	?	174
Weight Watchers							
apple raisin bar	1	?	3	?	?	?	100
shortbread cookies	3	?	2	?	?	?	80

	Portion	Chol (mg)	Total Fat(g)	Satur'd Fat(g)	Mono Fat(g)	Poly Fat(g)	Total Calor
chocolate cookies	3	?	3	?	?	?	80
oatmeal spice cookies	3	?	2	?	?	?	80

❏ CORNMEAL *See* FLOURS & CORNMEALS

❏ CRACKERS
See also SNACKS

	Portion	Chol (mg)	Total Fat(g)	Satur'd Fat(g)	Mono Fat(g)	Poly Fat(g)	Total Calor
bread sticks *See* BREADS, ROLLS, BISCUITS, & MUFFINS							
cheese, plain	10 (1" square)	6	3	1	?	?	50
cheese & peanut butter sandwich	1	1	2	tr	?	?	40
graham *See* COOKIES, BARS, & BROWNIES							
matzo	1	?	tr	?	?	?	117
melba toast, plain	1	0	tr	tr	?	?	20
oyster	33	?	3	?	?	?	120
rice wafers	3	?	0	?	?	?	31
rye crisp	2 triple crackers	?	tr	?	?	?	50
rye wafers, whole grain	2 (1⅞" × 3½")	0	1	tr	?	?	55
saltines	4	4	1	1	?	?	50
soda, unsalted tops	10	?	3	?	?	?	120
taco shells *See* BREADS, ROLLS, BISCUITS, & MUFFINS							
tortillas *See* BREADS, ROLLS, BISCUITS, & MUFFINS							
wheat, thin	4	0	1	1	?	?	35
whole-wheat wafers	2	0	2	1	?	?	35
zwieback *See* INFANT & TODDLER FOODS							

▪ BRAND NAME

Frito Lay

	Portion	Chol (mg)	Total Fat(g)	Satur'd Fat(g)	Mono Fat(g)	Poly Fat(g)	Total Calor
Cheddar Cracker Snacks	13-16	0	4	?	?	?	70
Cheese-filled Crackers	6	5	10	?	?	?	?
Peanut Butter-filled Crackers	6	0	10	?	?	?	210
Doritos							
Cool Ranch	1 oz	0	7	?	?	?	140
Nacho Cheese	1 oz	0	7	?	?	?	140

Hain

	Portion	Chol (mg)	Total Fat(g)	Satur'd Fat(g)	Mono Fat(g)	Poly Fat(g)	Total Calor
cheese	1 oz	?	6	?	?	?	130
onion	1 oz	?	6	?	?	?	130
onion, no salt added	1 oz	?	6	?	?	?	130
rich	1 oz	?	5	?	?	?	130
rich, no salt added	1 oz	?	5	?	?	?	130
rye	1 oz	?	4	?	?	?	120

	Portion	Chol (mg)	Total Fat(g)	Satur'd Fat(g)	Mono Fat(g)	Poly Fat(g)	Total Calor
rye, no salt added	1 oz	?	4	?	?	?	120
sesame	1 oz	?	7	?	?	?	140
sesame, no salt added	1 oz	?	7	?	?	?	140
sour cream & chive	1 oz	?	6	?	?	?	130
sour cream & chive, no salt added	1 oz	?	6	?	?	?	130
sourdough	½ oz	?	3	?	?	?	65
sourdough, no salt added	1 oz	?	5	?	?	?	130
vegetable	1 oz	?	5	?	?	?	130
vegetable, no salt added	1 oz	?	5	?	?	?	130
rice cakes (all varieties)	1	?	<1	?	?	?	40
mini rice cakes							
apple cinnamon	1	0	<1	?	?	?	60
barbeque	1	0	3	?	?	?	70
cheese	1	<5	2	?	?	?	60
honey nut	1	0	<1	?	?	?	60
nacho cheese	1	<5	2	?	?	?	70
plain	1	0	<1	?	?	?	60
ranch	1	0	3	?	?	?	70
teriyaki	1	0	<1	?	?	?	50
Health Valley							
herb, regular or no salt	13	0	6	?	?	?	130
honey graham	13	0	6	?	?	?	130
sesame, regular or no salt	13	0	6	?	?	?	130
7-grain vegetable							
regular	1 oz	0	6	?	?	?	130
no salt	1 oz	0	5	?	?	?	130
stoned-wheat, regular or no salt	13	0	6	?	?	?	130
Nabisco							
AMERICAN CLASSIC							
cracked wheat	4	0	4	<1	?	<1	70
dairy butter	4	<2	3	<1	?	<1	70
golden sesame	4	0	3	<1	?	<1	70
toasted poppy	4	0	3	<1	?	<1	70
Bacon-flavored Thins	7	<2	4	1	?	<1	70
Better Cheddars							
regular	10	<2	4	<1	?	<1	70
low salt	10	<2	4	<1	?	<1	70
Chicken in a Bisket	7	<2	5	1	?	<1	80
Crown Pilot	1	<2	2	<1	?	<1	70
Dandy Soup & Oyster	20	<2	2	<1	?	<1	60
Escort	3	0	4	<1	?	<1	70
Harvest Crisps							
5 grain	6	0	2	<1	?	<1	60
oat	6	0	2	<1	?	<1	60
Meal Mates Sesame Bread Wafers	3	0	3	<1	?	<1	70
Nips Cheese	13	<2	3	<1	?	<1	70

	Portion	Chol (mg)	Total Fat(g)	Satur'd Fat(g)	Mono Fat(g)	Poly Fat(g)	Total Calor
Oysterettes Soup & Oyster	18	<2	1	<1	?	<1	60
Premium Saltine							
regular	5	<2	2	<1	?	<1	60
low salt	5	<2	2	<1	?	<1	60
unsalted tops	5	<2	2	<1	?	<1	60
bits	5	<2	2	<1	?	<1	60
whole wheat	5	0	2	<1	?	<1	60
Ritz							
regular	4	<2	4	<1	?	<1	70
low salt	4	<2	4	<1	?	<1	70
bits							
regular	22	0	4	<1	?	<1	70
cheese	22	<2	4	<1	?	<1	70
low salt	22	0	4	<1	?	<1	70
peanut butter sandwiches	6	0	4	<1	?	<1	80
Royal Lunch	1	<5	2	<1	?	<1	60
Sociables	6	<2	3	<1	?	<1	70
Swiss Cheese	7	<2	4	1	?	<1	70
Tid Bits	16	<2	4	1	?	<1	70
Triscuits							
regular	3	0	2	<1	?	<1	60
low salt	3	0	2	<1	?	<1	60
wheat n' bran	3	0	2	<1	?	<1	60
bits	8	0	2	<1	?	<1	60
Twigs	5	<2	4	<1	?	<1	70
Uneeda, unsalted tops	3	0	2	<1	?	<1	60
Vegetable Thins	7	<2	4	<1	?	<1	70
Wavery							
regular	4	0	3	<1	?	<1	70
low salt	4	0	3	<1	?	<1	70
Wheat Thins							
regular	8	0	3	<1	?	<1	70
low salt	8	0	3	<1	?	<1	70
nutty	7	0	4	<1	?	<1	70
Oat Thins	8	0	3	<1	?	<1	70
Wheatsworth	4	0	3	<1	?	<1	70
Zwieback	2	<2	1	<1	?	<1	70
Pepperidge Farm							
butter-flavored thin crackers	4	<5	3	1	?	?	70
English Water Biscuits	4	0	1	0	?	?	70
Hearty wheat crackers	4	0	5	1	?	?	100
sesame crackers	4	0	4	1	?	?	80
Snack Sticks See SNACKS							
three cracker assortment	4	?	4	?	?	?	100
Tiny Goldfish See SNACKS							
Pillsbury							
Bread Sticks See BREADS, BISCUITS, & MUFFINS							

	Portion	Chol (mg)	Total Fat(g)	Satur'd Fat(g)	Mono Fat(g)	Poly Fat(g)	Total Calor
Quaker Oats							
rice cakes							
plain, lightly salted or salt free	1	0	<1	<1	<1	<1	35
sesame, lightly salted or salt free	1	0	<1	<1	<1	<1	35
multigrain, lightly salted	1	?	<1	<1	<1	<1	35
corn, lightly salted	1	0	<1	<1	<1	<1	35
corn cakes	1	?	<1	?	?	?	34
rye cakes	1	0	<1	<1	<1	<1	35
wheat cakes	1	0	<1	<1	<1	<1	34
Rykrisp							
natural	1/2 oz	0	0	?	?	?	40
seasoned	1/2 oz	0	1	?	?	?	48
sesame	1/2 oz	0	2	?	?	?	50

❑ CREAM & CREAM SUBSTITUTES
See MILK, MILK SUBSTITUTES, & MILK PRODUCTS

❑ CROUTONS *See* BREADCRUMBS, CROUTONS, STUFFINGS, & SEASONED COATINGS

❑ CUSTARDS *See* DESSERTS: CUSTARDS, GELATINS, PUDDINGS, & PIE FILLINGS

❑ DELI MEATS *See* PROCESSED MEAT & POULTRY PRODUCTS

❑ DESSERTS: CAKES, PASTRIES, & PIES

Cake & Coffee Cake

	Portion	Chol (mg)	Total Fat(g)	Satur'd Fat(g)	Mono Fat(g)	Poly Fat(g)	Total Calor
angel food							
from mix	whole (9¾" diam tube)	0	2	tr	?	?	1,510
from mix	1/12 cake	0	tr	tr	?	?	125
homemade	2.1 oz	?	tr	?	?	?	161
applesauce spice, from mix	1/12 cake	?	11	?	?	?	250

	Portion	Chol (mg)	Total Fat(g)	Satur'd Fat(g)	Mono Fat(g)	Poly Fat(g)	Total Calor
banana, from mix	1/12 cake	?	11	?	?	?	260
w/buttercream icing	1.8 oz	?	7	?	?	?	181
Boston cream pie	3.9 oz	?	10	?	?	?	332
butter brickle, from mix	1/12 cake	?	11	?	?	?	260
butter pecan, from mix	1/8 cake	?	15	?	?	?	310
butter pecan, from mix	1/12 cake	?	11	?	?	?	250
carrot							
from mix	1/12 cake	?	11	?	?	?	250
homemade, w/cream cheese icing	whole (10" diam tube)	1183	328	66	?	?	6,175
homemade, w/cream cheese icing	1/16 cake	74	21	4	?	?	385
cheesecake							
commercial	whole (9" diam)	2053	213	120	?	?	3,350
commercial	1/12 cake	170	18	10	?	?	280
from mix	1/8 cake	30	14	9	?	?	300
chocolate	1/12 cake	?	11	?	?	?	250
chocolate chip, from mix	1/12 cake	?	4	?	?	?	190
chocolate w/icing, from mix	1.3 oz cupcake	?	5	?	?	?	129
chocolate fudge bundt ring, from mix	1/16 cake	?	12	?	?	?	270
chocolate fudge w/vanilla icing, from mix	1/6 cake	?	10	?	?	?	280
chocolate pudding, from mix	1/6 cake	?	5	?	?	?	230
cinnamon streusel, from mix	1/8 cake	?	8	?	?	?	250
coffee cake, crumb, from mix	whole 15.1 oz	279	41	12	?	?	1385
coffee cake, crumb, from mix	1/6 cake	47	7	2	?	?	230
devil's food, w/chocolate icing							
from mix, made w/margarine, w/chocolate frosting	whole, 2-layer (8" or 9" diam)	598	136	56	?	?	3,755
from mix, made w/margarine	1/16 cake	37	8	4	?	?	235
from mix, made w/margarine	1.2 oz cupcake	19	4	2	?	?	120
homemade	2.1 oz	?	11	?	?	?	227
fruitcake							
dark, homemade	3 lb	640	228	48	?	?	5,185
dark, homemade	1½ oz	20	7	2	?	?	165
light	1.4 oz	?	7	?	?	?	156

	Portion	Chol (mg)	Total Fat(g)	Satur'd Fat(g)	Mono Fat(g)	Poly Fat(g)	Total Calor
German chocolate							
from mix	1/12 cake	?	11	?	?	?	260
gingerbread							
from mix	whole (8" square)	6	39	10	?	?	1,575
from mix	1/9 cake	1	4	1	?	?	175
lemon, from mix	1/12 cake	?	11	?	?	?	260
lemon bundt ring, from mix	1/16 cake	?	10	?	?	?	270
lemon pudding, from mix	1/6 cake	?	5	?	?	?	230
pineapple upside down							
from mix	1/9 cake	?	10	?	?	?	270
homemade	2.6 oz	?	9	?	?	?	236
plum pudding, canned	2" wedge	?	1	?	?	?	270
pound							
commercial	1.1 lb loaf	1100	94	52	?	?	1,935
commercial	1 oz	64	5	3	?	?	110
from mix	1/12 cake	?	9	?	?	?	200
homemade	1.1 lb loaf	555	94	21	?	?	2,025
homemade	1 oz	32	5	1	?	?	120
sheet, plain, homemade, w/vegetable oil							
unfrosted	whole (9" square)	552	108	30	?	?	2,830
unfrosted	1/9 cake	61	12	3	?	?	315
w/uncooked white icing	whole (9" square)	636	129	42	?	?	4,020
w/uncooked white icing	1/9 cake	70	14	5	?	?	445
shortcake	0.9 oz	?	2	?	?	?	86
snack cake, small, commercial							
devil's food w/cream filling	1 oz	15	4	2	?	?	105
sponge w/cream filling	1 oz	7	5	2	?	?	155
sour cream, from mix	1/8 cake	?	12	?	?	?	270
sour cream chocolate, from mix	1/12 cake	?	11	?	?	?	260
sour cream white, from mix	1/12 cake	?	3	?	?	?	180
spice, from mix	1.8 oz	?	6	?	?	?	175
w/vanilla icing	1.8 oz	?	5	?	?	?	176
sponge, homemade	2.3 oz	?	3	?	?	?	188
streusel swirl, from mix	1/16 cake	?	11	?	?	?	260
white cake							
commercial, w/white icing	whole, 2-layer (8" or 9" diam)	46	148	33	?	?	4,170
commercial, w/white icing	1/16 cake	3	9	2	?	?	260

	Portion	Chol (mg)	Total Fat(g)	Satur'd Fat(g)	Mono Fat(g)	Poly Fat(g)	Total Calor
from mix	2½ oz	?	10	?	?	?	219
homemade	0.7 oz	?	12	?	?	?	285
w/chocolate icing	2.7 oz	?	12	?	?	?	298
yellow, homemade	2.6 oz	?	12	?	?	?	283
yellow, w/chocolate icing							
commercial	whole, 2-layer (8" or 9" diam)	609	175	92	?	?	3,895
commercial	¹/₁₆ cake	38	11	6	?	?	245
from mix	whole, 2-layer (8" or 9" diam)	576	125	48	?	?	3,735
from mix	¹/₁₆ cake	36	8	3	?	?	235
homemade	1 piece	?	12	?	?	?	292
yellow cupcake							
w/chocolate icing	1	?	5	?	?	?	155
w/vanilla icing	1.4 oz	?	6	?	?	?	160

Cake Icing

	Portion	Chol (mg)	Total Fat(g)	Satur'd Fat(g)	Mono Fat(g)	Poly Fat(g)	Total Calor
caramel	1.4 oz	?	5	?	?	?	140
chocolate	1.4 oz	?	6	?	?	?	148
chocolate double dark	1.3 oz	?	4	?	?	?	150
chocolate fudge	1.4 oz	?	4	?	?	?	150
coconut	1.4 oz	?	3	?	?	?	140
coconut almond	1.2 oz	?	10	?	?	?	170
coconut pecan	1.2 oz	?	8	?	?	?	150
lemon	1.2 oz	?	5	?	?	?	140
milk chocolate	1.1 oz	?	5	?	?	?	150
strawberry	1.1 oz	?	5	?	?	?	140
vanilla	1.3 oz	?	5	?	?	?	150
white, fluffy	0.6 oz	?	0	?	?	?	70

Danish, Doughnuts, Sweet Rolls, & Toaster Pastries

	Portion	Chol (mg)	Total Fat(g)	Satur'd Fat(g)	Mono Fat(g)	Poly Fat(g)	Total Calor
Danish pastry							
plain, w/out fruit or nuts	12 oz ring	292	71	29	?	?	1,305
plain, w/out fruit or nuts	1 (4¼" diam)	49	12	4	?	?	220
plain, w/out fruit or nuts	1 oz	24	6	2	?	?	110
cinnamon raisin, refrigerator dough	2	?	11	?	?	?	270
fruit	1 round	56	13	4	?	?	235
doughnut							
cale type, plain	1.8 oz	20	12	3	?	?	210

	Portion	Chol (mg)	Total Fat(g)	Satur'd Fat(g)	Mono Fat(g)	Poly Fat(g)	Total Calor
yeast-leavened, glazed	2.1 oz	21	13	5	?	?	235
sweet roll	1	?	7	?	?	?	154
cinnamon w/icing, from refrigerator dough	2	?	8	?	?	?	230
toaster pastries	1	0	6	2	?	?	210

Fruit Bettys, Cobblers, Crisps, & Turnovers

apple brown Betty	½ c	?	5	?	?	?	211
apple crisp	½ c	?	8	?	?	?	302
apple dumpling	1	?	17	?	?	?	280
peach cobbler	⅓ c	?	6	?	?	?	160
turnover, from mix, apple, blueberry, or cherry	1	?	8	?	?	?	173

Pastry

brownies *See* COOKIES, BARS, & BROWNIES							
cream puff w/custard filling	1	?	15	?	?	?	245
éclair							
w/chocolate icing & custard filling	1	?	15	?	?	?	316
lady finger, w/whipped cream filling	1	?	17	?	?	?	326
pastry shells & pie crusts *See* BAKING INGREDIENTS							

Pie

apple, w/vegetable shortening crust	whole (9″ diam)	0	105	27	?	?	2,420
apple, w/vegetable shortening crust	⅙ pie	2	18	5	?	?	405
banana custard, homemade	5.6 oz piece	?	15	?	?	?	353
blueberry, w/vegetable shortening crust	whole (9″ diam)	0	102	26	?	?	2,285
blueberry, w/vegetable shortening crust	⅙ pie	0	17	4	?	?	380
cherry, w/vegetable shortening crust	whole (9″ diam)	0	107	28	?	?	2,465
cherry, w/vegetable shortening crust	⅙ pie	0	18	5	?	?	410
chocolate chiffon, homemade	2.8 oz piece	?	12	?	?	?	262
chocolate cream, homemade	4 oz piece	?	17	?	?	?	301
coconut custard, homemade	5½ oz piece	?	19	?	?	?	365

	Portion	Chol (mg)	Total Fat(g)	Satur'd Fat(g)	Mono Fat(g)	Poly Fat(g)	Total Calor
cream, w/vegetable shortening crust	whole (9" diam)	46	139	90	?	?	2,710
creme, w/vegetable shortening crust	⅙ pie	8	23	15	?	?	455
custard, w/vegetable shortening crust	whole (9" diam)	1010	101	34	?	?	1,985
custard, w/vegetable shortening crust	⅙ pie	169	17	6	?	?	330
fried							
apple	3 oz	14	14	6	?	?	255
cherry	3 oz	13	14	6	?	?	250
lemon chiffon, homemade	3.8 oz piece	?	10	?	?	?	288
lemon meringue, w/vegetable shortening crust	whole (9" diam)	857	86	26	?	?	2,140
lemon meringue, w/vegetable shortening crust	⅙ pie	143	14	4	?	?	355
mincemeat, homemade	5.6 oz piece	?	18	?	?	?	434
peach, w/vegetable shortening crust	whole (9" diam)	0	101	25	?	?	2,410
peach, w/vegetable shortening crust	⅙ pie	0	17	4	?	?	405
pecan, w/vegetable shortening crust	whole (9" diam)	569	189	28	?	?	3,450
pecan, w/vegetable shortening crust	⅙ pie	95	32	5	?	?	575
pineapple cheese, homemade	5.6 oz piece	?	10	?	?	?	270
pumpkin, w/vegetable shortening crust	whole (9" diam)	655	102	38	?	?	1,920
pumpkin, w/vegetable shortening crust	⅙ pie	109	17	6	?	?	320
sweet potato, homemade	5.6 oz piece	?	18	?	?	?	342

Pie Fillings *See* DESSERTS: CUSTARDS, GELATINS, PUDDINGS, & PIE FILLINGS

■ BRAND NAME

Banquet
FROZEN PIES

	Portion	Chol (mg)	Total Fat(g)	Satur'd Fat(g)	Mono Fat(g)	Poly Fat(g)	Total Calor
cream pies							
banana	⅙ pie	?	10	?	?	?	180
chocolate	⅙ pie	?	10	?	?	?	190
coconut	⅙ pie	?	11	?	?	?	190
lemon	⅙ pie	?	9	?	?	?	170

	Portion	Chol (mg)	Total Fat(g)	Satur'd Fat(g)	Mono Fat(g)	Poly Fat(g)	Total Calor
family size fruit pies							
apple	⅙ pie	?	11	?	?	?	250
blueberry	⅙ pie	?	11	?	?	?	270
cherry	⅙ pie	?	11	?	?	?	250
mincemeat	⅙ pie	?	11	?	?	?	260
pumpkin	⅙ pie	?	8	?	?	?	200
Kellogg's							
FROSTED POP-TARTS							
blueberry	1	0	6	?	?	?	210
brown sugar cinnamon	1	0	7	?	?	?	210
cherry	1	0	5	?	?	?	200
chocolate fudge	1	0	5	?	?	?	200
chocolate-vanilla creme	1	0	5	?	?	?	200
Dutch apple	1	0	6	?	?	?	210
grape	1	0	5	?	?	?	200
raspberry	1	0	5	?	?	?	200
strawberry	1	0	5	?	?	?	200
POP-TARTS							
blueberry	1	?	5	?	?	?	210
brown sugar cinnamon	1	?	8	?	?	?	210
cherry	1	0	6	?	?	?	210
strawberry	1	0	6	?	?	?	210
Pepperidge Farm Frozen Cakes & Pastries							
FROZEN PRODUCTS							
puffy pastry							
apple turnovers	1	?	17	?	?	?	300
blueberry turnovers	1	?	19	?	?	?	310
cherry turnovers	1	?	19	?	?	?	310
peach turnovers	1	?	18	?	?	?	310
raspberry turnovers	1	?	17	?	?	?	310
patty shells	1	?	15	?	?	?	210
apple dumplings	3 oz	?	13	?	?	?	260
dough sheets	¼ sheet	?	17	?	?	?	260
mini puff pastry shell	1	?	4	?	?	?	50
American collection desserts							
Amherst apple crumb coffee cake	1	20	11	7	3	1	220
Berkshire apple crisp	1	40	8	4	2	1	250
Charleston peach melba shortcake	1	135	5	3	1	0	220
Hyannis Boston cream pie	1	70	10	4	3	1	230
Manhattan strawberry cheesecake	1	150	9	5	2	0	300
Mississippi mud pie	1	60	23	12	6	1	310
Monterey hot fudge chocolate chunk brownie	1	65	26	14	7	1	480

	Portion	Chol (mg)	Total Fat(g)	Satur'd Fat(g)	Mono Fat(g)	Poly Fat(g)	Total Calor
Newport hot fudge brownie	1	80	20	10	5	1	400
San Francisco chocolate mousse	1	150	34	18	9	2	490
dessert lights							
apple 'n spice	4¼ oz	10	2	0	1	0	170
cherries supreme	3¼ oz	80	2	0	1	0	170
chocolate mousse cake	2½ oz	5	9	3	0	2	190
lemon cake supreme	2¾ oz	50	5	1	2	1	170
peach parfait	4¼ oz	10	5	1	2	1	150
raspberry vanilla swirl	3¼ oz	15	5	1	2	1	160
strawberry shortcake	3 oz	70	5	1	2	1	170
large layer cake							
chocolate fudge	1⅝ oz	20	10	3	3	2	180
chocolate fudge stripe	1⅝ oz	20	9	3	3	2	170
coconut	1⅝ oz	20	8	3	2	1	180
devil's food	1⅝ oz	20	9	3	2	2	180
German chocolate cake	1⅝ oz	20	10	4	3	2	180
golden	1⅝ oz	20	9	3	2	2	180
strawberry stripe	1½ oz	20	8	3	2	1	160
tropical guava	1¾ oz	20	?	?	?	?	?
vanilla	1⅝ oz	20	8	3	2	1	190
supreme cakes							
Boston cream	2⅞ oz	50	14	6	4	2	290
chocolate	2⅞ oz	25	16	7	5	3	300
lemon coconut	3 oz	30	13	6	3	2	280
lemon cream	1⅝ oz	20	9	3	2	2	170
peach melba	3⅛ oz	35	7	3	2	1	270
pineapple cream	2 oz	20	7	2	2	1	190
strawberry cream	2 0z	20	7	3	2	1	190
classic cakes							
carrot	1 cake	50	16	6	6	2	260
coconut	1 cake	20	11	4	4	2	230
double chocolate	1 cake	35	13	4	5	2	250
fudge golden	1 cake	40	14	4	6	2	260
German chocolate	1 cake	45	13	4	4	2	250
lemon coconut	1 cake	40	10	4	2	0	220
vanilla fudge swirl	1 cake	35	11	4	4	2	250
old-fashioned cakes							
butter pound	1 oz	60	7	3	2	1	130
carrot w/cream cheese icing	1½ oz	15	9	3	3	2	150
cholesterol-free pound	1 oz	0	6	1	?	2	110
fruit squares							
apple	1 sq.	?	12	?	?	?	200
cherry	1 sq.	?	12	?	?	?	230
Pillsbury							
SWEET ROLLS							
caramel Danish w/nuts	1 roll	0	8	2	?	<1	160
cinnamon w/icing	1 roll	0	5	1	?	<1	110
cinnamon raisin Danish w/icing	1 roll	0	7	2	?	<1	150

	Portion	Chol (mg)	Total Fat(g)	Satur'd Fat(g)	Mono Fat(g)	Poly Fat(g)	Total Calor
orange Danish w/icing	1 roll	0	7	2	?	<1	150
TURNOVERS							
all flavors	1 roll	0	8	2	?	<1	170
COFFEE CAKES							
cinnamon swirl	1 slice	0	9	2	?	<1	180
pecan struesel	1 slice	0	9	2	?	<1	180
Sara Lee							
ALL BUTTER COFFEE CAKES							
butter streusel	1/8 cake	?	7	?	?	?	160
pecan	1/8 cake	?	8	?	?	?	160
ALL BUTTER POUND CAKE							
original	1/10 cake	35	7	?	?	?	130
family size	1/15 cake	35	7	?	?	?	130
CLASSICS							
French cheesecake							
plain	1/10 pkg	20	16	?	?	?	250
strawberry	1/10 pkg	20	13	?	?	?	240
mousse cake							
chocolate	1/10 pkg	20	17	?	?	?	260
ELEGANT ENDINGS							
FREE & LIGHT							
apple Danish	1 slice	0	0	?	?	?	130
apple pie	1 slice	0	4	?	?	?	190
cherry pie	1 slice	0	5	?	?	?	200
pound cake	1 slice	0	0	?	?	?	70
INDIVIDUAL DANISH							
apple	1	?	6	?	?	?	120
cheese	1	?	8	?	?	?	130
cinnamon raisin	1	?	8	?	?	?	150
INDIVIDUALLY WRAPPED COFFEE CAKE							
apple cinnamon	1	?	13	?	?	?	290
butter streusel	1	?	12	?	?	?	230
pecan	1	?	16	?	?	?	280
LIGHTS							
apple crisp cake	1 cake	5	2	?	?	?	150
carrot cake	1 cake	5	4	?	?	?	170
chocolate mousse	1 cake	10	8	?	?	?	170
double chocolate cake	1 cake	10	5	?	?	?	150
fiend cheesecake	1 cake	15	4	?	?	?	150
lemon cream cake	1 cake	10	6	?	?	?	180
strawberry fiend cheesecake	1 cake	5	2	?	?	?	150

	Portion	Chol (mg)	Total Fat(g)	Satur'd Fat(g)	Mono Fat(g)	Poly Fat(g)	Total Calor
ORIGINAL CHEESECAKE							
cherry cream	1 slice	?	8	?	?	?	243
plain cream	1 slice	?	11	?	?	?	230
strawberry cream	1 slice	?	8	?	?	?	222
SINGLE-LAYER ICED CAKES							
banana	1 slice	?	6	?	?	?	170
carrot	1 slice	25	13	?	?	?	250
SNACK CAKES							
all butter pound	1	?	11	?	?	?	200
chocolate fudge	1	?	10	?	?	?	190
classic cheesecake	1	?	14	?	?	?	200
THREE-LAYER CAKES							
double chocolate	1 slice	20	11	?	?	?	220
flaky coconut	1 slice	20	12	?	?	?	220
German chocolate	1 slice	30	13	?	?	?	240
TWO-LAYER CAKES							
black forest	1 slice	25	10	?	?	?	250
strawberry shortcake	1 slice	?	8	?	?	?	190
9″ HOMESTYLE PIES							
apple	1 slice	0	12	?	?	?	280
blueberry	1 slice	0	12	?	?	?	300
cherry	1 slice	0	13	?	?	?	270
Dutch apple	1 slice	0	12	?	?	?	300
mince	1 slice	0	13	?	?	?	300
peach	1 slice	0	12	?	?	?	280
pecan	1 slice	55	18	?	?	?	400
10″ HOMESTYLE PIES							
apple	1 slice	0	23	?	?	?	400
Weight Watchers							
apple crisp	3½ oz	5	5	<1	3	1	190
apple pie	3½ oz	5	5	1	2	2	200
Boston cream pie	3 oz	5	4	1	1	2	160
brownie cheesecake	3½ oz	10	5	1	3	1	200
carrot cake	3 oz	5	5	<1	3	2	170
cheesecake	3.9 oz	20	7	2	4	1	210
cherries & cream cake	3 oz	5	6	1	1	3	190
chocolate brownie	1.25 oz	5	3	<1	2	1	100
chocolate cake	2½ oz	5	5	<1	3	2	180
chocolate mocha pie	2¾ oz	5	5	3	2	<1	160
double fudge cake	2¾ oz	5	5	<1	3	2	200
German chocolate cake	2½ oz	5	7	<1	4	3	200
strawberry cheesecake	3.9 oz	20	4	2	1	1	180
pastries							
apple sweet roll	2½ oz	5	4	<1	3	1	160

	Portion	Chol (mg)	Total Fat(g)	Satur'd Fat(g)	Mono Fat(g)	Poly Fat(g)	Total Calor
cheese sweet roll	2½ oz	5	4	5	<1	2	180
coffee cakes w/cinnamon streusel	2½ oz	5	7	1	5	1	190
strawberry sweet roll	2½ oz	20	5	20	1	3	170

❏ DESSERTS: CUSTARDS, GELATINS, PUDDINGS, & PIE FILLINGS

Custard

	Portion	Chol (mg)	Total Fat(g)	Satur'd Fat(g)	Mono Fat(g)	Poly Fat(g)	Total Calor
plain							
baked, homemade	½ c	?	7	?	?	?	153
boiled, homemade	½ c	?	7	?	?	?	164
from mix	½ c	80	5	3	?	?	161
banana	½ c	?	5	?	?	?	143
chocolate	½ c	?	4	?	?	?	142
coconut	½ c	?	4		?	?	144
lemon	½ c	?	5	?	?	?	143
vanilla	½ c	?	5	?	?	?	143

Gelatin

	Portion	Chol (mg)	Total Fat(g)	Satur'd Fat(g)	Mono Fat(g)	Poly Fat(g)	Total Calor
dry	1 envelope	0	tr	tr	?	?	25
made w/water, all flavors	½ c	0	tr	tr	?	?	81

Pie Filling

	Portion	Chol (mg)	Total Fat(g)	Satur'd Fat(g)	Mono Fat(g)	Poly Fat(g)	Total Calor
pumpkin pie mix, canned	½ c	0	tr	tr	?	?	141

Pudding

	Portion	Chol (mg)	Total Fat(g)	Satur'd Fat(g)	Mono Fat(g)	Poly Fat(g)	Total Calor
butterscotch, homemade	½ c	?	5	?	?	?	207
chocolate							
canned	5 oz	1	11	10	?	?	205
from mix, prepared w/whole milk							
regular	½ c	15	4	2	?	?	150
instant	½ c	14	4	2	?	?	155
homemade	½ c	?	7	?	?	?	219
lemon snow, homemade	½ c	?	tr	?	?	?	114
rice, from mix, prepared w/whole milk	½ c	15	4	2	?	?	155
tapioca							
canned	5 oz	tr	5	5	?	?	160
from mix, prepared w/whole milk	½ c	15	4	2	?	?	145
homemade	½ c	?	5	?	?	?	133

	Portion	Chol (mg)	Total Fat(g)	Satur'd Fat(g)	Mono Fat(g)	Poly Fat(g)	Total Calor
vanilla							
canned	5 oz	1	10	10	?	?	220
from mix, prepared w/whole milk							
regular	½ c	15	4	2	?	?	145
instant	½ c	15	4	2	?	?	150
homemade	½ c	?	5	?	?	?	152

Rennin Dessert

homemade	½ c	?	4	?	?	?	113
chocolate, from mix							
w/skim milk	½ c	?	1	?	?	?	95
w/whole milk	½ c	?	18	?	?	?	127
fruit vanilla, from mix							
w/skim milk	½ c	?	tr	?	?	?	88
w/whole milk	½ c	?	5	?	?	?	140

■ BRAND NAME

D-Zerta

gelatin, low-cal	½ c	0	0	0	?	?	8
pudding, reduced-calorie, w/skim milk							
butterscotch	½ c	0	0	?	?	?	70
chocolate	½ c	0	0	0	?	?	60
vanilla	½ c	0	0	0	?	?	70

Jell-O

AMERICAN DESSERTS (PREPARED W/WHOLE MILK)

golden egg custard	½ c	80	5	?	?	?	160
rice pudding	½ c	15	4	?	?	?	170
tapioca pudding							
vanilla	½ c	15	4	?	?	?	160

GELATIN

all flavors	½ c	0	0	0	?	?	80
fudge	½ c	10	6	?	?	?	150

PUDDING & PIE FILLING

Regular (prepared w/whole milk)

butterscotch	½ c	15	4	?	?	?	170
chocolate	½ c	15	4	?	?	?	160
chocolate fudge	½ c	15	4	?	?	?	160
coconut cream	½ c	10	4	?	?	?	110
flan	½ c	15	4	?	?	?	150
French vanilla	½ c	15	4	?	?	?	170
milk chocolate	½ c	15	4	?	?	?	160
vanilla	½ c	15	4	?	?	?	160

	Portion	Chol (mg)	Total Fat(g)	Satur'd Fat(g)	Mono Fat(g)	Poly Fat(g)	Total Calor
Instant (prepared w/whole milk)							
banana cream	½ c	15	4	?	?	?	160
butter pecan	½ c	15	5	?	?	?	170
butterscotch	½ c	15	4	?	?	?	160
chocolate	½ c	15	4	?	?	?	180
chocolate fudge	½ c	15	5	?	?	?	180
coconut cream	½ c	15	6	?	?	?	180
French vanilla	½ c	15	4	?	?	?	160
lemon	½ c	15	4	?	?	?	170
milk chocolate	½ c	15	5	?	?	?	180
vanilla	½ c	15	4	?	?	?	160
Sugar-free (prepared w/2% low-fat milk)							
chocolate	½ c	10	3	?	?	?	90
vanilla	½ c	10	2	?	?	?	80
Sugar-free Instant (prepared w/2% low-fat milk)							
banana	½ c	10	2	?	?	?	80
butterscotch	½ c	10	2	?	?	?	90
chocolate	½ c	10	3	?	?	?	90
chocolate fudge	½ c	10	3	?	?	?	100
pistachio	½ c	10	3	?	?	?	90
vanilla	½ c	10	2	?	?	?	90
Pudding Snacks							
butterscotch/chocolate/ vanilla swirl	4 oz c	0	6	?	?	?	180
chocolate	4 oz c	0	6	?	?	?	170
chocolate fudge	4 oz c	0	6	?	?	?	170
chocolate/caramel swirl	4 oz c	0	6	?	?	?	170
chocolate fudge/milk chocolate swirl	4 oz c	0	6	?	?	?	170
chocolate/vanilla swirl	4 oz c	0	6	?	?	?	170
milk chocolate	4 oz c	0	6	?	?	?	170
milk chocolate/ chocolate fudge swirl	4 oz c	0	6	?	?	?	170
tapioca	4 oz c	0	4	?	?	?	170
vanilla	4 oz c	0	7	?	?	?	180
vanilla/chocolate swirl	4 oz c	0	6	?	?	?	180
chocolate	5.5 oz c	0	8	?	?	?	230
vanilla	5.5 oz c	0	9	?	?	?	250
chocolate/vanilla swirl	5.5 oz c	0	8	?	?	?	240
Microwave Pudding (prepared w/whole milk)							
banana cream	½ c	15	4	?	?	?	150
butterscotch	½ c	15	4	?	?	?	170
chocolate	½ c	15	5	?	?	?	170
milk chocolate	½ c	15	5	?	?	?	160
vanilla	½ c	15	4	?	?	?	160

	Portion	Chol (mg)	Total Fat(g)	Satur'd Fat(g)	Mono Fat(g)	Poly Fat(g)	Total Calor
Light Pudding Snacks							
chocolate	4 oz c	5	2	?	?	?	100
chocolate fudge	4 oz c	5	1	?	?	?	100
chocolate vanilla combo	4 oz c	5	2	?	?	?	100
vanilla	4 oz c	5	2	?	?	?	100
No Bake Desserts, 8" pie or cake (prepared w/whole milk)							
banana cream pie	1/8	30	14	?	?	?	240
cheesecake	1/8	30	13	?	?	?	280
lemon cheesecake	1/8	25	13	?	?	?	270
New York style cheesecake	1/8	30	12	?	?	?	280
chocolate mousse pie	1/8	30	17	?	?	?	260
coconut cream pie	1/8	30	16	?	?	?	260
pumpkin pie	1/8	30	13	?	?	?	250
Rich & Luscious Mousse (prepared w/whole milk)							
chocolate	1/2 c	10	6	?	?	?	150
chocolate fudge	1/2 c	10	6	?	?	?	140
My-T-Fine							
PUDDINGS							
butterscotch	makes 1/2 c	?	0	0	?	0	90
chocolate	dry mix to make 1/2 c	0	0	0	?	0	100
chocolate almond	dry mix to make 1/2 c	0	1	0	?	0	100
chocolate fudge	dry mix to make 1/2 c	?	0	0	?	0	100
lemon	dry mix to make 1 serving	0	0	0	?	0	90
vanilla	makes 1/2 c	0	0	0	?	0	90
vanilla tapioca	dry mix to make 1 serving	0	0	0	?	0	80
Royal							
GELATIN							
all flavors	1/2 c	0	0	0	?	?	80
sugar-free	1/2 c	0	0	0	?	?	8-10
banana cream, dry mix to make	1 serving	0	0	0	?	?	80
butterscotch, dry mix to make	1/2 c	0	0	0	?	?	90
chocolate, dry mix to make	1/2 c	0	0	0	?	?	90

	Portion	Chol (mg)	Total Fat(g)	Satur'd Fat(g)	Mono Fat(g)	Poly Fat(g)	Total Calor
custard, dry mix to make	½ c	?	0	?	?	?	60
Dark 'n Sweet, dry mix to make	½ c	0	0	0	?	?	90
flan w/caramel sauce, dry mix to make	½ c	0	0	?	?	?	60
key lime, dry mix to make	1 serving	0	0	0	?	?	50
lemon, dry mix to make	1 serving	0	0	0	?	?	50
vanilla, dry mix to make	1 serving	0	0	0	?	?	80
Instant							
banana cream, dry mix to make	1 serving	0	0	0	?	?	90
butterscotch, dry mix to make	1 serving	0	0	0	?	?	90
cherry vanilla, dry mix to make	1 serving	0	0	0	?	?	90
chocolate, dry mix to make	1 serving	0	0	0	?	?	160
chocolate almond	½ c	0	1	0	?	?	120
chocolate chocolate chip, dry mix to make	1 serving	0	1	0	?	?	110
chocolate peanut butter chip, dry mix to make	1 serving	0	1	0	?	?	110
Dark 'n Sweet, dry mix to make	1 serving	0	0	0	?	?	110
lemon, dry mix to make	1 serving	0	0	0	?	?	90
pistachio nut, dry mix to make	1 serving	0	1	0	?	?	90
strawberry, dry mix to make	1 serving	0	0	0	?	?	100
toasted coconut, dry mix to make	1 serving	0	2	0	?	?	100
vanilla, dry mix to make	1 serving	0	1	0	?	?	90
vanilla chocolate, dry mix to make	1 serving	0	1	0	?	?	90
Instant Sugar-free							
chocolate, dry mix to make	½ c	?	0	?	?	?	50
Snack Pack							
banana pudding	4.25 oz	1	6	1	?	1	145
butterscotch pudding	4.25 oz	1	6	1	?	1	170
chocolate pudding	4.25 oz	1	6	1	?	1	170
chocolate fudge pudding	4.25 oz	1	6	1	?	1	165
chocolate marshmallow pudding	4.25 oz	1	6	1	?	1	165
lemon pudding	4.25 oz	0	4	1	?	1	150
tapioca pudding	4.25 oz	1	5	1	?	1	150

	Portion	Chol (mg)	Total Fat(g)	Satur'd Fat(g)	Mono Fat(g)	Poly Fat(g)	Total Calor
vanilla	4.25 oz	1	6	1	?	1	170
light tapioca pudding	4 oz	1	2	<1	?	<1	100
light chocolate pudding	4 oz	1	2	<1	?	<1	100
Swiss Miss							
butterscotch pudding	4 oz	1	6	1	?	1	180
chocolate pudding	4 oz	1	6	1	?	<1	180
chocolate fudge pudding	4 oz	1	6	2	?	1	220
tapioca pudding	4 oz	1	5	1	?	<1	160
vanilla pudding	4 oz	1	7	1	?	<1	190
chocolate parfait	4 oz	1	6	1	?	<1	170
vanilla parfait	4 oz	1	6	1	?	1	180
chocolate pudding sundae	4 oz	1	7	2	?	1	220
vanilla pudding sundae	4 oz	1	7	2	?	1	220
light chocolate pudding	4 oz	1	2	<1	?	<1	100
light chocolate fudge pudding	4 oz	1	1	<1	?	<1	100
light vanilla pudding	4 oz	<1	1	<1	?	<1	100
light vanilla/chocolate parfait	4 oz	<1	1	<1	?	<1	100
Weight Watchers							
MOUSSE MIXES (PREPARED W/SKIM MILK)							
cheesecake	½ c	?	2	?	?	?	60
chocolate	½ c	?	3	?	?	?	60
raspberry	½ c	?	3	?	?	?	60
white chocolate almond	½ c	?	3	?	?	?	60
INSTANT PUDDING (PREPARED W/SKIM MILK)							
butterscotch	½ c	?	?	?	?	?	90
chocolate	½ c	?	1	?	?	?	90
vanilla	½ c	?	?	?	?	?	90

❏ DESSERTS, FROZEN: ICE CREAM, ICE MILK, ICES, & SHERBETS, FROZEN JUICE, PUDDING, TOFU, & YOGURT

Frozen Pudding on a Stick

banana	1		1	3	3	?	?	94
butterscotch	1		1	3	3	?	?	94
chocolate	1		1	3	3	?	?	99
vanilla	1		1	3	3	?	?	93

Yogurt

IN A CUP

fruit varieties	½ c	?	1	?	?	?	108

	Portion	Chol (mg)	Total Fat(g)	Satur'd Fat(g)	Mono Fat(g)	Poly Fat(g)	Total Calor
ON A STICK							
plain	1	5	1	?	?	?	65
carob/chocolate coated	1	5	8	?	?	?	135
raspberry, chocolate coated	1	?	7	?	?	?	127
strawberry	1	?	1	?	?	?	69
Ice Cream							
chocolate	1 c	?	16	?	?	?	295
French custard	1 c	?	14	?	?	?	257
French vanilla, soft serve	1 c	153	23	14	?	?	377
strawberry	1 c	?	12	?	?	?	250
vanilla							
10% fat	1 c	59	14	9	?	?	269
16% fat	1 c	88	24	15	?	?	349
Ice Cream & Ice Novelties & Cones							
creamsicle	1	?	3	?	?	?	103
drumstick	1	?	10	?	?	?	186
fudgsicle	1	?	tr	?	?	?	91
ice cream cone (cone only)	1	?	tr	?	?	?	45
ice cream sandwich	1	?	6	?	?	?	167
popsicle	1	0	0	0	?	?	65
vanilla ice cream bar w/chocolate coating	1	?	11	?	?	?	162
vanilla ice milk bar w/chocolate coating	1	?	8	?	?	?	144
Ice Milk							
chocolate	⅔ c	?	5	?	?	?	137
strawberry	⅔ c	?	3	?	?	?	133
vanilla							
regular	1 c	18	6	4	?	?	184
soft serve	1 c	13	5	3	?	?	223
Ices & Sherbets							
lemon sherbet	¾ c	?	5	?	?	?	241
lime/orange ice	1 c	?	tr	?	?	?	247
lime/orange ice	⅔ c	?	tr	?	?	?	165
orange sherbet	1 c	14	4	2	?	?	270
various sherbet	1 c	?	0	0	?	?	236

	Portion	Chol (mg)	Total Fat (g)	Satur'd Fat (g)	Mono Fat (g)	Poly Fat (g)	Total Calor
■ **BRAND NAME**							
Baskin-Robbins							
CONES							
sugar	1	0	1	?	?	?	60
waffle	1	0	2	?	?	?	140
DELUXE ICE CREAM							
butter pecan	1 scoop	40	18	?	?	?	280
chocolate	1 scoop	37	14	?	?	?	270
chocolate chip	1 scoop	40	15	?	?	?	260
chocolate almond	1 scoop	34	18	?	?	?	300
chocolate fudge	1 scoop	41	15	?	?	?	290
chocolate mousse	1 scoop	32	16	?	?	?	320
cookies 'n cream	1 scoop	39	17	?	?	?	280
French vanilla	1 scoop	90	18	?	?	?	320
fudge brownie	1 scoop	36	18	?	?	?	310
German chocolate cake	1 scoop	32	15	?	?	?	240
jamoca almond fudge	1 scoop	32	14	?	?	?	260
mint chocolate chip	1 scoop	40	15	?	?	?	330
peanut butter 'n chocolate	1 scoop	33	20	?	?	?	290
pistachio almond	1 scoop	39	18	?	?	?	280
Rocky Road	1 scoop	32	14	?	?	?	300
vanilla	1 scoop	52	14	?	?	?	240
very berry	1 scoop	30	10	?	?	?	220
world-class chocolate	1 scoop	36	14	?	?	?	280
INTERNATIONAL ICE CREAM							
chocolate-raspberry truffle	1 scoop	45	17	?	?	?	310
kaluha 'n cream	1 scoop	15	14	?	?	?	270
ICES & SHERBERTS							
daiquiri ice	1 scoop	0	0	?	?	?	140
orange sherbert	1 scoop	6	2	?	?	?	160
rainbow sherbert	1 scoop	6	2	?	?	?	160
SUGAR FREE							
cherry cordial	½ c	3	1	?	?	?	100
chocolate chip	½ c	4	2	?	?	?	100
chunky banana	½ c	3	1	?	?	?	80
jamoca Swiss almond	½ c	4	2	?	?	?	90
strawberry	½ c	3	2	?	?	?	80
thin mint	½ c	4	2	?	?	?	90
FAT FREE							
twist	½ c	0	0	?	?	?	100
just peachy	½ c	0	0	?	?	?	100

	Portion	Chol (mg)	Total Fat(g)	Satur'd Fat(g)	Mono Fat(g)	Poly Fat(g)	Total Calor
LIGHT							
almond buttercrunch	½ c	12	6	?	?	?	130
chocolate caramel nut	½ c	8	5	?	?	?	130
espresso 'n cream	½ c	12	5	?	?	?	120
strawberry royal	½ c	9	3	?	?	?	110
vanilla fudge	½ c	11	4	?	?	?	110
FROZEN YOGURT							
nonfat							
chocolate	½ c	0	0	?	?	?	110
strawberry	½ c	0	0	?	?	?	110
vanilla	½ c	0	0	?	?	?	100
lowfat							
chocolate	½ c	6	2	?	?	?	140
raspberry	½ c	5	2	?	?	?	120
vanilla	½ c	6	2	?	?	?	120
NOVELTIES							
chilly burgers							
chocolate chip	1	26	12	?	?	?	270
vanilla	1	29	11	?	?	?	240
very berry strawberry	1	23	9	?	?	?	230
sundae bars							
jamoca almond fudge	1	24	13	?	?	?	300
pralines 'n cream	1	30	13	?	?	?	310
strawberry royal	1	21	9	?	?	?	280
light sundae bars							
vanilla/chocolate	1	10	4	?	?	?	155
chocolate/caramel	1	11	5	?	?	?	150
tiny toon bars							
chocolate chip	1	17	15	?	?	?	230
mint chocolate	1	17	15	?	?	?	230
strawberry	1	15	13	?	?	?	210
vanilla	1	18	14	?	?	?	210
Ben & Jerry's							
PINT ORIGINALS							
cherry garcia	4 oz	81	16	?	?	?	260
chocolate	4 oz	52	15	?	?	?	250
chocolate chip cookie dough	4 oz	52	15	?	?	?	300
chocolate fudge brownie	4 oz	45	15	?	?	?	270
chunky monkey	4 oz	70	18	?	?	?	290
coffee Heath bar crunch	4 oz	79	18	?	?	?	280
Heath bar crunch	4 oz	83	19	?	?	?	290
mint chocolate cookie	4 oz	84	18	?	?	?	280
New York super fudge chunk	4 oz	44	20	?	?	?	300
peach	4 oz	73	13	?	?	?	270
rainforest crunch	4 oz	81	21	?	?	?	300
strawberry	4 oz	74	14	?	?	?	220

	Portion	Chol (mg)	Total Fat(g)	Satur'd Fat(g)	Mono Fat(g)	Poly Fat(g)	Total Calor
vanilla	4 oz	93	17	?	?	?	250
vanilla chocolate chunk	4 oz	82	17	?	?	?	270
wild Maine blueberry	4 oz	78	14	?	?	?	220

PINT LIGHTS

	Portion	Chol (mg)	Total Fat(g)	Satur'd Fat(g)	Mono Fat(g)	Poly Fat(g)	Total Calor
chocolate fudge brownie	4 oz	23	9	?	?	?	220
coffee almond fudge	4 oz	22	10	?	?	?	240
Heath bar crunch ·	4 oz	26	9	?	?	?	230
peach	4 oz	23	8	?	?	?	230
reverse chocolate chunk	4 oz	25	10	?	?	?	230
sweet cream & cookie	4 oz	26	8	?	?	?	220
vanilla fudge	4 oz	24	7	?	?	?	210
vanilla Swiss chocolate almond	4 oz	25	12	?	?	?	250

PINT YOGURTS

	Portion	Chol (mg)	Total Fat(g)	Satur'd Fat(g)	Mono Fat(g)	Poly Fat(g)	Total Calor
banana strawberry	3 oz	5	1	?	?	?	130
blueberry cheesecake	3 oz	5	1	?	?	?	120
cherry garcia	3 oz	5	1	?	?	?	120
chocolate	3 oz	6	2	?	?	?	130
chocolate fudge brownie	3 oz	5	3	?	?	?	150
coffee almond fudge	3 oz	5	4	?	?	?	150
Heath bar crunch	3 oz	5	5	?	?	?	160
raspberry	3 oz	5	1	?	?	?	130

NOVELTIES

	Portion	Chol (mg)	Total Fat(g)	Satur'd Fat(g)	Mono Fat(g)	Poly Fat(g)	Total Calor
brownie bar							
vanilla	4 oz	58	19	?	?	?	360
chocolate	4 oz	34	17	?	?	?	350
peace pop							
cherry garcia	4 oz	57	14	?	?	?	260
Heath bar crunch	4 oz	55	17	?	?	?	310
New York super fudge	4 oz	33	19	?	?	?	310
rainforest	4 oz	53·	21	?	?	?	340
vanilla	4 oz	70	16	?	?	?	260

Colombo

	Portion	Chol (mg)	Total Fat(g)	Satur'd Fat(g)	Mono Fat(g)	Poly Fat(g)	Total Calor
nonfat frozen yogurt	4 oz	0	0	?	?	?	100
lowfat frozen yogurt	4 oz	7	2	?	?	?	110
sugar-free nonfat frozen yogurt	4 oz	0	0	?	?	?	60

Crystal Light

COOL 'N CREAMY BARS

	Portion	Chol (mg)	Total Fat(g)	Satur'd Fat(g)	Mono Fat(g)	Poly Fat(g)	Total Calor
chocolate/vanilla	1	0	2	?	?	?	50
double chocolate fudge	1	0	2	?	?	?	50
orange vanilla	1	0	2	?	?	?	30
amaretto chocolate swirl	1	0	2	?	?	?	60

	Portion	Chol (mg)	Total Fat(g)	Satur'd Fat(g)	Mono Fat(g)	Poly Fat(g)	Total Calor
BARS							
average values, all flavors	1	0	0	?	?	?	14
Dole							
FRESH LITES							
all flavors	1 bar	0	<1	?	?	?	25
FRUIT & CREAM BARS							
blueberry	1	5	1	?	?	?	90
Peach	1	?	1	5	?	?	90
strawberry	1	5	1	?	?	?	90
FRUIT 'N JUICE BARS							
all flavors	1	0	<1	?	?	?	60-70
SUN TOPS							
all flavors	1 bar	0	<1	?	?	?	40
SORBETS							
strawberry	4 oz	0	<1	?	?	?	100
all other flavors	4 oz	0	<1	?	?	?	110
YOGURT BARS							
chocolate	1	2	<1	?	?	?	70
strawberry	1	2	<1	?	?	?	70
strawberry	1	2	<1	?	?	?	60
GELATIN POPS							
all flavors	1	0	0	0	?	?	35
PUDDING POPS							
chocolate	1	0	2	?	?	?	80
Häagen-Dazs							
ICE CREAM							
vanilla	4 fl oz	120	17	8	?	<1	260
chocolate	4 fl oz	120	17	8	?	<	270
coffee	4 fl oz	120	17	8	?	<1	270
strawberry	4 fl oz	95	15	8	?	<1	250
rum raisin	4 fl oz	110	17	8	?	<1	250
honey vanilla	4 fl oz	135	16	8	?	<1	250
vanilla Swiss almond	4 fl oz	?	19	?	?	?	290
vanilla fudge	4 fl oz	?	17	?	?	?	270
deep chocolate	4 fl oz	?	14	?	?	?	290
chocolate chocolate chip	4 fl oz	105	20	10	?	<1	290
vanilla peanut butter swirl	4 fl oz	110	21	8	?	2	280
butter pecan	4 fl oz	110	24	9	?	3	390

	Portion	Chol (mg)	Total Fat(g)	Satur'd Fat(g)	Mono Fat(g)	Poly Fat(g)	Total Calor
chocolate chocolate mint	4 fl oz	?	20	?	?	?	300
deep chocolate fudge	4 fl oz	?	14	?	?	?	290
deep chocolate peanut butter	4 fl oz	?	19	?	?	?	330
macadamia brittle	4 fl oz	?	18	?	?	?	280
caramel nut sundae	4 fl oz	?	21	?	?	?	310

SORBETS & CREAM

	Portion	Chol (mg)	Total Fat(g)	Satur'd Fat(g)	Mono Fat(g)	Poly Fat(g)	Total Calor
blueberry	4 fl oz	?	2	?	?	?	190
key lime	4 fl oz	?	7	?	?	?	190
orange	4 fl oz	?	8	?	?	?	190
raspberry	4 fl oz	?	8	?	?	?	180

FROZEN YOGURT

	Portion	Chol (mg)	Total Fat(g)	Satur'd Fat(g)	Mono Fat(g)	Poly Fat(g)	Total Calor
chocolate	3 fl oz	25	3	2	?	<1	130
peach	3 fl oz	31	3	1.5	?	<1	120
strawberry	3 fl oz	30	3	1.6	?	<1	120
vanilla	3 fl oz	40	3	1.7	?	<1	130
vanilla almond crunch	3 fl oz	65	5	1.5	?	<1	150

CRUNCH BARS & ICE CREAM POPS

	Portion	Chol (mg)	Total Fat(g)	Satur'd Fat(g)	Mono Fat(g)	Poly Fat(g)	Total Calor
caramel almond	1	40	18	7	?	2	240
peanut butter	1	35	21	7	?	3	270
vanilla	1	40	18	7	?	2	220
fudge bar pop	1	?	14	?	?	?	210
orange & cream pop	1	?	6	?	?	?	130

ICE CREAM BARS

	Portion	Chol (mg)	Total Fat(g)	Satur'd Fat(g)	Mono Fat(g)	Poly Fat(g)	Total Calor
chocolate/dark chocolate	1	85	27	?	?	?	390
vanilla/dark chocolate	1	90	27	?	?	?	390
vanilla/milk chocolate	1	90	27	?	?	?	360
vanilla/milk chocolate almond	1	90	27	?	?	?	370
vanilla/milk chocolate brittle	1	?	25	?	?	?	370

Jell-O

GELATIN POPS

	Portion	Chol (mg)	Total Fat(g)	Satur'd Fat(g)	Mono Fat(g)	Poly Fat(g)	Total Calor
all flavors	1	0	0	0	?	?	35

PUDDING POPS

	Portion	Chol (mg)	Total Fat(g)	Satur'd Fat(g)	Mono Fat(g)	Poly Fat(g)	Total Calor
chocolate	1	0	2	?	?	?	80
chocolate fudge	1	0	2	?	?	?	80
chocolate/peanut butter swirl	1	0	3	?	?	?	80
chocolate/vanilla swirl	1	0	2	?	?	?	80
double chocolate swirl	1	0	2	?	?	?	80
milk chocolate	1	0	2	?	?	?	80
vanilla	1	0	2	?	?	?	80

	Portion	Chol (mg)	Total Fat(g)	Satur'd Fat(g)	Mono Fat(g)	Poly Fat(g)	Total Calor
SUNBURST BARS							
lemon, orange	1	0	0	?	?	?	45
Kool-Aid							
CREAM POPS							
average values, all flavors	1	5	2	?	?	?	50
KOOL POPS							
average values, all flavors	1	0	0	?	?	?	40
Nestlé							
Crunch Lite Frozen Dairy Dessert	2.5 oz	?	10	?	?	?	150
ICE CREAM BARS							
Nestlé Quick	1	?	11	?	?	?	210
milk chocolate w/almonds premium	1	?	23	?	?	?	250
Oh Henry!	1	?	20	?	?	?	320
Nestlé Crunch chocolate	1	?	12	?	?	?	190
Nestlé Crunch vanilla	1	?	12	?	?	?	180
Alpine white candy tops	1	?	18	?	?	?	250
Tofutti							
PINTS							
vanilla	4 oz	0	11	2	3	7	200
chocolate supreme	4 oz	0	13	3	4	6	210
wild berry	4 oz	0	12	2	3	6	210
vanilla almond bark	4 oz	0	14	3	4	6	230
vanilla love drops	4 oz	0	12	3	3	6	220
cappucino love drops	4 oz	0	12	3	4	6	230
chocolate love drops	4 oz	0	13	5	4	4	230
SOFT SERVE							
regular	4 oz	0	8	2	3	4	158
hi-lite vanilla	4 oz	0	1	?	?	?	90
hi-lite chocolate	4 oz	0	1	?	?	?	100
SINGLE-SERVE NOVELTIES							
vanilla cuties	?	0	5	1	2	2	130
chocolate cuties	?	0	5	2	2	2	140
LAND OF THE FREE							
three berry	4 oz	0	0	?	?	?	90
vanilla apple orchard	4 oz	0	0	?	?	?	90
Fruittis	2 fl oz	0	?	?	?	?	120

	Portion	Chol (mg)	Total Fat(g)	Satur'd Fat(g)	Mono Fat(g)	Poly Fat(g)	Total Calor
LITE LITE							
deep chocolate fudge	4 fl oz	0	<1	?	?	?	100
special strawberry	4 fl oz	0	<1	?	?	?	90
Swiss mocha coffee	4 fl oz	0	<1	?	?	?	90
vanilla chocolate strawberry	4 fl oz	0	<1	?	?	?	90
Weight Watchers							
ICE MILK							
chocolate chip	½ c	10	4	2	?	?	120
chocolate premium	½ c	10	3	2	?	?	110
Neopolitan premium	½ c	10	3	1	?	?	110
vanilla premium	½ c	10	3	1	?	?	100
pecans pralines & creme	½ c	10	4	3	?	?	120
FAT-FREE FROZEN DESSERT							
chocolate	½ c	5	?	?	?	?	80
chocolate swirl	½ c	5	?	?	?	?	90
vanilla	½ c	5	?	?	?	?	80
FROZEN NOVELTIES							
chocolate dip bar	1.7 oz	5	7	3	?	1	110
double fudge bar	1.75 oz	5	1	?	?	?	60
English toffee crunch bar	1.75 oz	5	8	4	?	3	120
sugar-free chocolate mousse bar	1.75 oz	5	<1	?	?	?	35
sugar-free orange vanilla bar	1.75 oz	5	<1	?	?	?	30
sandwich snacks	1.5 oz	?	2	?	?	?	90
vanilla sandwich bars	2.75 oz	5	3	2	?	?	150
One-ders chocolate chip	4 oz	10	4	?	?	?	120
One-ders heavenly hash	4 oz	10	3	?	?	?	120
One-ders pralines 'n creme	4 oz	10	4	?	?	?	120
One-ders strawberry	4 oz	10	3	?	?	?	110

❏ DESSERT SAUCES, SYRUPS, & TOPPINGS

See also NUTS & NUT-BASED BUTTERS, FLOURS, MEALS, MILKS, PASTES, & POWDERS

Sauces, Syrups, & Flavored Toppings

butterscotch sauce, homemade	2 T	?	7	?	?	?	203

	Portion	Chol (mg)	Total Fat(g)	Satur'd Fat(g)	Mono Fat(g)	Poly Fat(g)	Total Calor
butterscotch topping	3 T	?	tr	?	?	?	156
caramel topping	3 T	?	tr	?	?	?	155
chocolate-flavored syrup or topping							
fudge type	2 T	0	5	3	?	?	125
thin type	2 T	0	tr	tr	?	?	85
custard sauce, homemade	4 T	?	4	?	?	?	85
hard sauce, homemade	4 T	?	11	?	?	?	193
honey *See* SUGARS & SWEETENERS							
lemon sauce, homemade	4 T	?	3	?	?	?	133
walnuts in syrup topping	3 T	?	1	?	?	?	169

Whipped Cream-type Toppings

	Portion	Chol (mg)	Total Fat(g)	Satur'd Fat(g)	Mono Fat(g)	Poly Fat(g)	Total Calor
nondairy							
powdered, prepared w/whole milk	1 T	tr	1	tr	?	?	8
powdered, prepared w/whole milk	1 c	8	10	9	?	?	151
pressurized, containing lauric acid oil & sodium caseinate	1 T	0	1	1	?	?	11
pressurized, containing lauric acid oil & sodium caseinate	1 c	0	16	13	?	?	184
semisolid, frozen, containing lauric acid oil & sodium caseinate	1 T	0	1	1	?	?	13
semisolid, frozen, containing lauric acid oil & sodium caseinate	1 c	0	19	16	?	?	239
whipped cream topping, pressurized	1 T	2	1	4	?	?	8
whipped cream topping, pressurized	1 c	46	13	8	?	?	159

■ BRAND NAME

Cool Whip

	Portion	Chol (mg)	Total Fat(g)	Satur'd Fat(g)	Mono Fat(g)	Poly Fat(g)	Total Calor
extra creamy dairy recipe whipped topping	1 T	0	1	?	?	?	16
lite whipped topping	1 T	0	<1	?	?	?	8

	Portion	Chol (mg)	Total Fat(g)	Satur'd Fat(g)	Mono Fat(g)	Poly Fat(g)	Total Calor
nondairy whipped topping	1 T	0	1	?	?	?	12
Dream Whip							
whipped topping mix prepared w/whole milk	1 T	0	0	0	?	?	10
D-Zerta							
reduced cal whipped topping	1 T	0	1	?	?	?	8
Hershey							
chocolate fudge topping	2 T	5	4	?	?	?	100
Kraft							
artificially flavored butterscotch topping	1 T	0	1	0	?	0	60
caramel topping	1 T	0	0	0	?	0	60
chocolate topping	1 T	0	0	0	?	0	50
hot fudge topping	1 T	0	2	1	?	0	70
pineapple topping	1 T	0	0	0	?	0	50
strawberry topping	1 T	0	0	0	?	0	50
Nestlé							
ICE CREAM TOPPINGS							
Nestlé Crunch candy tops	1.25 oz	?	17	?	?	?	220
milk chocolate w/almonds candy tops	1.25 oz	?	18	?	?	?	230
Alpine White w/almonds candy tops	1.25 oz	?	20	?	?	?	240
Oh Henry! candy tops	1.25 oz	?	18	?	?	?	230
Smucker's							
butterscotch	2 T	?	1	?	?	?	140
caramel	2 T	?	1	?	?	?	140
chocolate	2 T	?	1	?	?	?	130
chocolate fudge	2 T	?	1	?	?	?	130
hot caramel	2 T	?	4	?	?	?	150
hot fudge	2 T	?	4	?	?	?	110
hot toffee fudge	2 T	?	4	?	?	?	110
light hot fudge	2 T	?	<1	?	?	?	70
Magic Shell							
chocolate & chocolate fudge	2 T	?	15	?	?	?	190
chocolate nut	2 T	?	16	?	?	?	200
marshmallow	2 T	?	0	?	?	?	120
peanut butter caramel	2 T	?	2	?	?	?	150
pecans in syrup	2 T	?	1	?	?	?	130
pineapple	2 T	?	0	0	?	?	130
Special Recipe							
hot fudge	2 T	?	5	?	?	?	150
butterscotch	2 T	?	3	?	?	?	160
dark chocolate	2 T	?	1	?	?	?	130

	Portion	Chol (mg)	Total Fat(g)	Satur'd Fat(g)	Mono Fat(g)	Poly Fat(g)	Total Calor
strawberry	2 T	?	0	0	?	?	120
Swiss milk chocolate fudge	2 T	?	1	?	?	?	140

❏ DINNERS, FROZEN

▪ BRAND NAMES

Banquet
DINNERS

	Portion	Chol (mg)	Total Fat(g)	Satur'd Fat(g)	Mono Fat(g)	Poly Fat(g)	Total Calor
beef & frankfurters	10 oz	35	25	?	?	?	520
beef enchilada	12 oz	?	15	?	?	?	500
cheese enchilada	12 oz	?	19	?	?	?	550
chicken & dumplings	10 oz	45	24	?	?	?	430
chopped beef	11 oz	80	32	?	?	?	420
fried chicken	10 oz	?	?	?	?	?	400
macaroni & cheese	10 oz	30	20	?	?	?	420
meat loaf	11 oz	85	27	?	?	?	440
Mexican style	12 oz	?	18	?	?	?	490
Mexican style combination	12 oz	?	17	?	?	?	520
noodles & chicken	10 oz	45	15	?	?	?	350
Salisbury steak	11 oz	80	34	?	?	?	500
spaghetti & meatballs	10 oz	30	10	?	?	?	290
turkey	10.5 oz	40	20	?	?	?	390
western	11 oz	90	41	?	?	?	630

EXTRA HELPING DINNERS

	Portion	Chol (mg)	Total Fat(g)	Satur'd Fat(g)	Mono Fat(g)	Poly Fat(g)	Total Calor
beef	16 oz	120	61	?	?	?	870
chicken nuggets w/barbeque sauce	10 oz	?	36	?	?	?	640
chicken nuggets w/sweet & sour sauce	10 oz	?	34	?	?	?	650
fried chicken	16 oz	?	28	?	?	?	570
Salisbury steak	18 oz	175	60	?	?	?	910
turkey	19 oz	65	42	?	?	?	750

Healthy Choice

	Portion	Chol (mg)	Total Fat(g)	Satur'd Fat(g)	Mono Fat(g)	Poly Fat(g)	Total Calor
breast & turkey	10½ oz	45	5	?	?	?	290
beef & pepper steak	11 oz	65	6	?	?	?	290
chicken oriental	11¼ oz	55	2	?	?	?	220
chicken parmigiana	11½ oz	60	3	?	?	?	280
chicken & pasta divan	11½ oz	60	4	?	?	?	310
herb roasted chicken	11 oz	40	3	?	?	?	260
mesquite chicken	10½ oz	45	2	?	?	?	310
Salisbury steak	11½ oz	50	7	?	?	?	300
shrimp creole	11¼ oz	65	1	?	?	?	210
shrimp marmara	10½ oz	50	1	?	?	?	220
sirloin tips	11¾ oz	70	6	?	?	?	290

	Portion	Chol (mg)	Total Fat(g)	Satur'd Fat(g)	Mono Fat(g)	Poly Fat(g)	Total Calor
sole au gratin	11 oz	55	5	?	?	?	270
sweet & sour chicken	11½ oz	50	2	?	?	?	280
Yankee pot roast	11 oz	45	4	?	?	?	260
Hungry-Man Dinners See Swanson, below							
Le Menu							
beef sirloin Tips	11½ oz	?	18	?	?	?	400
beef Stroganoff	10 oz	?	24	?	?	?	430
chicken la king	10¼ oz	?	13	?	?	?	330
chicken in wine sauce	10 oz	?	7	?	?	?	280
chicken parmigiana	11¾ oz	?	20	?	?	?	410
chopped sirloin beef	12¼ oz	?	24	?	?	?	430
ham steak	10 oz	?	11	?	?	?	300
manicotti w/three cheeses	11¾ oz	?	15	?	?	?	390
Salisbury steak	10½ oz	?	20	?	?	?	370
sliced breast of turkey w/mushroom gravy	10½ oz	?	7	?	?	?	300
sweet & sour chicken	11¼ oz	?	18	?	?	?	400
veal parmigiana	11½ oz	?	17	?	?	?	390
Yankee pot roast	10 oz	?	13	?	?	?	330
Le Menu Health Dinners (Light Style)							
cheese tortellini	10 oz	?	6	?	?	?	230
glazed chicken breast	10 oz	?	3	?	?	?	230
herb roasted chicken	10 oz	?	7	?	?	?	240
Salisbury steak	10 oz	?	9	?	?	?	280
3-cheese stuffed shells	10 oz	?	8	?	?	?	280
sliced turkey	10 oz	?	5	?	?	?	210
sweet & sour chicken	10 oz	7	?	?	?	?	250
turkey divan	10 oz	?	7	?	?	?	260
veal marsala	10 oz	?	3	?	?	?	230
Patio							
MEXICAN DINNERS							
beef enchilada	13¼ oz	40	24	?	?	?	520
cheese enchilada	12¼ oz	20	10	?	?	?	380
fiesta	12¼ oz	30	20	?	?	?	470
tamale	13 oz	35	21	?	?	?	470
Mexican style	13¼ oz	45	25	?	?	?	540
Swanson							
3-COMPARTMENT DINNERS							
beans & franks	10½ oz	?	19	?	?	?	440
macaroni & cheese	12¼ oz	?	15	?	?	?	370
noodles & chicken	10½ oz	?	8	?	?	?	280
spaghetti & meatballs	12½ oz	?	17	?	?	?	390
4-COMPARTMENT DINNERS							
beef	11¼ oz	?	6	?	?	?	310
beef in barbeque sauce	11 oz	?	17	?	?	?	460
beef enchiladas	13¾ oz	?	21	?	?	?	480

	Portion	Chol (mg)	Total Fat(g)	Satur'd Fat(g)	Mono Fat(g)	Poly Fat(g)	Total Calor
chicken nuggets	8¾ oz	?	23	?	?	?	470
chopped sirloin beef	10¾ oz	?	16	?	?	?	340
fish 'n chips	10 oz	?	21	?	?	?	500
fried chicken, white meat	10¼ oz	?	25	?	?	?	550
fried chicken, dark meat	9 ¾ oz	?	28	?	?	?	560
loin of pork	10¾ oz	?	12	?	?	?	280
meatloaf	10¾ oz	?	15	?	?	?	360
Mexican style combination	14¼ oz	?	18	?	?	?	490
Salisbury steak	10¾ oz	?	17	?	?	?	400
Swiss steak	10 oz	?	11	?	?	?	350
turkey	11½ oz	?	11	?	?	?	350
veal parmigiana	12¼ oz	?	20	?	?	?	450
western style	11½ oz	?	19	?	?	?	430

HUNGRY MAN DINNERS

	Portion	Chol (mg)	Total Fat(g)	Satur'd Fat(g)	Mono Fat(g)	Poly Fat(g)	Total Calor
chopped beef steak	16¾ oz	?	37	?	?	?	640
fried chicken, white meat	14¼ oz	?	46	?	?	?	870
fried chicken, dark meat	14¼ oz	?	45	?	?	?	860

Tyson

GOURMET SELECTION DINNERS

	Portion	Chol (mg)	Total Fat(g)	Satur'd Fat(g)	Mono Fat(g)	Poly Fat(g)	Total Calor
sweet & sour	11 oz	?	15	?	?	?	420
parmigiana	11¼ oz	36	17	?	?	?	380
Français	9½ oz	54	14	?	?	?	280
marsala	10½ oz	52	4	?	?	?	200
picatta	9 oz	63	10	?	?	?	240
Kiev	9¼ oz	78	33	?	?	?	520
mesquite	9½ oz	54	8	?	?	?	320
beef champignon	10½ oz	51	15	?	?	?	370
short ribs	11 oz	70	24	?	?	?	470
turkey	11½ oz	35	11	?	?	?	380
Salisbury supreme	10 oz	62	26	?	?	?	430
grilled chicken	7¾ oz	55	3	?	?	?	220
chicken w/gravy	9 oz	50	6	?	?	?	230
chicken pie	9½ oz	?	18	?	?	?	360

LOONEY TUNES MEALS

	Portion	Chol (mg)	Total Fat(g)	Satur'd Fat(g)	Mono Fat(g)	Poly Fat(g)	Total Calor
Road Runner chicken sandwich	6.7 oz	?	11	?	?	?	300
Wile E. Coyote hamburger pizza	6 oz	?	11	?	?	?	320
Bugs Bunny chicken chunks	7.7 oz	?	11	?	?	?	290
Yosemite Sam BBQ glazed chicken	8.3 oz	?	12	?	?	?	280
Tweety macaroni & cheese	9¾ oz	?	8	?	?	?	280
Daffy Duck spaghetti & meatballs	8.65 oz	?	10	?	?	?	320

	Portion	Chol (mg)	Total Fat(g)	Satur'd Fat(g)	Mono Fat(g)	Poly Fat(g)	Total Calor
Speedy Gonzales beef enchilada	9.5 oz	?	15	?	?	?	390
Foghorn Leghorn pepperoni pizza	6.45 oz	?	13	?	?	?	410
Elmer Fudd turkey & dressing	6.45 oz	?	7	?	?	?	240

❑ EGGS & EGG SUBSTITUTES

Chicken Eggs

COOKED

egg dishes, prepared *See* BREAKFAST FOODS, PREPARED; FAST FOODS

	Portion	Chol (mg)	Total Fat(g)	Satur'd Fat(g)	Mono Fat(g)	Poly Fat(g)	Total Calor
fried in butter	1 large	246	6	2	?	?	83
hard boiled	1 large	274	6	2	?	?	79
omelet, cooked w/butter & milk	1 egg (large)	248	7	3	?	?	95
poached	1 large	273	6	2	?	?	79
scrambled w/butter & milk	1 large	248	7	3	?	?	95

DRIED

	Portion	Chol (mg)	Total Fat(g)	Satur'd Fat(g)	Mono Fat(g)	Poly Fat(g)	Total Calor
whole	1 c sifted	1,631	36	11	?	?	505
stabilized (glucose-reduced)	1 c sifted	1,714	37	11	?	?	523
white only							
flakes stabilized (glucose reduced)	½ lb	0	tr	0	?	?	796
powder, stabilized (glucose reduced)	1 c sifted	0	tr	0	?	?	402
yolk only	1 c sifted	1,962	41	12	?	?	460

UNCOOKED

	Portion	Chol (mg)	Total Fat(g)	Satur'd Fat(g)	Mono Fat(g)	Poly Fat(g)	Total Calor
whole, fresh & frozen	1	274	6	2	?	?	79
white only, fresh & frozen	1	0	tr	0	?	?	16
yolk only, fresh	1	272	6	2	?	?	63

Eggs, Other

	Portion	Chol (mg)	Total Fat(g)	Satur'd Fat(g)	Mono Fat(g)	Poly Fat(g)	Total Calor
duck	1	619	10	3	?	?	130
goose	1	?	19	5	?	?	267
quail	1	76	1	tr	?	?	14
turkey	1	737	9	3	?	?	135

	Portion	Chol (mg)	Total Fat(g)	Satur'd Fat(g)	Mono Fat(g)	Poly Fat(g)	Total Calor
Egg Substitute							
frozen, containing egg white, corn oil, nonfat dry milk	¼ c	1	7	1	?	?	96
liquid, containing egg white, soybean oil, soy protein	1 c	3	8	2	?	?	211
powder, containing egg white solids, whole egg solids, sweet whey solids, nonfat dry milk, soy protein	0.7 oz	113	3	1	?	?	88

▪ BRAND NAME

Fleischmann's

	Portion	Chol (mg)	Total Fat(g)	Satur'd Fat(g)	Mono Fat(g)	Poly Fat(g)	Total Calor
Egg Beaters (cholesterol-free egg product)	¼ c	0	0	?	?	0	25
Egg Beaters cheese omelette mix	approx. ½ c	5	5	2	?	0	110
Egg Beaters vegetable omelette mix	approx. ½ c	0	0	0	?	0	50

❏ ENTREES & MAIN COURSES, CANNED & BOXED

chili & bean products, canned & boxed *See* LEGUMES & LEGUME PRODUCTS; SOYBEANS & SOYBEAN PRODUCTS

▪ BRAND NAME

Chun King

DIVIDER PAK ENTREES, CANNED

4 servings
42 oz pkg

	Portion	Chol (mg)	Total Fat(g)	Satur'd Fat(g)	Mono Fat(g)	Poly Fat(g)	Total Calor
beef chow mein	7 oz	15	2	1	?	0	100
chicken chow mein	7 oz	15	4	2	?	1	110
pork chow mein	7 oz	25	4	0	?	1	120
shrimp chow mein	7 oz	30	2	0	?	1	100
beef pepper oriental	7 oz	15	4	1	?	0	110

STIR-FRY ENTREES, CANNED

	Portion	Chol (mg)	Total Fat(g)	Satur'd Fat(g)	Mono Fat(g)	Poly Fat(g)	Total Calor
egg foo young	5 oz	140	8	2	?	4	140

	Portion	Chol (mg)	Total Fat(g)	Satur'd Fat(g)	Mono Fat(g)	Poly Fat(g)	Total Calor
pepper steak	6 oz	50	17	4	?	2	250
sukiyaki	6	50	17	3	?	2	260
chow mein w/beef	6	50	19	4	?	4	290
chow mein w/chicken	6	45	11	6	?	6	220
Featherweight							
beef stew	7½ oz	35	3	?	?	?	160
chicken stew	7½ oz	20	1	?	?	?	140
spaghetti w/meatballs	7½ oz	20	3	?	?	?	160
Franco-American							
beef ravioli in meat sauce	7½ oz	?	8	?	?	?	250
Circuso's pasta in tomato & cheese sauce	7⅜ oz	?	2	?	?	?	170
Circuso's pasta w/meatballs in tomato sauce	7⅜ oz	?	8	?	?	?	210
macaroni & cheese	7⅜ oz	?	5	?	?	?	170
spaghetti in tomato sauce w/cheese	7⅜ oz	?	2	?	?	?	180
spaghetti w/meatballs in tomato sauce	7⅜ oz	?	8	?	?	?	220
SpaghettiO's w/meatballs	7⅜ oz	?	9	?	?	?	220
SpaghettiO's w/sliced franks	7⅜ oz	?	9	?	?	?	220
SportyO's in tomato & cheese sauce	7½ oz	?	2	?	?	?	170
SportyO's pasta w/meatballs in tomato sauce	7⅜ oz	?	8	?	?	?	210
TeddyO's in tomato & cheese sauce	7½ oz	?	2	?	?	?	170
TeddyO's pasta w/meatballs	7⅜ oz	?	8	?	?	?	210
Hain							
CHILI							
spicy w/chicken	7½ oz	40	2	?	?	?	130
spicy tempeh	7½ oz	0	4	?	?	?	160
spicy vegetarian, reduced sodium	7½	0	1	?	?	?	160
PASTA & SAUCE MIXES							
creamy Parmesan	¼ pkg	10	3	?	?	?	150
creamy Swiss	⅕ pkg	?	4	?	?	?	170
fettucine Alfredo	¼ pkg	?	4	?	?	?	180
Italian herb	⅕ pkg	?	2	?	?	?	110
primavera	¼ pkg	10	4	?	?	?	140
tangy cheddar	¼ pkg	3	6	?	?	?	180

	Portion	Chol (mg)	Total Fat(g)	Satur'd Fat(g)	Mono Fat(g)	Poly Fat(g)	Total Calor
Kraft							
MACARONI & CHEESE DINNERS							
regular	¾ c	5	13	3	?	1	290
deluxe	¾ c	20	8	4	?	1	260
Dinomac	¾ c	10	14	3	?	2	310
spirals	¾ c	10	18	4	?	3	340
teddy bears	¾ c	10	14	3	?	2	310
wild wheels	¾ c	10	14	3	?	2	310
SHELLS & CHEESE							
Velveeta							
regular	½ c	20	8	4	?	1	210
bits of bacon	½ c	25	10	5	?	1	240
touch of Mexico	½ c	20	8	4	?	1	210
EGG NOODLE							
w/cheese	¾ c	50	17	4	?	2	340
w/chicken	¾ c	45	9	2	?	2	240
SPAGHETTI							
mild American	1 c	0	7	2	?	1	300
w/meat sauce	1 c	15	14	4	?	3	360
tangy Italian style	1 c	5	8	2	?	2	310
PASTA & CHEESE							
cheddar broccoli	½ c	30	8	3	?	1	180
chicken w/herbs	½ c	25	7	2	?	1	170
fettucini Alfredo	½ c	30	9	3	?	1	180
Parmesan	½ c	30	8	2	?	1	180
sour cream w/chives	½ c	25	8	2	?	1	180
3-cheese w/vegetables	½ c	25	8	3	?	1	180
Noodle-Roni Pasta							
macaroni & cheddar	1.8 ox dry mix	4	2	1	<1	<1	190
chicken & mushroom	1.2 oz dry mix	19	2	1	1	1	134
fettucini	1.5 oz dry mix	27	5	2	1	1	181
creamy garlic	1.5 oz dry mix	29	4	2	1	1	172
herb & butter	1 oz dry mix	19	3	1	1	<1	114
Parmesano	1.2 oz dry mix	19	3	1	1	1	135
Romanoff	1.5 oz	23	4	2	1	1	168
Stroganoff	2 oz dry mix	42	6	2	1	1	225
Old El Paso							
burrito dinner w/filling	1 burrito	23	13	4	?	2	299

	Portion	Chol (mg)	Total Fat(g)	Satur'd Fat(g)	Mono Fat(g)	Poly Fat(g)	Total Calor
enchilada dinner w/filling	1 ench.	21	8	3	?	1	145
chili con carne	1 c	47	7	?	?	?	162
chili w/beans	1 c	32	10	?	?	?	217
menado	½ can	176	52	21	3	?	476
tamales	2	20	12	?	?	?	190
Swanson							
chicken à la king	5¼ oz	?	12	?	?	?	190
chicken & dumplings	7½ oz	?	11	?	?	?	220
Van Camp's							
Chilee Weenee	1 c	?	16	?	?	?	307
Spaghetee Weene	1 c	?	7	?	?	?	243
Walt Brand							
beef stew	?	?	8	?	?	?	179
chili-mac	?	?	20	?	?	?	317
tamales	?	?	25	?	?	?	328

❏ ENTREES & MAIN COURSES, FROZEN

▪ BRAND NAME

Armour
CLASSICS

chicken & noodles	1	50	7	?	?	?	230
chicken fettucini	1	50	9	?	?	?	260
chicken mesquite	1	55	16	?	?	?	370
chicken parmegiana	1	75	19	?	?	?	370
glazed chicken	1	60	16	?	?	?	300
meat loaf	1	65	17	?	?	?	360
Salisbury steak	1	55	17	?	?	?	350
Swedish meatballs	1	80	18	?	?	?	330
turkey w/dressing & gravy	1	50	12	?	?	?	320
veal parmegiana	1	55	22	?	?	?	400

CLASSIC LITE

baby bay shrimp	1	105	6	?	?	?	220
beef pepper steak	1	35	4	?	?	?	220
beef Stroganoff	1	55	6	?	?	?	250
chicken à la king	1	55	7	?	?	?	290
chicken Burgundy	1	45	2	?	?	?	210
chicken oriental	1	35	1	?	?	?	180
Salisbury steak	1	40	11	?	?	?	300
sweet & sour chicken	1	35	2	?	?	?	240

Banquet
BONELESS CHICKEN HOT BITES

breast patties	1	?	13	?	?	?	200
breast tenders	1	?	6	?	?	?	150

	Portion	Chol (mg)	Total Fat(g)	Satur'd Fat(g)	Mono Fat(g)	Poly Fat(g)	Total Calor
chicken drum snackers	1	?	15	?	?	?	220
chicken nuggets	1	?	14	?	?	?	210
chicken sticks	1	?	15	?	?	?	220
hot 'n spicy chicken nuggets	1	?	19	?	?	?	250
southern fried breast tenders	1	?	7	?	?	?	160
southern fried chicken nuggets	1	?	14	?	?	?	220

MICROWAVE CHICKEN HOT BITES

breast pattie & bun	1	?	14	?	?	?	310
southern fried breast pattie & biscuit	1	?	14	?	?	?	320
breast tenders	1	?	10	?	?	?	260
chicken nuggets w/sweet & sour sauce	1	?	21	?	?	?	360
hot 'n spicy chicken nuggets w/bbq sauce	1	?	21	?	?	?	360

CHICKEN PRODUCTS

fried chicken	1	?	19	?	?	?	330
fried chicken breast portions	1	?	11	?	?	?	220
fried chicken thighs & drumsticks	1	?	14	?	?	?	250
hot 'n spicy fried chicken	1	?	19	?	?	?	330

COOKIN' BAGS

bbq sauce & sliced beef	1	?	2	?	?	?	100
breaded veal parmigiana	1	?	11	?	?	?	230
chicken à la king	1	?	5	?	?	?	230
chicken vegetables primavera	1	?	2	?	?	?	100
creamed chipped beef	1	?	4	?	?	?	100
gravy & Salisbury steak	1	?	14	?	?	?	190
gravy & sliced turkey	1	?	6	?	?	?	100
meat loaf	1	?	44	?	?	?	200
mushroom gravy & charbroiled beef patty	1	?	15	?	?	?	210

CASSEROLES

macaroni & cheese	1	?	17	?	?	?	350
spaghetti w/meat sauce	1	?	8	?	?	?	270

PLATTERS

all white meat fried chicken	1	105	22	?	?	?	430
all white meat hot 'n spicy fried chicken	1	105	22	?	?	?	430

	Portion	Chol (mg)	Total Fat(g)	Satur'd Fat(g)	Mono Fat(g)	Poly Fat(g)	Total Calor
beef	1	75	34	?	?	?	460
boneless chicken pattie	1	?	21	?	?	?	380
fish	1	95	22	?	?	?	450
ham	1	50	17	?	?	?	400
FAMILY ENTREES							
beef stew	1	?	5	?	?	?	140
chicken & dumplings	1	?	14	?	?	?	280
chicken & vegetables primavera	1	?	3	?	?	?	140
chili gravy & beef enchiladas	1	?	13	?	?	?	270
gravy & Salisbury steak	1	?	22	?	?	?	300
gravy & sliced turkey	1	?	8	?	?	?	150
lasagna w/meat sauce	1	?	10	?	?	?	270
mushroom gravy & charbroiled beef patties	1	?	21	?	?	?	240
noodles & beef w/gravy	1	?	7	?	?	?	200
onion gravy & beef patties	1	?	21	?	?	?	300
MEAT PIES							
beef	1	25	33	?	?	?	510
chicken	1	35	36	?	?	?	550
turkey	1	40	31	?	?	?	510
SUPREME MICROWAVE MEAT PIES (SINGLE CRUST)							
beef	1	35	29	?	?	?	440
chicken	1	40	28	?	?	?	430
turkey	1	27	27	?	?	?	430
Celentano							
baked pasta & cheese	6 oz	35	7	?	?	?	280
broccoli stuffed shells	6.75 oz	64	14	?	?	?	270
cannelloni Florentine	12 oz	88	8	?	?	?	350
chicken parmigiana	9 oz	87	21	?	?	?	400
chicken primavera	11.5 oz	30	7	?	?	?	260
eggplant parmigiana	10 oz	40	19	?	?	?	350
eggplant rollettes	11 oz	122	14	?	?	?	320
lasagna	10 oz	92	24	?	?	?	460
lasagna primavera	11 oz	90	14	?	?	?	330
manicotti	10 oz	82	14	?	?	?	380
ravioli	6.5 oz	111	11	?	?	?	380
mini ravioli	4 oz	50	5	?	?	?	250
stuffed shells	10 oz	74	14	?	?	?	410
COUNTRY PRIDE							
chicken chunks	1	?	15	?	?	?	240
chicken nuggets	1	?	16	?	?	?	250
chicken patties	1	?	16	?	?	?	250
chicken sticks	1	?	15	?	?	?	240

	Portion	Chol (mg)	Total Fat(g)	Satur'd Fat(g)	Mono Fat(g)	Poly Fat(g)	Total Calor
southern fried chicken chunks	1	?	20	?	?	?	280
southern fried chicken patties	1	?	16	?	?	?	240
Contadina Fresh Pasta & Cheese							
spinach tortellini w/cheese	3 oz	45	6	2	?	<1	260
Italian sausage tortellini	3 oz	35	8	2	?	1	260
rigatoni	3½ oz	125	5	1	?	<1	300
agnolotti w/basil & cheese	3 oz	40	7	2	?	2	270
tortellini w/cheese	3 oz	40	6	2	?	<1	270
chicken ravioli	3 oz	85	10	2	?	1	260
tortellini w/meat	3 oz	45	6	2	?	<1	260
ravioli w/cheese	3 oz	75	11	6	?	<1	270
Dining Lite							
beef teriyaki	1	45	5	?	?	?	270
cheese cannelloni	1	70	9	?	?	?	310
chicken à la king	1	40	7	?	?	?	240
chicken w/noodles	1	50	7	?	?	?	240
fettucini w/broccoli	1	35	12	?	?	?	290
glazed chicken	1	45	4	?	?	?	220
lasagna w/meat sauce	1	25	5	?	?	?	240
oriental pepper steak	1	40	6	?	?	?	260
Salisbury steak	1	55	8	?	?	?	200
spaghetti w/beef	1	20	8	?	?	?	220
Healthy Choice							
beef pepper steak	9½ oz	40	4	?	?	?	250
chicken chow mein	8½ oz	45	3	?	?	?	220
fettucini Alfredo	8 oz	45	7	?	?	?	240
glazed chicken	8½ oz	50	3	?	?	?	220
lasagna w/meat sauce	9 oz	20	5	?	?	?	260
seafood Newburg	8 oz	55	3	?	?	?	200
sole w/lemon butter	8¼ oz	45	4	?	?	?	230
spaghetti w/meat sauce	10 oz	15	6	?	?	?	310
Kid Cuisine							
beef patty sandwich w/cheese	1	?	22	?	?	?	430
cheese pizza	1	?	12	?	?	?	380
chicken nuggets	1	?	17	?	?	?	360
chicken sandwiches	1	?	17	?	?	?	470
fish sticks	1	?	14	?	?	?	360
fried chicken	1	?	28	?	?	?	520
hamburger pizza	1	?	10	?	?	?	330
macaroni & cheese w/mini-franks	1	?	15	?	?	?	360
mini-cheese ravioli	1	?	8	?	?	?	290
spaghetti w/meat sauce	1	?	11	?	?	?	340
Le Menu Healthy Entrees (light style)							
chicken à la king	8¼ oz	?	5	?	?	?	240

	Portion	Chol (mg)	Total Fat (g)	Satur'd Fat (g)	Mono Fat (g)	Poly Fat (g)	Total Calor
chicken Dijon	8 oz	?	7	?	?	?	240
chicken enchiladas	8 oz	?	8	?	?	?	280
garden vegetables lasagna	10½ oz	?	5	?	?	?	210
glazed turkey	8¼ oz	?	8	?	?	?	260
herb roasted chicken	7¾ oz	?	6	?	?	?	260
lasagna w/meat sauce	10 oz	?	8	?	?	?	290
meat sauce & cheese tortellini	8 oz	?	8	?	?	?	250
spaghetti w/beef sauce & mushrooms	9 oz	?	6	?	?	?	280
Swedish meatballs	8 oz	?	8	?	?	?	260
Minute							
MICROWAVE DISHES (FAMILY SIZE)							
chicken-flavored noodles, prepared w/butter	½ c	35	5	?	?	?	160
noodles Alfredo, prepared w/butter	½ c	45	6	?	?	?	170
parmesan noodles, prepared w/butter	½ c	45	6	?	?	?	170
pasta & cheddar cheese, prepared w/butter	½ c	15	7	?	?	?	160
Morton							
MEAT PIES							
beef	1	30	31	?	?	?	430
chicken	1	35	28	?	?	?	420
turkey	1	40	28	?	?	?	420
Mrs. Paul's							
LIGHT FILLETS							
cod	1 oz	?	11	?	?	?	240
flounder	1 oz	?	10	?	?	?	240
haddock	1 oz	?	9	?	?	?	220
sole	1 oz	?	10	?	?	?	240
LIGHT SEAFOOD ENTREES							
fish Florentine	8 oz	?	8	?	?	?	220
fish Dijon	8¾ oz	?	5	?	?	?	200
fish Mornay	9 oz	?	10	?	?	?	230
seafood lasagna	9½ oz	?	8	?	?	?	290
seafood rotini	9 oz	?	6	?	?	?	240
shrimp & clams w/linguini	9 oz	?	5	?	?	?	240
PREPARED SEAFOODS							
batter-dipped fish fillets	2	?	17	?	?	?	330
battered-fish sticks	4	?	12	?	?	?	210
crispy crunchy breaded fish sticks	4	?	6	?	?	?	140
crispy crunchy fish fillets	2	?	9	?	?	?	220

	Portion	Chol (mg)	Total Fat(g)	Satur'd Fat(g)	Mono Fat(g)	Poly Fat(g)	Total Calor
crispy crunchy fish sticks	4	?	8	?	?	?	190
crunchy batter fish fillets	2	?	14	?	?	?	280
crunchy batter flounder fillets	2	?	5	?	?	?	220
crunchy batter haddock fillets	2	?	5	?	?	?	190
deviled crabs	3½ oz	?	12	?	?	?	240
fish cakes	2	?	7	?	?	?	190
fried clams	2½ oz	?	9	?	?	?	200
fried scallops	3 oz	?	7	?	?	?	160
light fillets in butter sauce	1	?	6	?	?	?	140

Old El Paso

FESTIVE DINNERS

	Portion	Chol (mg)	Total Fat(g)	Satur'd Fat(g)	Mono Fat(g)	Poly Fat(g)	Total Calor
beef & bean burrito	11 oz	?	9	?	?	?	470
beef chimichanga	11 oz	?	21	?	?	?	540
cheese enchilada	11 oz	?	31	?	?	?	590
chicken enchilada	11 oz	?	18	?	?	?	460
beef enchilada	11 oz	?	8	?	?	?	390

FROZEN ENTREES

	Portion	Chol (mg)	Total Fat(g)	Satur'd Fat(g)	Mono Fat(g)	Poly Fat(g)	Total Calor
beef & cheese chimichangas	11 oz	20	19	?	?	?	380
beef chimichangas	1	?	23	?	?	?	380
chicken chimichangas	1	?	21	?	?	?	370
beef enchiladas	1	10	13	?	?	?	210
cheese enchiladas	1	?	12	?	?	?	250
chicken enchiladas	1	?	12	?	?	?	220

INDIVIDUAL FROZEN

	Portion	Chol (mg)	Total Fat(g)	Satur'd Fat(g)	Mono Fat(g)	Poly Fat(g)	Total Calor
chicken chimichangas	1	?	20	?	?	?	360
beef chimichangas	1	?	21	?	?	?	370
bean & cheese burrito	1	?	11	?	?	?	330
hot beef & bean burrito	1	?	11	?	?	?	310

Patio

BRITOS

	Portion	Chol (mg)	Total Fat(g)	Satur'd Fat(g)	Mono Fat(g)	Poly Fat(g)	Total Calor
beef & bean	1	15	10	?	?	?	250
green chili	1	15	10	?	?	?	250
nacho beef	1	25	13	?	?	?	270
nacho cheese	1	20	10	?	?	?	250
red chili	1	15	10	?	?	?	240
spicy chicken	1	25	10	?	?	?	250

BURRITOS

	Portion	Chol (mg)	Total Fat(g)	Satur'd Fat(g)	Mono Fat(g)	Poly Fat(g)	Total Calor
beef & bean	1	?	16	?	?	?	370
beef & bean red chili	1	?	13	?	?	?	340
red hot	1	?	15	?	?	?	360

	Portion	Chol (mg)	Total Fat(g)	Satur'd Fat(g)	Mono Fat(g)	Poly Fat(g)	Total Calor

Stouffer's
ENTREES

	Portion	Chol (mg)	Total Fat(g)	Satur'd Fat(g)	Mono Fat(g)	Poly Fat(g)	Total Calor
baked chicken breast & vegetable medley	7³/₈ oz	?	6	?	?	?	190
beef chop suey w/rice	12 oz	?	9	?	?	?	300
beef pie	10 oz	?	32	?	?	?	500
beef Stroganoff w/parsley noodles	9³/₄ oz	?	20	?	?	?	390
cashew chicken in sauce w/rice	9¹/₂ oz	?	16	?	?	?	380
cheese enchiladas	9¹/₂ oz	?	40	?	?	?	590
chicken à la king w/rice	9¹/₂ oz	?	9	?	?	?	290
chicken chow mein w/o noodles	8 oz	?	4	?	?	?	130
chicken divan	8¹/₂ oz	?	20	?	?	?	320
chicken parmigiana & pasta Alfredo	9⁷/₈ oz	?	15	?	?	?	360
chicken pie	10 oz	?	33	?	?	?	530
chili con carne w/beans	8³/₄ oz	?	10	?	?	?	260
creamed chipped beef	5¹/₂ oz	?	16	?	?	?	230
escalloped chicken & noodles	10 oz	?	25	?	?	?	420
fettucini Alfredo	5 oz	?	19	?	?	?	270
fiesta lasagna	10¹/₄ oz	?	22	?	?	?	430
fried chicken breast & whipped potatoes	7¹/₈ oz	?	18	?	?	?	350
green pepper steak w/rice	10¹/₂ oz	?	11	?	?	?	330
ham & asparagus crêpes	6¹/₄ oz	?	18	?	?	?	310
homestyle beef & noodles & vegetable medley	8³/₈ oz	?	7	?	?	?	230
homestyle chicken & noodles	10 oz	?	13	?	?	?	290
homestyle meatloaf & whipped potatoes	9⁷/₈ oz	?	20	?	?	?	360
lasagna	10¹/₂ oz	?	13	?	?	?	360
lobster Newburg	6¹/₂ oz	?	32	?	?	?	380
macaroni & beef w/tomatoes	11¹/₂ oz	?	7	?	?	?	170
macaroni & cheese	6 oz	?	13	?	?	?	250
noodles Romanoff	4 oz	?	9	?	?	?	170
pasta primavera	10⁵/₈ oz	?	21	?	?	?	270
pasta shells, cheese & tomato sauce	9¹/₄ oz	?	15	?	?	?	330
roast turkey breast & homestyle stuffing	7⁷/₈ oz	?	13	?	?	?	300
Salisbury steak & macaroni & cheese	8⁵/₈ oz	?	18	?	?	?	350
spaghetti w/meatballs	12⁵/₈ oz	?	15	?	?	?	380
spaghetti w/meat sauce	12⁷/₈ oz	?	11	?	?	?	370

	Portion	Chol (mg)	Total Fat(g)	Satur'd Fat(g)	Mono Fat(g)	Poly Fat(g)	Total Calor
stuffed green peppers w/beef in tomato sauce	7¾ oz	?	9	?	?	?	200
Swedish meatballs in gravy w/parsley noodles	11 oz	?	26	?	?	?	480
tortellini							
beef w/marinara sauce	10 oz	?	12	?	?	?	360
cheese in Alfredo sauce	8⅞ oz	?	40	?	?	?	600
tortilla grande	9⅝ oz	?	33	?	?	?	530
turkey casserole w/gravy & dressing	9¾ oz	?	17	?	?	?	360
turkey pie	10 oz	?	36	?	?	?	540
veal parmigiana & pasta Alfredo	9¼ oz	?	15	?	?	?	350
vegetable lasagna	10½ oz	?	24	?	?	?	420
Welsh rarebit	5 oz	?	30	?	?	?	350

LEAN CUISINE

	Portion	Chol (mg)	Total Fat(g)	Satur'd Fat(g)	Mono Fat(g)	Poly Fat(g)	Total Calor
baked cheese ravioli	8½ oz	55	8	3	?	<1	240
beef & bean enchanadas	9¼ oz	45	6	3	?	1	240
beef canneloni w/mornay sauce	9⅝ oz	25	4	2	?	<1	210
beefsteak ranchero	9¼ oz	30	8	2	?	1	260
breaded breast of chicken parmesan	10⅞ oz	35	9	2	?	2	270
broccoli & cheddar baked potato	10⅜ oz	20	9	4	?	<1	290
cheese canneloni w/tomato sauce	9⅛ oz	25	8	4	?	<1	270
chicken à l'orange w/almond rice	8 oz	55	4	1	?	<1	280
chicken & vegetables w/vermicelli	11¾ oz	35	6	3	?	2	250
chicken cacciatore w/vermicelli	10⅞ oz	45	7	2	?	1	280
chicken chow mein w/rice	9 oz	30	5	1	?	1	240
chicken enchanadas	9⅞ oz	55	9	3	?	2	290
chicken in barbeque sauce	8¾ oz	50	6	1	?	2	260
chicken fettucini	9 oz	45	8	4	?	1	280
chicken oriental w/vegetables & vermicelli	9 oz	35	7	2	?	2	280
chicken tenderloins in herb cream sauce	9½ oz	60	5	2	?	1	240
fiesta chicken	8½ oz	40	5	2	?	1	240
filet of fish divan	10⅜ oz	65	5	2	?	1	210
filet of fish Florentine	9⅝ oz	65	7	3	?	2	220
glazed chicken w/vegetable rice	8½ oz	55	8	2	?	3	260

	Portion	Chol (mg)	Total Fat(g)	Satur'd Fat(g)	Mono Fat(g)	Poly Fat(g)	Total Calor
homestyle turkey w/vegetables & pasta	9³/₈ oz	50	5	2	?	<1	230
lasagna w/meat sauce	10¹/₄ oz	25	5	2	?	<1	260
linguini w/clam sauce	9⁵/₈ oz	30	8	2	?	2	280
macaroni & beef in tomato sauce	10 oz	40	6	1	?	2	240
oriental beef w/vegetables & rice	8⁵/₈ oz	40	9	2	?	<1	290
rigatoni bake w/meat sauce & cheese	9³/₄ oz	25	8	3	?	1	250
Salisbury steak w/gravy & scalloped potatoes	9¹/₂ oz	45	7	2	?	<1	240
sliced turkey breast w/dressing	7⁷/₈ oz	25	5	1	?	2	200
spaghetti w/meat sauce	11¹/₂ oz	20	6	2	?	2	290
spaghetti w/meatballs	9¹/₂ oz	35	7	2	?	1	280
stuffed cabbage w/meat in tomato sauce	10³/₄ oz	40	6	1	?	1	210
Swedish meatballs in gravy w/pasta	9¹/₈ oz	50	8	3	?	1	290
tuna lasagna w/spinach noodles & vegetables	9³/₄ oz	20	7	2	?	<1	240
turkey Dijon	9¹/₂ oz	45	5	2	?	<1	230
Swanson							
CHICKEN							
chicken nibbles	3¹/₄ oz	?	19	?	?	?	300
chicken nuggets	3 oz	?	14	?	?	?	230
fried chicken, breast portions	4¹/₂ oz	?	20	?	?	?	360
thighs & drumsticks	3¹/₄ oz	?	18	?	?	?	290
HOMESTYLE RECIPE ENTREES							
chicken cacciatore	10.95 oz	?	8	?	?	?	260
chicken pie	8 oz	?	21	?	?	?	410
fish & fries	6¹/₂ oz	?	16	?	?	?	340
fried chicken	7 oz	?	21	?	?	?	390
lasagna w/meat sauce	10¹/₂ oz	?	15	?	?	?	400
macaroni & cheese	10 oz	?	19	?	?	?	390
Salisbury steak	10 oz	?	16	?	?	?	320
scalloped potatoes & ham	9 oz	?	13	?	?	?	300
HOMESTYLE RECIPE ENTREES							
seafood Creole w/rice	9 oz	?	6	?	?	?	240
sirloin tips in Burgundy sauce	7 oz	?	5	?	?	?	160
spaghetti w/Italian style meatballs	8¹/₂	?	20	?	?	?	360
Swedish meatballs	8¹/₂	?	20	?	?	?	360
turkey w/dressing & potatoes	9 oz	?	11	?	?	?	290

	Portion	Chol (mg)	Total Fat(g)	Satur'd Fat(g)	Mono Fat(g)	Poly Fat(g)	Total Calor
HUNGRY-MAN POT PIES							
beef	16 oz	?	31	?	?	?	610
chicken	16 oz	?	35	?	?	?	630
turkey	16 oz	?	36	?	?	?	650
POT PIES							
beef	7 oz	?	19	?	?	?	370
chicken	7 oz	?	22	?	?	?	380
macaroni & cheese	7 oz	?	8	?	?	?	200
turkey	7 oz	?	21	?	?	?	380
Weight Watchers							
imperial chicken	9¼ oz	35	3	1	<1	1	240
chicken à la king	9 oz	20	6	3	1	2	240
sweet 'n sour chicken tenders	10 oz	40	1	<1	<1	<1	240
spaghetti w/meat sauce	10½ oz	25	7	3	3	1	280
beef Stroganoff	8½ oz	25	9	4	3	2	290
beef sirloin tips & mushrooms in wine sauce	7½ oz	50	7	3	2	2	220
London broil in mushroom sauce	7 oz	40	3	1	1	1	140
pasta primavera	8½ oz	5	11	<1	8	3	210
chicken fettucini	8¼ oz	40	9	3	4	2	280
fettucini Alfredo	9 oz	35	8	3	3	1	210
cheese tortellini	9 oz	15	6	1	4	1	310
homestyle chicken & noodles	9 oz	30	7	2	3	1	240
angel hair pasta	10 oz	20	5	1	2	2	210
pasta rigat	10½ oz	25	9	2	6	1	300
lasagna w/meat sauce	11 oz	45	10	4	4	2	320
Italian cheese lasagna	11 oz	30	12	4	4	4	350
garden lasagna	11 oz	20	7	2	3	2	290
baked cheese ravioli	9 oz	85	9	4	3	1	290
cheese manicotti	9½	75	8	4	3	1	280
chicken divan & baked potato	11 oz	40	4	2	1	1	280
broccoli & cheese & baked potato	10½ oz	25	8	2	4	2	290
homestyle turkey & baked potato	12 oz	60	6	3	1	2	300
ham Lorraine & baked potato	11 oz	15	4	2	2	<1	250
chicken nuggets	6 oz	50	12	4	6	2	270
fillet of fish au gratin	9¼ oz	60	6	1	4	1	200
oven fried fish	7 oz	15	7	<1	5	2	240
southern fried chicken	6½ oz	65	16	7	7	2	320
stuffed turkey breast	8½ oz	80	10	4	5	1	260
veal patty parmigiana	8½ oz	55	6	3	2	1	190
beef Salisbury steak Romana	8¾ oz	40	7	2	3	1	190

	Portion	Chol (mg)	Total Fat(g)	Satur'd Fat(g)	Mono Fat(g)	Poly Fat(g)	Total Calor
chicken cordon bleu	8 oz	50	9	5	3	1	220
chicken Kiev	7 oz	30	9	3	4	1	230
chicken burrito	7½ oz	60	13	4	6	3	310
beef enchiladas ranchero	9 oz	40	10	3	4	2	230
chicken enchiladas suiza	9 oz	30	11	2	7	2	280
cheese enchiladas ranchero	9 oz	60	18	5	11	2	360
beef fajitas	6¾ oz	20	7	2	3	1	250
chicken fajitas	6¾ oz	30	5	2	2	1	230

❏ FAST FOODS

■ BRAND NAME

Arby's
BREAKFAST ITEMS

	Portion	Chol (mg)	Total Fat(g)	Satur'd Fat(g)	Mono Fat(g)	Poly Fat(g)	Total Calor
Toastix	1 serving	20	25	5	17	3	420
cinnamon nut danish	1	0	10	2	6	2	340
plain biscuit	1	0	15	3	11	1	280
bacon biscuit	1	8	18	4	12	1	318
sausage biscuit	1	60	32	9	20	3	460
ham biscuit	1	21	17	4	12	1	323
plain croissant	1	49	16	10	5	1	260
bacon/egg croissant	1	221	26	14	10	2	389
ham/cheese croissant	1	90	21	12	7	1	345
mushroom/cheese croissant	1	116	38	15	13	8	493
sausage/egg croissant	1	271	40	19	17	4	519
ham platter	1	374	26	8	122	5	518
sausage platter	1	406	41	13	20	7	640
egg platter	1	346	24	7	11	5	460
bacon platter	1	366	32	10	15	6	860
blueberry muffin	1	22	6	2	3	1	200

ROAST BEEF SANDWICHES

	Portion	Chol (mg)	Total Fat(g)	Satur'd Fat(g)	Mono Fat(g)	Poly Fat(g)	Total Calor
regular roast beef	1	39	15	7	5	2	353
beef 'n cheddar	1	52	20	7	8	4	451
junior roast beef	1	23	11	4	5	2	218
giant roast beef	1	78	27	11	13	4	530
super roast beef	1	47	28	8	11	9	529
philly beef 'n Swiss	1	91	26	6	11	9	498
bac 'n cheddar deluxe	1	83	33	8	14	11	532
light roast beef deluxe	1	42	10	?	?	?	294
French dip	1	5	12	6	6	1	345
French dip 'n Swiss	1	87	18	8	9	2	425

	Portion	Chol (mg)	Total Fat(g)	Satur'd Fat(g)	Mono Fat(g)	Poly Fat(g)	Total Calor
CHICKEN SANDWICHES							
chicken breast	1	45	26	4	8	14	489
roast chicken club	1	75	29	5	8	14	513
roast chicken deluxe	1	2	20	3	7	10	373
chicken cordon bleu	1	65	37	9	14	14	658
grilled chicken deluxe	1	44	21	5	6	10	426
grilled chicken barbeque	1	44	14	4	2	7	378
light roast chicken deluxe	1	39	6	?	?	?	263
OTHER SANDWICHES							
sub deluxe	1	45	26	5	7	11	482
fish fillet	1	79	29	6	12	11	537
turkey deluxe	1	39	20	4	4	12	399
ham 'n cheese	1	45	15	4	7	3	330
light roast turkey deluxe	1	30	5	?	?	?	260
SALADS (PREPACKED)							
cashew chicken salad	1	65	37	9	13	15	590
chef salad	1	115	11	5	4	2	210
garden salad	1	74	9	4	3	2	149
side salad	1	0	0	0	0	0	25
honey French dressing	1	0	27	4	6	16	322
light Italian	1	0	1	<1	<1	1	23
thousand island dressing	1	24	29	4	7	17	298
blue cheese dressing	1	50	31	6	8	16	295
buttermilk ranch dressing	1	6	39	6	9	22	349
croutons	1	1	2	<1	<1	2	59
SOUPS							
Boston clam chowder	8 oz	28	11	4	5	2	244
cream of broccoli	8 oz	3	8	5	2	<1	244
pilgrim's corn chowder	8 oz	28	11	4	5	2	244
Wisconsin cheese	8 oz	31	19	8	8	<1	244
French onion	8 oz	0	3	1	2	1	244
lumberjack mixed salad	8 oz	4	4	2	1	<1	244
old fashion chicken noodle	8 oz	25	2	1	1	<1	244
split pea w/ham	8 oz	30	10	5	4	1	244
beef w/vegetables & barley	8 oz	10	3	1	1	<1	244
tomato Florentine	8 oz	2	2	1	<1	<1	244
POTATOES							
french fries	1 serving	0	13	3	6	5	246
potato cakes	1 serving	0	12	2	6	4	204
curly fries	1 serving	0	18	7	8	2	337
cheddar fries	1 serving	9	22	9	10	2	399
plain baked potato	1	0	2	0	1	1	240

	Portion	Chol (mg)	Total Fat(g)	Satur'd Fat(g)	Mono Fat(g)	Poly Fat(g)	Total Calor
baked potato w/butter/ margarine & sour cream	1	40	25	12	8	3	463
broccoli 'n cheddar baked potato	1	22	18	7	7	3	417
deluxe baked potato	1	58	36	18	11	4	621
mushroom 'n cheese baked potato	1	47	27	6	11	9	515

DESSERTS

apple turnover	1	0	18	7	8	3	303
cherry turnover	1	0	18	5	9	4	280
blueberry turnover	1	0	19	6	8	3	320
cheese cake	1	95	23	7	8	8	306
chocolate chip cookie	1	0	4	2	2	20	130
chocolate shake	1	36	12	3	7	2	451
vanilla shake	1	32	12	4	5	2	330
jamocha shake	1	35	11	3	6	2	368
peanut butter cup polar swirl	1	34	24	8	11	5	517
Oreo polar swirl	1	35	10	10	7	2	482
Snickers polar swirl	1	33	19	7	9	4	511
Heath polar swirl	1	39	22	5	13	3	543
Butterfinger polar swirl	1	28	18	8	6	4	457

Burger King

BURGERS

Whopper sandwich	1	90	36	12	11	13	614
Whopper w/cheese sandwich	1	115	44	16	13	13	706
double Whopper sandwich	1	169	53	19	19	13	844
double Whopper w/cheese sandwich	1	194	61	24	22	14	935
cheeseburger	1	50	15	7	6	1	318
cheeseburger deluxe	1	56	23	8	7	7	390
hamburger	1	37	11	4	5	1	272
hamburger deluxe	1	43	19	6	6	7	344
bacon double cheeseburger	1	105	31	14	13	2	515
bacon double cheeseburger deluxe	1	111	39	16	14	8	592
barbeque bacon double cheeseburger	1	105	31	14	13	2	536
mushroom Swiss double cheeseburger	1	25	27	12	11	2	473
double cheeseburger	1	100	27	13	11	2	483
burger buddies	1	52	17	7	8	1	349

	Portion	Chol (mg)	Total Fat(g)	Satur'd Fat(g)	Mono Fat(g)	Poly Fat(g)	Total Calor
SANDWICHES AND SIDE ORDERS							
bk broiler chicken sandwich	1	53	18	3	7	8	349
chicken sandwich	1	82	40	8	11	20	685
ocean catch fish filet	1	57	25	4	6	13	495
chicken tenders	1 serving	46	13	3	5	3	236
chef salad	1	103	9	4	3	1	178
chunky chicken salad	1	49	4	1	1	1	142
garden salad	1	15	5	3	1	0	95
side salad	1	0	0	0	0	0	25
french fries (medium salted)	1 serving	0	20	5	12	2	372
onion rings	1 serving	0	19	5	9	5	339
apple pie	1 slice	4	14	4	8	1	311
SHAKES							
vanilla	1	33	10	6	3	0	334
chocolate	1	31	10	6	4	0	326
chocolate (syrup added)	1	33	11	6	3	0	403
strawberry	1	33	10	6	3	0	394
BREAKFAST							
croissant"wich" w/egg & cheese	1	22	20	7	10	2	315
croissant"wich" w/bacon, egg & cheese	1	227	24	8	12	3	361
croissant"wich" w/sausage, egg & cheese	1	268	40	13	20	5	534
croissant"wich" w/ham, egg & cheese	1	241	21	7	11	2	346
croissant	1	4	10	2	7	1	180
bagel sandwich w/egg & cheese	1	247	16	5	5	4	407
bagel sandwich w/bacon, egg & cheese	1	252	20	7	7	4	453
bagel sandwich w/sausage, egg & cheese	1	293	36	12	15	6	626
bagel sandwich w/ham, egg & cheese	1	266	17	6	6	4	438
bagel w/cream cheese	1	58	16	6	5	3	370
bagel	1	29	6	1	1	3	272
biscuit w/bacon	1	8	20	5	11	2	378
biscuit w/sausage	1	33	29	8	15	4	478
biscuit w/bacon & egg	1	213	27	7	13	4	467
biscuit w/sausage & egg	1	238	36	10	18	5	568
biscuit	1	2	17	3	9	2	332

	Portion	Chol (mg)	Total Fat(g)	Satur'd Fat(g)	Mono Fat(g)	Poly Fat(g)	Total Calor
scrambled egg platter	1	365	34	9	18	6	549
scrambled egg platter w/bacon	1	373	39	11	20	7	610
scrambled egg platter w/sausage	1	412	53	15	30	8	768
French toast sticks	1 serving	80	32	5	15	11	538
tater tenders	1 serving	0	12	3	6	3	213
mini muffins							
blueberry	1	72	14	3	4	8	292
lemon poppyseed	1	72	18	3	5	11	318
raisin oat bran	1	0	12	2	3	7	291
Danish							
apple cinnamon	1	19	13	3	8	2	390
cinnamon raisin	1	15	18	4	10	3	449
cheese	1	7	16	5	9	2	406

Hardee's
BREAKFAST MENU

	Portion	Chol (mg)	Total Fat(g)	Satur'd Fat(g)	Mono Fat(g)	Poly Fat(g)	Total Calor
rise 'n shine biscuit	1	0	18	3	11	4	320
cinnamon 'n raisin	1	0	17	5	10	2	320
sausage biscuit	1	25	28	7	16	5	440
sausage & egg biscuit	1	170	31	8	18	6	490
bacon biscuit	1	10	21	4	13	4	360
bacon & egg biscuit	1	155	24	5	14	5	410
bacon, egg & cheese biscuit	1	165	28	8	15	5	460
ham biscuit	1	15	16	2	10	4	320
ham & egg biscuit	1	160	19	4	12	4	370
ham, egg & cheese biscuit	1	170	23	6	13	4	420
country ham biscuit	1	25	18	3	11	4	350
country ham & egg biscuit	1	175	22	4	13	4	400
Canadian rise 'n shine biscuit	1	180	27	8	15	5	470
steak biscuit	1	30	29	7	16	6	500
steak & egg biscuit	1	175	32	8	17	7	550
chicken biscuit	1	45	22	4	13	5	430
big country breakfast							
sausage	1	340	57	16	31	11	850
bacon	1	305	40	10	22	8	660
ham	1	325	33	7	19	8	620
country ham	1	345	38	9	21	8	670
muffins							
blueberry	1	80	19	4	5	10	400
oat bran	1	55	18	3	7	8	440

HAMBURGERS & SANDWICHES

	Portion	Chol (mg)	Total Fat(g)	Satur'd Fat(g)	Mono Fat(g)	Poly Fat(g)	Total Calor
hamburger	1	20	10	4	4	2	270
cheeseburger	1	30	14	7	5	2	320
quarter-pound cheeseburger	1	70	29	14	12	2	500

	Portion	Chol (mg)	Total Fat(g)	Satur'd Fat(g)	Mono Fat(g)	Poly Fat(g)	Total Calor
big deluxe burger	1	70	30	12	12	5	500
bacon cheeseburger	1	80	39	16	17	6	610
mushroom 'n Swiss burger	1	70	27	13	12	2	490
big twin	1	55	25	11	9	5	450
regular roast beef	1	35	9	4	4	2	260
big roast beef	1	45	11	5	5	2	300
hot ham 'n cheese	1	65	12	5	4	2	330
turkey club	1	70	16	4	6	5	390
fisherman's fillet	1	70	24	6	7	11	500
chicken fillet	1	55	13	2	4	6	370
grilled chicken sandwich	1	60	9	1	3	5	310
all-beef hot dog	1	25	17	8	8	2	300

DELI SANDWICHES SUPREME

ham 'n cheese	1	50	17	?	?	?	390
chicken fillet	1	55	14	3	5	6	380
roast beef	1	55	17	6	7	4	370
grilled chicken	1	55	10	2	3	5	320
turkey club	1	70	16	4	6	5	390

BONE-IN-CHICKEN

leg	1	115	12	5	6	2	220
breast	1	140	26	10	13	3	460
wing	1	65	18	7	9	2	280
thigh	1	180	37	13	19	6	520

SALADS & SPECIAL ITEMS

side salad	1	0	?	?	?	?	20
garden salad	1	105	14	8	5	1	210
chef salad	1	115	15	9	5	1	240
chicken 'n pasta salad	1	55	3	1	1	1	230
chicken stix							
6 piece	1 serving	35	9	2	4	3	210
9 piece	1 serving	55	14	3	6	5	310
french fries							
regular	1 serving	0	11	2	5	4	230
large	1 serving	0	17	3	8	6	360
big fry	1 serving	0	23	5	11	8	500
crispy curls	1 serving	0	16	3	8	5	300

SHAKES & DESSERTS

shakes							
vanilla	1	50	9	6	3	?	400
chocolate	1	45	8	5	2	?	460
strawberry	1	40	8	5	2	?	440
cool twist cone							
vanilla	1	15	6	4	2	?	190
chocolate	1	20	6	4	2	?	200
vanilla/chocolate	1	20	6	4	2	?	190

	Portion	Chol (mg)	Total Fat(g)	Satur'd Fat(g)	Mono Fat(g)	Poly Fat(g)	Total Calor
cool twist sundae							
hot fudge	1	25	12	6	4	1	320
caramel	1	20	10	5	3	1	330
strawberry	1	15	8	5	3	1	260
cool twist yogurt							
vanilla	1	10	4	3	1	0	160
chocolate	1	10	4	3	1	0	170
apple turnover	1	0	12	4	5	3	270
big cookie	1	5	13	4	7	2	250

Jack-in-the Box

BREAKFASTS

scrambled egg packet	1	354	21	8	7	2	431
supreme crescent	1	178	40	13	19	8	547
sausage crescent	1	187	43	16	22	6	584
breakfast jack	1	203	13	5	5	3	307
scrambled egg platter	1	378	32	9	17	4	559
hash browns	1 serving	0	11	3	7	<1	156
pancake platter	1	99	22	9	8	4	612

HAMBURGERS

hamburger	1	26	11	4	5	2	267
cheeseburger	1	41	14	6	6	2	315
double cheeseburger	1	72	27	12	12	3	467
jumbo jack	1	73	34	11	13	8	584
jumbo jack w/cheese	1	102	40	14	15	9	677
bacon cheeseburger	1	113	45	15	16	9	705
grilled sourdough burger	1	109	50	16	18	8	712
ultimate cheeseburger	1	127	69	26	24	18	942

SANDWICHES

sirloin cheesecake	1	79	30	9	9	10	621
ham & turkey melt	1	79	36	11	11	9	592
chicken fajita pita	1	34	8	3	4	1	292
grilled chicken fillet	1	64	17	4	5	6	408
chicken supreme	1	85	39	10	15	11	641
fish supreme	1	55	27	6	11	8	510

SALADS

chef salad	1	142	18	8	5	1	325
taco salad	1	92	31	13	12	2	503
side salad	1	<1	3	2	1	0	51
buttermilk house dressing	1 serving	21	36	6	8	22	362
thousand island	1 serving	23	30	5	7	18	312
reduced-calorie French dressing	1 serving	0	8	1	2	5	176

FINGER FOOD

egg rolls	3 pieces	29	24	7	13	3	437

	Portion	Chol (mg)	Total Fat(g)	Satur'd Fat(g)	Mono Fat(g)	Poly Fat(g)	Total Calor
egg rolls	5 pieces	49	41	12	22	5	753
chicken strips	4 pieces	52	13	3	8	1	285
chicken strips	6 pieces	82	20	5	13	1	451
taquitos	5 pieces	24	15	3	8	2	362
taquitos	7 pieces	34	21	5	12	3	511
MEXICAN FOOD							
guacamole	1 serving	0	5	?	?	?	55
salsa	1 serving	0	<1	<1	<1	<1	8
taco	1	18	11	4	5	1	187
super taco	1	29	17	6	8	1	281
SIDE DISHES & DESSERTS							
french fries							
small	1 serving	0	11	3	7	<1	219
regular	1 serving	0	17	4	7	1	351
jumbo	1 serving	0	19	5	13	1	396
onion rings	1 serving	0	23	6	15	1	380
sesame breadsticks	1 serving	<1	2	?	?	?	70
tortilla chips	1 serving	<1	6	?	?	?	139
hot apple turnover	1	7	19	6	11	2	348
cheesecake	1 serving	63	18	9	7	1	309
double fudge cake	1 serving	20	9	?	?	?	288
DRINKS							
milk shakes							
vanilla	1	<1	6	4	2	<1	320
chocolate	1	<1	7	3	2	<1	330
strawberry	1	<1	7	3	2	<1	320
Kentucky Fried Chicken							
ORIGINAL RECIPE							
wing	1	64	12	3	?	2	178
side breast	1	77	17	4	?	2	267
center breast	1	93	15	4	?	2	283
drumstick	1	67	9	2	?	1	146
thigh	1	123	20	5	?	3	294
EXTRA TASTY CRISPY							
wing	1	67	19	4	?	3	254
side breast	1	81	22	6	?	2	343
center breast	1	114	18	5	?	2	342
drumstick	1	71	14	3	?	2	204
thigh	1	129	30	8	?	4	406
LITE 'N CRISPY							
side breast	1	53	12	3	?	?	204
center breast	1	57	12	3	?	?	220
drumstick	1	51	7	2	?	?	121
thigh	1	80	17	4	?	?	246

	Portion	Chol (mg)	Total Fat (g)	Satur'd Fat (g)	Mono Fat (g)	Poly Fat (g)	Total Calor
NUGGETS & SAUCES							
nuggets	1	12	3	1	?	<1	46
barbeque	1 oz	<1	1	<1	?	<1	35
sweet 'n sour	1 oz	<1	1	<1	?	<1	58
honey	½ oz	<1	<1	<1	?	<1	58
mustard	1 oz	<1	1	<1	?	1	36
MISCELLANEOUS							
hot wings	1	148	24	5	?	4	376
Chicken Littles sandwich	1	18	10	2	?	3	169
buttermilk biscuits	1	1	12	3	?	2	235
mashed potatoes & gravy	1 serving	<1	2	<1	?	<1	71
french fries	1 serving	2	12	3	?	1	244
corn-on-the-cob	1 piece	<1	3	1	?	2	176
cole slaw	1 serving	5	7	1	?	3	119
Colonel's chicken sandwich	1	47	27	6	?	9	482
McDonald's							
BREAKFAST FOODS							
biscuit							
w/bacon, cheese & egg	1	240	26	16	2	8	440
w/spread	1	1	13	9	1	3	260
w/sausage	1	44	28	17	3	8	420
w/sausage & egg	1	260	33	20	3	10	505
danish							
apple	1	25	17	11	2	4	390
iced-cheese	1	47	21	13	2	6	390
cinnamon raisin	1	34	21	13	2	5	440
raspberry	1	26	16	11	2	3	410
muffins							
fat-free apple bran	1	0	0	0	0	0	180
fat-free blueberry	1	0	0	0	0	0	170
egg McMuffin	1	235	11	6	1	4	280
sausage McMuffin	1	57	20	11	2	7	345
sausage McMuffin w/egg	1	270	25	14	3	8	430
English McMuffin w/spread	1	0	4	2	1	1	170
sausage	1	43	15	8	2	5	160
scrambled eggs	1 serving	425	10	5	2	3	140
hash brown potatoes	1 serving	0	7	4	2	1	130
hotcakes w/margarine & syrup	1 serving	8	12	5	5	2	440
Cherrios	¾ c	0	1	<1	<1	<1	80
Wheaties	¾ c	0	1	<1	<1	<1	90
SANDWICHES							
hamburger	1	37	9	5	1	3	225
cheeseburger	1	50	13	7	1	5	305

	Portion	Chol (mg)	Total Fat(g)	Satur'd Fat(g)	Mono Fat(g)	Poly Fat(g)	Total Calor
quarter-pounder	1	85	20	11	1	8	410
quarter-pounder w/cheese	1	115	28	16	1	11	510
McLean deluxe	1	60	10	5	1	4	320
McLean deluxe w/cheese	1	75	14	8	1	5	370
Big Mac	1	100	26	16	1	9	500
Fillet-o-Fish	1	50	18	8	6	4	370
McChicken	1 serving	50	19	9	7	4	415
chicken McNuggets	6 pieces	55	15	10	1.5	3.5	270

DESSERTS

	Portion	Chol (mg)	Total Fat(g)	Satur'd Fat(g)	Mono Fat(g)	Poly Fat(g)	Total Calor
vanilla lowfat frozen yogurt cone	1	3	1	<1	<1	1	105
strawberry lowfat frozen yogurt sundae	1	5	1	<1	<1	1	210
hot fudge frozen yogurt sundae	1	6	3	1	1	2	240
hot caramel lowfat frozen yogurt sundae	1	13	3	1	1	2	270
apple pie	1 serving	6	15	10	1	4	260

SALADS

	Portion	Chol (mg)	Total Fat(g)	Satur'd Fat(g)	Mono Fat(g)	Poly Fat(g)	Total Calor
chef salad	1 serving	111	9	4	1	4	260
garden salad	1 serving	65	2	1	<1	1	50
chunky chicken salad	1 serving	78	4	2	1	1	150
side salad	1 serving	33	1	<1	<1	<1	30
croutons	1 serving	0	1	<1	1	2	50
bacon bits	1 serving	1	1	<1	<1	1	15

COOKIES & MILK SHAKES

	Portion	Chol (mg)	Total Fat(g)	Satur'd Fat(g)	Mono Fat(g)	Poly Fat(g)	Total Calor
McDonald's cookies	2 oz	1	9	7	1	1	290
chocolate chip cookies	2 oz	4	15	10	1	4	330
vanilla lowfat milk shake	10.4 oz	10	1.3	.6	.1	.6	290
chocolate lowfat milk shake	10.4 oz	10	1.7	.9	.1	.7	320
strawberry lowfat milk shake	10.4 oz	10	1.3	.6	.1	.6	320

FRENCH FRIES

	Portion	Chol (mg)	Total Fat(g)	Satur'd Fat(g)	Mono Fat(g)	Poly Fat(g)	Total Calor
small	1 serving	0	12	8	1	2.5	220
medium	1 serving	0	17	12	1.5	3.5	320
large	1 serving	0	22	15	2	5	400

Pizza Hut

PAN PIZZA

	Portion	Chol (mg)	Total Fat(g)	Satur'd Fat(g)	Mono Fat(g)	Poly Fat(g)	Total Calor
cheese	2 slices	49	24	?	?	?	640
pepperoni	2 slices	31	25	?	?	?	668
supreme	2 slices	73	32	?	?	?	722
super supreme	2 slices	73	33	?	?	?	694

	Portion	Chol (mg)	Total Fat(g)	Satur'd Fat(g)	Mono Fat(g)	Poly Fat(g)	Total Calor
PERSONAL PAN PIZZA							
pepperoni	whole pizza	47	21	?	?	?	593
supreme	whole pizza	55	23	?	?	?	679
THIN 'N CRISPY PIZZA							
cheese	2 slices	41	13	?	?	?	444
pepperoni	2 slices	50	22	?	?	?	503
supreme	2 slices	53	26	?	?	?	624
super supreme	2 slices	39	26	?	?	?	605
Wendy's							
SANDWICHES							
quarter-pound hamburger patty	1	65	12	5	7	0	180
plain single	1	65	15	6	7	2	340
single w/everything	1	70	21	6	7	2	420
Wendy's big classic	1	80	33	6	7	3	570
Jr. hamburger	1	35	9	3	4	2	260
Jr. cheeseburger	1	35	13	3	4	2	310
Jr. bacon cheeseburger	1	50	25	5	7	3	430
Jr. Swiss deluxe	1	40	18	3	4	2	360
kids' meal hamburger	1	35	9	3	4	2	260
kids' meal cheeseburger	1	35	13	3	4	2	300
grilled chicken fillet	1	55	3	<1	1	1	100
grilled chicken sandwich	1	60	19	3	5	4	340
chicken breast fillet	1	55	10	2	4	2	220
chicken sandwich	1	60	19	3	5	4	440
chicken club sandwich	1	70	25	5	8	4	506
fish fillet sandwich	1	50	25	5	10	10	460
country fried steak sandwich	1	35	25	6	8	4	440
POTATOES, CHILI & NUGGETS							
french fries (small)	3.2 oz	0	12	3	8	1	240
chili (regular)	9 oz	?	45	7	3	?	220
crispy chicken nuggets	6 pieces	50	20	5	10	4	280
hot stuffed baked potatoes							
plain	1	0	<1	tr	tr	tr	270
bacon & cheese	1	20	18	5	4	8	520
broccoli & cheese	1	<1	16	3	4	7	400
cheese	1	10	15	4	3	7	420
chili & cheese	1	25	18	4	3	3	500
sour cream & chives	1	25	23	9	6	7	500
SALAD/SUPER BAR							
prepared salads							
chef salad	1	40	5	1	1	1	130

	Portion	Chol (mg)	Total Fat(g)	Satur'd Fat(g)	Mono Fat(g)	Poly Fat(g)	Total Calor
garden salad	1	0	2	0	0	<1	70
taco salad	1	35	23	<1	<1	<1	530
superbar/Mexican fiesta							
cheese sauce	56 gr	tr	2	1	1	<1	39
picante sauce	56 gr	n/a	<1	<1	<1	<1	18
refried beans	56 gr	tr	3	1	<1	1	70
rice, Spanish	56 gr	tr	1	<1	<1	1	70
sour topping (imitation)	28 gr	0	5	5	<1	<1	58
taco chips	40 gr	0	10	1	2	4	260
taco meat	56 gr	25	7	2	2	2	110
taco sauce	28 gr	tr	<1	<1	<1	<1	16
taco shells	11 gr	0	3	1	n/a	<1	45
tortilla, flour	37 gr	n/a	3	<1	1	1	110
superbar/pasta							
Alfredo sauce	56 gr	tr	1	1	1	<1	35
classic ravioli in spaghetti sauce	56 gr	5	1	<1	<1	<1	45
classic tortellini in spaghetti sauce	57 gr	5	1	<1	1	<1	60
fettucini	56 gr	10	3	1	1	1	190
garlic toast	18.3 gr	tr	3	1	1	1	70
pasta medley	56 gr	tr	2	<1	<1	1	60
rotini	56 gr	tr	2	<1	<1	1	90
spaghetti sauce	56 gr	tr	<1	<1	<1	<1	28
spaghetti meat sauce	56 gr	10	2	1	1	<1	60
garden spot salad bar							
alfalfa sprouts	28 gr	0	0	0	0	0	8
applesauce, chunky	28 gr	0	<1	tr	tr	tr	22
bacon bits	14 gr	10	2	1	?	<1	40
bananas	28 gr	0	<1	tr	tr	tr	26
breadsticks	8 gr	0	1	<1	<1	<1	30
cauliflower	57 gr	0	0	0	0	0	14
cheddar chips	28 gr	5	12	?	?	?	160
cheese, shredded (imitation)	28 gr	tr	6	4	?	0	90
chicken salad	56 gr	tr	8	2	?	3	120
chow mein noodles	14 gr	0	4	1	1	2	74
cole slaw	57 gr	5	5	1	?	4	70
cottage cheese	105 gr	15	4	3	1	<1	180
croutons	14 gr	n/a	3	?	?	?	60
egg (hard cooked)	20 gr	90	2	1	1	<1	30
garbanzo beans	28 gr	0	1	<1	<1	<1	46
green peas	28 gr	0	0	0	0	0	21
honeydew melon	57 gr	0	0	0	0	0	20
jalapeño peppers	14 gr	0	0	0	0	0	2
lettuce							
iceberg	55 gr	0	0	0	0	0	8
Romaine	55 gr	0	0	0	0	0	9
mushrooms	17 gr	0	0	0	0	0	4
oranges	56 gr	0	0	0	0	0	26

	Portion	Chol (mg)	Total Fat(g)	Satur'd Fat(g)	Mono Fat(g)	Poly Fat(g)	Total Calor
parmesan	28 gr	20	9	5	3	<1	130
parmesan (imitation)	28 gr	tr	3	3	<1	<1	80
pasta salad	57 gr	0	<	?	?	?	35
pepperoni, sliced	28 gr	35	12	5	?	?	140
pineapples chunks	100 gr	0	0	0	0	0	60
potato salad	57 gr	10	11	1	?	4	125
pudding, butterscotch	57 gr	tr	11	2	?	1	90
pudding, chocolate	57 gr	tr	11	2	?	1	90
red peppers, crushed	28 gr	0	4	?	?	?	120
seafood salad	56 gr	tr	7	<	?	4	110
sunflower seeds & raisins	28 gr	0	10	7	?	1	140
three-bean salad	57 gr	?	<1	tr	tr	tr	60
tomatoes	28 gr	0	0	0	0	0	8
tuna salad	56 gr	tr	6	1	?	3	100
turkey ham	28 gr	15	1	1	<1	<1	35
watermelon	57 gr	0	0	0	0	0	18

❏ FATS, OILS, & SHORTENINGS
See also BUTTER & MARGARINE SPREADS

Fats

		Chol (mg)	Total Fat(g)	Satur'd Fat(g)	Mono Fat(g)	Poly Fat(g)	Total Calor
butter oil, anhydrous	1 c	524	204	127	?	?	1,795
butter oil, anhydrous	1 T	33	13	8	?	?	112
chicken fat	1 T	11	13	4	?	?	115
duck fat	1 T	13	13	4	?	?	115
goose fat	1 T	13	13	4	?	?	115
lard (pork)	1 c	195	205	80	?	?	1,849
lard (pork)	1 T	12	13	5	?	?	116

Oils

		Chol (mg)	Total Fat(g)	Satur'd Fat(g)	Mono Fat(g)	Poly Fat(g)	Total Calor
almond	1 T	0	14	1	?	?	120
apricot kernel	1 T	0	14	1	?	?	120
cocoa butter	1 T	0	14	8	?	?	120
coconut	1 T	0	14	12	?	?	120
corn	1 T	0	14	2	?	?	120
cottonseed	1 T	0	14	4	?	?	120
hazelnut	1 T	0	14	1	?	?	120
olive	1 T	0	14	2	?	?	119
palm	1 T	0	14	7	?	?	120
palm kernel	1 T	0	14	11	?	?	120
peanut	1 T	0	14	2	?	?	119
poppyseed	1 T	0	14	2	?	?	120
rapeseed, erucic acid content, zero	1 T	0	14	1	?	?	120

	Portion	Chol (mg)	Total Fat(g)	Satur'd Fat(g)	Mono Fat(g)	Poly Fat(g)	Total Calor
rice bran	1 T	0	14	3	?	?	120
safflower							
linoleic (over 70%)	1 T	0	14	1	?	?	120
oleic (over 70%)	1 T	0	14	1	?	?	120
sesame	1 T	0	14	2	?	?	120
soybean	1 T	0	14	2	?	?	120
soybean (hydrogenated)	1 T	0	14	2	?	?	120
soybean (hydrogenated) & cottonseed	1 T	0	14	2	?	?	120
soybean lecithin (values for commercial products containing 70% soybean phosphatide in 30% soybean oil)	1 T	0	14	2	?	?	120
sunflower							
hydrogenated	1 T	0	14	2	?	?	120
linoleic (< 60%)	1 T	0	14	1	?	?	120
tomato seed	1 T	0	14	3	?	?	120
walnut	1 T	0	14	1	?	?	120
wheat germ	1 T	0	14	3	?	?	120

Shortenings

HOUSEHOLD

	Portion	Chol (mg)	Total Fat(g)	Satur'd Fat(g)	Mono Fat(g)	Poly Fat(g)	Total Calor
lard & vegetable oil	1 T	?	13	5	?	?	115
soybean (hydrogenated) & cottonseed (hydrogenated)	1 T	?	13	3	?	?	113
soybean (hydrogenated) & palm	1 T	0	13	4	?	?	113

INDUSTRIAL

	Portion	Chol (mg)	Total Fat(g)	Satur'd Fat(g)	Mono Fat(g)	Poly Fat(g)	Total Calor
lard & vegetable oil	1 T	?	13	5	?	?	115
soybean (hydrogenated) & cottonseed	1 T	0	13	3	?	?	113

SPECIAL FOR BREAD

	Portion	Chol (mg)	Total Fat(g)	Satur'd Fat(g)	Mono Fat(g)	Poly Fat(g)	Total Calor
soybean (hydrogenated) & cottonseed	1 T	0	13	3	?	?	113

SPECIAL FOR CAKE MIX

	Portion	Chol (mg)	Total Fat(g)	Satur'd Fat(g)	Mono Fat(g)	Poly Fat(g)	Total Calor
soybean (hydrogenated) & cottonseed (hydrogenated)	1 T	0	13	4	?	?	113

SPECIAL FOR CONFECTIONERY

	Portion	Chol (mg)	Total Fat(g)	Satur'd Fat(g)	Mono Fat(g)	Poly Fat(g)	Total Calor
coconut (hydrogenated) and/or palm kernel (hydrogenated)	1 T	0	13	12	?	?	113

	Portion	Chol (mg)	Total Fat(g)	Satur'd Fat(g)	Mono Fat(g)	Poly Fat(g)	Total Calor
fractionated palm	1 T	0	14	9	?	?	120

SPECIAL FOR FRYING

regular

soybean (hydrogenated) & cottonseed (hydrogenated)	1 T	0	13	2	?	?	113

heavy duty

beef tallow & cottonseed	1 T	?	13	6	?	?	115
palm (hydrogenated)	1 T	0	13	6	?	?	113
soybean (hydrogenated)							
linoleic (< 1%)	1 T	0	13	3	?	?	113
linoleic (about 30%) (stabilized w/silicones)	1 T	0	13	2	?	?	113

■ BRAND NAME

Arrowhead Mills

olive oil, unrefined	1 T	0	14	1	?	?	120
safflower oil, unrefined	1 T	0	14	2	?	?	120
sesame oil, unrefined	1 T	0	14	2	?	?	120

Hain

NON-VEGETABLE OILS

cod liver, plain, mint & cherry	1 T	0	14	?	?	?	120

UNREFINED OIL

safflower	1 T	0	?	1	?	11	120

VEGETABLE OILS

all blend	1 T	0	14	2	?	9	120
almond	1 T	0	14	1	?	4	120
apricot kernel	1 T	0	14	1	?	4	120
canola	1 T	0	14	1	?	5	120
coconut	1 T	0	14	12	?	0	120
corn	1 T	0	14	2	?	9	120
hi-oleic safflower	1 T	0	14	1	?	2	120
olive	1 T	0	14	2	?	1	120
peanut	1 T	0	14	2	?	5	120
safflower	1 T	0	14	1	?	11	120
sesame	1 T	0	14	1	?	11	120
soy	1 T	0	14	2	?	8	120
sunflower	1 T	0	14	2	?	9	120
walnut	1 T	0	14	2	?	9	120

Hollywood

canola oil	1 T	0	14	1	?	5	120
peanut oil	1 T	0	14	4	?	5	120
safflower oil	1 T	0	14	1	?	11	120

	Portion	Chol (mg)	Total Fat(g)	Satur'd Fat(g)	Mono Fat(g)	Poly Fat(g)	Total Calor
soy oil	1 T	0	14	3	?	8	120
sunflower oil	1 T	0	14	2	?	10	120
Mazola							
corn oil	1 T	2	14	2	4	8	125
No-stick	2½ second spray	0	<1	tr	tr	.1	2
Progresso							
imported olive oil	1 T	0	14	2	?	1	119
extra virgin olive oil	1 T	0	14	2	?	1	119
extra light olive oil	1 T	0	14	2	?	1	119
Wesson							
vegetable oil	1 T	0	14	2	?	8	120
cooking spray	.27 gr	0	<1	?	?	?	.4
shortening	1 T	0	12	4	?	3	110
sunflower oil	1 T	0	14	2	?	10	120
corn oil	1 T	0	14	2	?	8	120
canola oil	1 T	0	14	4	?	1	120
olive oil	1 T	0	14	1	?	2	120

❏ FISH *See* SEAFOOD & SEAFOOD PRODUCTS

❏ FLOURS & CORNMEALS

arrowroot flour	1 T	0	0	?	?	?	29
barley flour	1 T	0	tr	?	?	?	28
barley flour	1 c	0	2	?	?	?	401
buckwheat flour							
dark	1 oz	0	1	?	?	?	92
light	1 c	0	1	tr	?	?	340
carob flour	1 T	0	tr	tr	?	?	14
carob flour	1 c	0	1	tr	?	?	185
corn flour	1 c	0	3	?	?	?	405
masa harina	⅓ c	0	2	?	?	?	137
masa trigo	⅓ c	0	4	?	?	?	149
white, tortilla, lime-treated	1 oz	0	2	?	?	?	103
yellow, tortilla, untreated	1 oz	0	1	?	?	?	101
corn germ, toasted	1 oz	0	7	?	?	?	130
cornmeal							
whole-ground, dry							
unbolted	1 c	0	5	1	?	?	122
bolted	1 c	0	4	1	?	?	122
degermed, enriched							
dry	1 c	0	.2	tr	?	?	138
cooked	1 c	0	tr	tr	?	?	240
white, self-rising, dry	1 oz or ⅙ c	0	1	?	?	?	98

	Portion	Chol (mg)	Total Fat(g)	Satur'd Fat(g)	Mono Fat(g)	Poly Fat(g)	Total Calor
cornstarch	1 T	0	tr	?	?	?	35
manioc (casava) flour	3½ oz	0	1	?	?	?	320
nut flours *See* NUTS & NUT-BASED BUTTERS, FLOURS, MEALS, MILKS, PASTES, & POWDERS							
potato flour	1 c	0	1	tr	?	?	628
rice bran	1 oz	0	tr	?	?	?	80
rice flour	1 c	0	tr	?	?	?	479
rice polish	1 oz	0	2	?	?	?	101
rye flour							
dark	3½ oz	0	3	?	?	?	327
light	3½ oz	0	1	?	?	?	357
rye wheat flour	1 c	0	1	?	?	?	400
soy flour *See* SOYBEANS & SOYBEAN PRODUCTS							
wheat & gluten flour	1 c	0	3	?	?	?	529
wheat flour, enriched all-purpose							
sifted	1 c	0	1	tr	?	?	420
unsifted	1 c	0	1	tr	?	?	455
bread sifted	1 c	0	1	?	?	?	409
cake or pastry, sifted	1 c	0	1	tr	?	?	350
self-rising, unsifted	1 c	0	1	tr	?	?	440
whole-wheat & soy flour	3½ oz	0	7	?	?	?	365
whole-wheat flour, from hard wheats	1 c	0	2	tr	?	?	400
whole-wheat flour, straight, soft	3½ oz	0	1	?	?	?	364

▪ BRAND NAME

Argo

	Portion	Chol (mg)	Total Fat(g)	Satur'd Fat(g)	Mono Fat(g)	Poly Fat(g)	Total Calor
Argo & Kingsford's Corn Starch	1 T	0	0	0	?	?	30

Arrowhead Mills

	Portion	Chol (mg)	Total Fat(g)	Satur'd Fat(g)	Mono Fat(g)	Poly Fat(g)	Total Calor
barley flour	2 oz	0	1	?	?	?	200
brown rice flour	2 oz	0	1	?	?	?	200
buckwheat flour	2 oz	0	1	?	?	?	190
cornmeal							
blue	2 oz	0	3	?	?	?	210
hi-lysine	2 oz	0	2	?	?	?	210
yellow	2 oz	0	2	?	?	?	210
millet flour	2 oz	0	2	?	?	?	185
oat flour	2 oz	0	1	?	?	?	200
pastry flour	2 oz	0	1	?	?	?	180
rye flour	2 oz	0	1	?	?	?	190
unbleached white flour	2 oz	0	1	?	?	?	200
vital wheat gluten	1 oz	0	1	?	?	?	100
whole-wheat flour	2 oz	0	1	?	?	?	200

	Portion	Chol (mg)	Total Fat(g)	Satur'd Fat(g)	Mono Fat(g)	Poly Fat(g)	Total Calor
Aunt Jemima							
CORNMEAL							
bolted white mix	3 T	0	1	?	?	?	99
buttermilk self-rising white mix	3 T	0	1	?	?	?	101
enriched white	3 T	0	1	?	?	?	102
enriched yellow	3 T	0	1	?	?	?	102
self-rising white mix	3 T	0	1	?	?	?	98
self-rising white enriched bolted	3 T	0	1	?	?	?	99
FLOUR							
enriched self-rising	¼ c	?	tr	?	?	?	109
Gold Medal							
better for bread	4 oz (1 c)	?	1	?	?	?	400
all-purpose	4 oz (1 c)	?	1	?	?	?	400
oat flour blend	4 oz (1 c)	?	3	?	?	?	390
self-rising	4 oz (1 c)	?	1	?	?	?	380
unbleached	4 oz (1 c)	?	1	?	?	?	400
whole wheat	4 oz (1 c)	?	2	?	?	?	350
whole wheat blend	4 oz (1 c)	?	2	?	?	?	380
Heckers							
flour	about 1 c (4 oz)	0	1	?	?	?	380–400
Pillsbury's Best							
all purpose	1 c	?	1	?	?	?	400
bread	1 c	?	2	?	?	?	400
medium rye	1 c	?	2	?	?	?	400
self-rising unbleached or bleached	1 c	?	2	?	?	?	380
shake & blend	2 T	?	0	?	?	?	50
unbleached all-purpose	1 c	?	1	?	?	?	400
whole wheat	1 c	?	2	?	?	?	400
Quaker Oats							
grits							
enriched white hominy, regular & quick	3 T	?	tr	?	?	?	101
enriched yellow hominy quick	3 T	?	tr	?	?	?	101
instant grits							
white hominy	1 pkt	?	tr	?	?	?	79
w/imitation bacon bits	1 pkt	?	tr	?	?	?	101
w/red cheddar cheese flavor	1 pkt	0	1	?	?	?	104
masa harina de maiz	2–6" tortillas	?	2	?	?	?	137
masa trigo	2–6" tortillas	?	4	?	?	?	149

Portion	Chol (mg)	Total Fat(g)	Satur'd Fat(g)	Mono Fat(g)	Poly Fat(g)	Total Calor

❑ FRANKFURTERS *See* PROCESSED MEAT & POULTRY PRODUCTS

❑ FRUIT, FRESH & PROCESSED
See also PICKLES, OLIVES, RELISHES, & CHUTNEYS
See also SNACKS

	Portion	Chol (mg)	Total Fat(g)	Satur'd Fat(g)	Mono Fat(g)	Poly Fat(g)	Total Calor
apples							
raw							
w/skin	1 = 4.9 oz	0	21	tr	?	?	81
w/out skin	1 = 4½ oz	0	tr	tr	?	?	72
baked in microwave, w/out skin	½ c sliced	0	tr	tr	?	?	48
boiled, w/out skin	1½ c sliced	0	tr	tr	?	?	46
canned, sweetened, unheated	½ c sliced	0	1	tr	?	?	68
dehydrated, sulfured							
cooked	½ c	0	tr	tr	?	?	71
uncooked	½ c	0	tr	tr	?	?	104
dried, sulfured							
cooked, w/added sugar	½ c	0	tr	tr	?	?	116
cooked, w/out added sugar	½ c	0	tr	tr	?	?	72
uncooked	2¼ oz	0	tr	tr	?	?	155
uncooked	1 c	0	tr	tr	?	?	209
frozen, sliced, unsweetened							
heated	½ c sliced	0	tr	tr	?	?	48
unheated	½ c sliced	0	tr	tr	?	?	41
applesauce, canned							
sweetened	½ c	0	tr	tr	?	?	97
unsweetened	½ c	0	tr	tr	?	?	53
apricots							
raw	3 fruit = 3.7 oz	0	tr	tr	?	?	51
canned, w/skin							
in water	3 halves + 1¾ T liquid	0	tr	tr	?	?	22
in juice	3 halves + 1¾ T liquid	0	tr	tr	?	?	40
in extra light syrup	3 halves + 1¾ T liquid	0	tr	tr	?	?	41

	Portion	Chol (mg)	Total Fat(g)	Satur'd Fat(g)	Mono Fat(g)	Poly Fat(g)	Total Calor
in light syrup	3 halves + 1¾ T liquid	0	tr	tr	?	?	54
in heavy syrup	3 halves + 1¾ T liquid	0	tr	tr	?	?	70
canned, w/out skin							
in water	2 fruit + 2 T liquid	0	tr	tr	?	?	20
in heavy syrup	2 fruit + 2 T liquid	0	tr	tr	?	?	75
in extra heavy syrup	2 fruit + 2 T liquid	0	tr	tr	?	?	87
dehydrated (low-moisture), sulfured							
cooked	½ c	0	tr	tr	?	?	156
uncooked	½ c	0	tr	tr	?	?	192
dried, sulfured							
cooked, w/added sugar	½ c halves	0	tr	tr	?	?	153
cooked, w/out added sugar	½ c halves	0	tr	tr	?	?	106
uncooked	10 halves	0	tr	tr	?	?	83
frozen, sweetened	½ c	0	tr	tr	?	?	119
avocados, raw							
all commercial varieties	1 fruit = 7.1 oz	0	31	5	?	?	324
all commercial varieties	1 c puree	0	35	6	?	?	370
California	1 fruit = 6.1 oz	0	30	4	?	?	306
California	1 c puree	0	40	6	?	?	407
Florida	1 fruit = 10.7 oz	0	27	5	?	?	339
Florida	1 c puree	0	20	4	?	?	257
bananas							
raw	1 fruit = 4 oz	0	tr	1	?	?	105
dehydrated (banana powder)	1 T	0	tr	tr	?	?	21
blackberries							
raw	½ c	0	tr	?	?	?	37
canned, in heavy syrup	½ c	0	tr	?	?	?	118
frozen, unsweetened	1 c	0	1	?	?	?	97
blueberries							
raw	1 c	0	1	?	?	?	82
canned, in heavy syrup	½ c	0	tr	?	?	?	112
frozen							
sweetened	1 c	0	tr	?	?	?	187
unsweetened	1 c	0	1	?	?	?	78
boysenberries							
canned, in heavy syrup	½ c	0	tr	?	?	?	113

	Portion	Chol (mg)	Total Fat(g)	Satur'd Fat(g)	Mono Fat(g)	Poly Fat(g)	Total Calor
frozen, unsweetened	1 c	0	tr	?	?	?	66
breadfruit, raw	¼ small fruit = 3.4 oz	0	tr	?	?	?	99
candied fruit *See* BAKING INGREDIENTS							
cantaloupe *See* MELONS, below							
casaba *See* MELONS, below							
cherries, sour, red							
raw	1 c w/pits	0	tr	tr	?	?	51
canned							
in water	½ c	0	tr	tr	?	?	43
in light syrup	½ c	0	tr	tr	?	?	94
in heavy syrup	½ c	0	tr	tr	?	?	116
in extra heavy syrup	½ c	0	tr	tr	?	?	148
frozen, unsweetened	1 c	0	1	tr	?	?	72
cherries, sweet							
raw	10 fruit = 2.4 oz	0	1	tr	?	?	49
canned							
in water	½ c	0	tr	tr	?	?	57
in juice	½ c	0	tr	tr	?	?	68
in light syrup	½ c	0	tr	tr	?	?	85
in heavy syrup	½ c	0	tr	tr	?	?	107
in extra heavy syrup	½ c	0	tr	tr	?	?	133
frozen, sweetened	1 c	0	tr	tr	?	?	232
Chinese gooseberries *See* kiwi fruit, below							
coconut *See* BAKING INGREDIENTS; NUTS & NUT-BASED BUTTERS, FLOURS, MEALS, MILKS, PASTES, & POWDERS							
crabapples, raw	1 c sliced	0	tr	tr	?	?	83
cranberries, raw	1 c whole	0	tr	?	?	?	46
cranberry sauce, canned, sweetened	½ c	0	tr	?	?	?	209
currants							
European, black, raw	½ c	0	tr	tr	?	?	36
red & white, raw	½ c	0	tr	tr	?	?	31
zante, dried	½ c	0	tr	tr	?	?	204
custard-apple, raw	edible portion = 3½ oz	0	1	?	?	?	101
dates, domestic, dry	10 fruit = 2.9 oz	0	tr	?	?	?	228
figs							
raw	1 medium fruit = 1¾ oz	0	tr	tr	?	?	37
canned							
in water	3 fruit + 1¾ T liquid	0	tr	tr	?	?	42

	Portion	Chol (mg)	Total Fat(g)	Satur'd Fat(g)	Mono Fat(g)	Poly Fat(g)	Total Calor
in light syrup	3 fruit + 1¾ T liquid	0	tr	tr	?	?	58
in heavy syrup	3 fruit + 1¾ T liquid	0	tr	tr	?	?	75
in extra heavy syrup	3 fruit + 1¾ T liquid	0	tr	tr	?	?	91
dried							
cooked	½ c	0	1	tr	?	?	140
uncooked	10 fruit = 6.6 oz	0	2	tr	?	?	477
fruit cocktail, canned							
in water	½ c	0	tr	tr	?	?	40
in juice	½ c	0	tr	tr	?	?	56
in extra light syrup	½ c	0	tr	tr	?	?	55
in light syrup	½ c	0	tr	tr	?	?	72
in heavy syrup	½ c	0	tr	tr	?	?	93
in extra heavy syrup	½ c	0	tr	tr	?	?	115
fruit salad, canned							
in water	½ c	0	tr	tr	?	?	37
in juice	½ c	0	tr	tr	?	?	62
in light syrup	½ c	0	tr	tr	?	?	73
in heavy syrup	½ c	0	tr	tr	?	?	94
in extra heavy syrup	½ c	0	tr	tr	?	?	114
fruit salad, tropical, canned, in heavy syrup	½ c	0	tr	?	?	?	110
gooseberries							
raw	1 c	0	1	tr	?	?	67
canned, in light syrup	½ c	0	tr	tr	?	?	93
grandilla See passion fruit, belowgrapefruit							
raw, pink & red	½ fruit = 4.3 oz	0	tr	tr	?	?	37
raw, white	½ fruit = 4.2 oz	0	tr	tr	?	?	39
canned							
in water	½ c	0	tr	tr	?	?	44
in juice	½ c	0	tr	tr	?	?	46
in light syrup	½ c	0	tr	tr	?	?	76
grapes							
American type, raw	10 fruit = 0.8 oz	0	tr	tr	?	?	15
European type, raw	10 fruit = 1.8 oz	0	tr	tr	?	?	36

	Portion	Chol (mg)	Total Fat(g)	Satur'd Fat(g)	Mono Fat(g)	Poly Fat(g)	Total Calor
Thompson seedless, canned							
in water	½ c	0	tr	tr	?	?	48
in heavy syrup, solids & liquids	½ c	0	tr	tr	?	?	94
guava sauce, cooked	½ c	0	tr	tr	?	?	43
guavas							
common, raw	1 fruit = 3.2 oz	0	1	tr	?	?	45
strawberry, raw	1 fruit = 0.2 oz	0	tr	tr	?	?	4
honeydew *See* melons, below							
kiwi fruit, raw	1 medium fruit = 2.7 oz	0	tr	?	?	?	46
kumquats, raw	1 fruit = 0.7 oz	0	tr	?	?	?	12
lemon peel, raw	1 t	0	tr	tr	?	?	?
lemon peel, raw	1 T	0	tr	tr	?	?	?
lemons, raw							
w/peel	1 medium fruit = 2 oz	0	tr	tr	?	?	22
w/out peel	1 medium fruit = 3.8 oz	0	tr	tr	?	?	17
limes, raw	1 fruit = 2.4 oz	0	tr	tr	?	?	20
mangos, raw	1 fruit = 7.3 oz	0	1	tr	?	?	135
melon balls, frozen, cantaloupe & honeydew	1 c	0	tr	?	?	?	55
melons							
cantaloupe, raw	½ = 9.4 oz	22	1	?	?	?	94
cantaloupe, raw	1 c cubed	13	tr	?	?	?	57
cassaba, raw	⅒ = 5.8 oz	0	tr	?	?	?	43
cassaba, raw	1 c cubed	0	tr	?	?	?	45
honeydew, raw	⅒ = 4½ oz	0	tr	?	?	?	46
honeydew, raw	1 c cubed	0	tr	?	?	?	60
musk *See* Cantaloupe, above							
mixed fruit							
canned, in heavy syrup, solids & liquids	½ c	0	tr	tr	?	?	92
dried	11 oz pkg	0	1	tr	?	?	712
frozen, sweetened	1 c	0	tr	tr	?	?	245
mulberries, raw	10 fruit = 15g	0	tr	?	?	?	7

	Portion	Chol (mg)	Total Fat(g)	Satur'd Fat(g)	Mono Fat(g)	Poly Fat(g)	Total Calor
muskmelons *See* MELONS, above							
nectarines, raw	1 fruit = 4.8 oz	0	1	?	?	?	67
orange peel, raw	1 t	0	0	0	?	?	?
orange peel, raw	1 T	0	tr	tr	?	?	?
oranges, raw							
w/peel	1 fruit = 5.6 oz	0	tr	tr	?	?	64
w/out peel							
all commercial varieties	1 fruit = 4.6 oz	0	tr	tr	?	?	62
California, navels	1 fruit = 4.9 oz	0	tr	tr	?	?	65
California, Valencias	1 fruit = 4.3 oz	0	tr	tr	?	?	59
Florida	1 fruit = 5.3 oz	0	tr	tr	?	?	69
papayas, raw	1 fruit = 10.7 oz	0	tr	tr	?	?	117
passion-fruit, purple, raw	1 fruit = 0.6 oz	0	tr	?	?	?	18
peaches							
raw	1 fruit = 3.1 oz	0	tr	tr	?	?	37
canned, clingstone							
in water	1 half + 1⅔ T liquid	0	tr	tr	?	?	18
in extra light syrup	1 half + 1⅔ T liquid	0	tr	tr	?	?	32
in light syrup	1 half + 1¾ T liquid	0	tr	tr	?	?	44
canned, clingstone & freestone							
in juice	1 half + 1⅔ T liquid	0	tr	tr	?	?	34
in heavy syrup	1 half + 1¾ T liquid	0	tr	tr	?	?	60
canned, freestone in extra heavy syrup	1 half + 1¾ T liquid	0	tr	tr	?	?	77
dehydrated (low-moisture), sulfured							
cooked	½ c	0	1	tr	?	?	161
uncooked	½ c	0	1	tr	?	?	188

	Portion	Chol (mg)	Total Fat(g)	Satur'd Fat(g)	Mono Fat(g)	Poly Fat(g)	Total Calor
dried, sulfured							
cooked, w/added sugar	½ c halves	0	tr	tr	?	?	139
cooked, w/out added sugar	½ c halves	0	tr	tr	?	?	99
uncooked	10 halves	0	1	tr	?	?	311
frozen, sliced, sweetened	1 c sliced, thawed	0	tr	tr	?	?	235
peaches, spiced, canned, in heavy syrup	1 fruit + 2 T liquid	0	tr	tr	?	?	66
pears							
raw	1 fruit 5.8 oz	0	1	tr	?	?	98
canned							
in water	1 half + 1²/₃ T liquid	0	tr	tr	?	?	22
in juice	1 half + 1²/₃ T liquid	0	tr	tr	?	?	38
in extra light syrup	1 half + 1²/₃ T liquid	0	tr	tr	?	?	36
in light syrup	1 half + 1³/₄ T liquid	0	tr	tr	?	?	45
in heavy syrup	1 half + 1³/₄ T liquid	0	tr	tr	?	?	58
in extra heavy syrup	1 half + 1³/₄ T liquid	0	tr	tr	?	?	77
dried, sulfured							
cooked, w/added sugar	½ c halves	0	tr	tr	?	?	196
cooked, w/out added sugar	½ c halves	0	tr	tr	?	?	163
uncooked	10 halves	0	1	tr	?	?	459
pineapple							
raw	1 slice = 3 oz	0	tr	tr	?	?	42
raw	1 c diced	0	1	tr	?	?	77
canned							
in water	1 slice + 1¼ T liquid	0	tr	tr	?	?	19
in water	1 c tidbits	0	tr	tr	?	?	79

	Portion	Chol (mg)	Total Fat(g)	Satur'd Fat(g)	Mono Fat(g)	Poly Fat(g)	Total Calor
in juice	1 slice + 1¼ T liquid	0	tr	tr	?	?	35
in juice	1 c chunks or tidbits	0	tr	tr	?	?	150
in light syrup	1 slice + 1¼ T liquid	0	tr	tr	?	?	30
in light syrup	1 c	0	tr	tr	?	?	131
in heavy syrup	1 slice + 1¼ T liquid	0	tr	tr	?	?	45
in heavy syrup	1 c chunks, tidbits, or crushed	0	tr	tr	?	?	199
in extra heavy syrup	1 slice + 1¼ T liquid	0	tr	tr	?	?	48
in extra heavy syrup	1 c chunks or crushed	0	tr	tr	?	?	217
frozen, sweetened	½ c chunks	0	tr	tr	?	?	104
plantains							
raw	1 fruit = 6.3 oz	0	1	?	?	?	218
cooked	½ c sliced	0	tr	?	?	?	89
plums, purple							
raw	1 fruit = 2.3 oz	0	tr	tr	?	?	36
canned							
in water	3 fruit + 2 T liquid	0	tr	tr	?	?	39
in water	1 c	0	tr	tr	?	?	102
in juice	3 fruit + 2 T liquid	0	tr	tr	?	?	55
in juice	1 c	0	tr	tr	?	?	146
in light syrup	3 fruit + 2¾ T liquid	0	tr	tr	?	?	83
in light syrup	1 c	0	tr	tr	?	?	158
in heavy syrup	3 fruit + 2¾ T liquid	0	tr	tr	?	?	119
in heavy syrup	1 c	0	tr	tr	?	?	230
in extra heavy syrup	3 fruit + 2¾ T liquid	0	tr	tr	?	?	135
in extra heavy syrup	1 c	0	tr	tr	?	?	265

	Portion	Chol (mg)	Total Fat(g)	Satur'd Fat(g)	Mono Fat(g)	Poly Fat(g)	Total Calor
pomegranates, raw	1 fruit = 5.4 oz	0	tr	?	?	?	104
prickly pears, raw	1 fruit = 3.6 oz	0	1	?	?	?	42
prunes							
canned, in heavy syrup	5 fruit + 2 T liquid	0	tr	tr	?	?	90
canned, in heavy syrup	1 c	0	tr	tr	?	?	245
dehydrated (low moisture)							
cooked	½ c	0	tr	tr	?	?	158
uncooked	½ c	0	tr	tr	?	?	224
dried							
cooked, w/added sugar	½ c	0	tr	tr	?	?	147
cooked, w/out added sugar	½	0	tr	tr	?	?	113
uncooked	10 fruit = 3 oz	0	tr	tr	?	?	201
uncooked	1 c	0	1	tr	?	?	385
raisins							
golden seedless	1 c not packed	0	1	tr	?	?	437
golden seedless	1 c packed	0	1	tr	?	?	498
seeded	1 c not packed	0	1	tr	?	?	428
seeded	1 c packed	0	1	tr	?	?	488
seedless	1 c not packed	0	1	tr	?	?	434
seedless	1 c packed	0	1	tr	?	?	494
raspberries, red							
raw	1 c	0	1	tr	?	?	61
canned, in heavy syrup, solids & liquids	½ c	0	tr	tr	?	?	117
frozen, sweetened	1 c	0	tr	tr	?	?	256
frozen, sweetened	10 oz	0	tr	tr	?	?	291
rhubarb							
raw	½ c diced	0	tr	?	?	?	13
frozen							
cooked, w/added sugar	½ c	0	tr	?	?	?	139
uncooked	½ c	0	tr	?	?	?	14
rose-apples, raw	edible portion = 3½ oz	0	tr	?	?	?	25
strawberries							
raw	1 c	0	1	tr	?	?	45
canned, in heavy syrup	½ c	0	tr	tr	?	?	117
frozen, sweetened	1 c sliced	0	tr	tr	?	?	245
frozen, sweetened	10 oz sliced	0	tr	tr	?	?	273
frozen, sweetened	1 c whole	0	tr	tr	?	?	200

	Portion	Chol (mg)	Total Fat(g)	Satur'd Fat(g)	Mono Fat(g)	Poly Fat(g)	Total Calor
frozen, sweetened	10 oz whole	0	tr	tr	?	?	223
frozen, unsweetened	1 c	0	tr	tr	?	?	52
sugar-apples, raw	1 fruit = 5½oz	?	?	?	?	?	146
sweetsop *See* SUGAR-APPLES, above							
tamarinds, raw	1 fruit = 0.1 oz	0	tr	tr	?	?	5
tangerines							
raw	1 fruit = 3 oz	0	tr	tr	?	?	37
canned							
in juice, solids & liquids	½ c	0	tr	tr	?	?	46
in light syrup, solids & liquids	½ c	0	tr	tr	?	?	76
watermelon, raw	1/16 fruit = 17 oz	0	2	?	?	?	152
watermelon, raw	1 c diced	0	1	?	?	?	50

▪ BRAND NAME

Birds Eye
fruit in quick thaw pouch

	Portion	Chol (mg)	Total Fat(g)	Satur'd Fat(g)	Mono Fat(g)	Poly Fat(g)	Total Calor
mixed fruit in syrup	5 oz	0	0	?	?	?	120
red raspberries in lite syrup	5 oz	0	1	?	?	?	100
strawberries, halved in lite syrup	5 oz	0	0	?	?	?	90
strawberries, halved in syrup	5 oz	0	0	?	?	?	120
whole strawberries in lite syrup	4 oz	0	0	?	?	?	80

Dole

	Portion	Chol (mg)	Total Fat(g)	Satur'd Fat(g)	Mono Fat(g)	Poly Fat(g)	Total Calor
raisins, seedless & golden	½ c	0	0	?	?	?	260
dates, pitted & chopped	½ c	0	0	?	?	?	280
canned fruit							
pineapple							
juice pack	½ c	0	<1	?	?	?	70
syrup pack	½ c	0	<1	?	?	?	90
mandarin orange segments	½ c	0	<1	?	?	?	70
pineapple, mandarin & orange segments	½ c	0	<1	?	?	?	60
tropical fruit salad	½ c	0	<1	?	?	?	70

Dromedary

	Portion	Chol (mg)	Total Fat(g)	Satur'd Fat(g)	Mono Fat(g)	Poly Fat(g)	Total Calor
chopped dates	¼ c	?	0	?	?	?	130

	Portion	Chol (mg)	Total Fat(g)	Satur'd Fat(g)	Mono Fat(g)	Poly Fat(g)	Total Calor
Motts							
APPLESAUCE							
single serve							
regular sweetened	4 oz	<1	<1	?	?	?	88
cinnamon	4 oz	<1	<1	?	?	?	92
natural	4 oz	<1	<1	?	?	?	48
Dutch apple spice	4 oz	<1	<1	?	?	?	84
chunky applesauce & cherries fruit pak	3.9 oz	<1	<1	?	?	?	68
chunky applesauce & peaches fruit pak	3.9 oz	<1	<1	?	?	?	72
multiserve							
regular sweetened	4 oz	<1	<1	?	?	?	88
cinnamon	4 oz	<1	<1	?	?	?	92
natural	4 oz	<1	<1	?	?	?	48
chunky	4 oz	<1	<1	?	?	?	88
Dutch apple spice	4 oz	<1	<1	?	?	?	84
Mrs Paul's							
apple fritters	2	?	13	?	?	?	270
Stouffer							
escalloped apples	4 oz	?	2	?	?	?	130

❑ **FRUIT & NUT SNACK MIXES** *See* SNACKS

❑ **FRUIT SPREADS**

Fruit Butters

	Portion	Chol (mg)	Total Fat(g)	Satur'd Fat(g)	Mono Fat(g)	Poly Fat(g)	Total Calor
apple	1 T	0	tr	?	?	?	37
guava	1 T	?	0	0	?	?	39

Jams

	Portion	Chol (mg)	Total Fat(g)	Satur'd Fat(g)	Mono Fat(g)	Poly Fat(g)	Total Calor
all varieties							
regular	1 T	0	tr	?	?	?	55
low-cal	1 T	0	tr	?	?	?	29
grape	1 T	0	tr	?	?	?	59
plum	1 T	0	tr	0	?	?	59

Jellies

	Portion	Chol (mg)	Total Fat(g)	Satur'd Fat(g)	Mono Fat(g)	Poly Fat(g)	Total Calor
all varieties							
regular	1 T	0	tr	?	?	?	55
low-cal	1 T	0	0	0	?	?	27
blackberry	1 T	0	0	0	?	?	51
boysenberry	1 T	0	0	0	?	?	52
cherry	1 T	0	tr	?	?	?	52

	Portion	Chol (mg)	Total Fat(g)	Satur'd Fat(g)	Mono Fat(g)	Poly Fat(g)	Total Calor
currant	1 T	0	0	0	?	?	52
grape	1 T	0	tr	?	?	?	55
strawberry	1 T	0	0	?	?	?	51

Marmalades

citrus	1 T	0	tr	?	?	?	51
orange	1 T	0	tr	?	?	?	56
papaya	1 T	0	0	0	?	?	57

Preserves

apricot	1 T	0	tr	?	?	?	51
apricot-pineapple	1 T	0	tr	?	?	?	51
blackberry	1 T	0	tr	?	?	?	55
boysenberry	1 T	0	tr	?	?	?	54
peach	1 T	0	0	0	?	?	51

▪ BRAND NAME

Kraft

jam, all varieties	1 t	0	0	0	?	0	17
jelly, all varieties	1 t	0	0	0	?	0	17
perserves, all varieties	1 t	0	0	0	?	0	17
reduced calorie, all varieties	1 t	0	0	0	?	0	6

Smucker's

FRUIT BUTTER

apple	2 t	0	0	0	?	?	24
apple harvest pumpkin	2 t	?	0	?	?	?	24
peach	2 t	0	0	0	?	?	30

JAMS, JELLIES, MARMALADES, & PRESERVES

all flavors							
regular	2 t	0	0	0	?	?	36
low sugar	2 t	0	0	0	?	?	16
Slenderella	2 t	?	0	?	?	?	14
simply fruit spread	2 t	?	0	?	?	?	32

❏ **FRUIT CHUTNEYS & RELISHES** *See* **PICKLES, OLIVES, RELISHES, & CHUTNEYS**

❏ **FRUIT SAUCES** *See* **FRUITS, FRESH & PROCESSED**

	Portion	Chol (mg)	Total Fat(g)	Satur'd Fat(g)	Mono Fat(g)	Poly Fat(g)	Total Calor

❑ **GELATIN & GELATIN DESSERTS**
See **DESSERTS: CUSTARDS, GELATINS, PUDDINGS, & PIE FILLINGS**

❑ **GRAINS** *See* **RICE & GRAINS, PLAIN & PREPARED**

❑ **GRAVIES** *See* **SAUCES, GRAVIES, & CONDIMENTS**

❑ **HAM** *See* **PORK, FRESH & CURED; PROCESSED MEAT & POULTRY PRODUCTS**

❑ **HERBS & SPICES** *See* **SEASONINGS**

❑ **HONEY** *See* **SUGARS & SWEETENERS**

❑ **HOTDOGS** *See* **PROCESSED MEAT & POULTRY PRODUCTS**

❑ **ICE CREAM & ICE MILK** *See* **DESSERTS, FROZEN**

❑ **INFANT & TODDLER FOODS**

Baked Products

	Portion	Chol (mg)	Total Fat(g)	Satur'd Fat(g)	Mono Fat(g)	Poly Fat(g)	Total Calor
arrowroot cookies	1		tr	1	tr	?	?	24
arrowroot cookies	1 oz		tr	4	1	?	?	125
cookies	1		?	1	tr	?	?	28
cookies	1 oz		?	4	1	?	?	123
pretzels	1		?	tr	?	?	?	24
pretzels	1 oz		?	1	?	?	?	113
teething biscuits	1		?	1	?	?	?	43
teething biscuits	1 oz		?	1	?	?	?	111
zwieback	1		1	1	tr	?	?	30
zwieback	1 oz		6	3	1	?	?	121

Cereals, Hot & Cold

	Portion	Chol (mg)	Total Fat(g)	Satur'd Fat(g)	Mono Fat(g)	Poly Fat(g)	Total Calor
barley dry	½ oz		?	tr	?	?	?	52

	Portion	Chol (mg)	Total Fat(g)	Satur'd Fat(g)	Mono Fat(g)	Poly Fat(g)	Total Calor
w/whole milk	1 oz	?	1	?	?	?	31
cereal & eggs, strained	about 4½ oz	66	2	1	?	?	112
cereal & egg yolks							
strained	about 4½ oz	81	2	1	?	?	66
junior	about 7½ oz	?	4	1	?	?	110
cereal, egg yolks, & bacon							
strained	about 4½ oz	?	7	?	?	?	101
junior	about 7½ oz	?	11	?	?	?	178
grits & egg yolks, strained	about 4½ oz	?	3	?	?	?	?
high protein							
dry	½ oz	?	1	?	?	?	51
w/whole milk	1 oz	?	1	?	?	?	31
high protein w/apple & orange							
dry	½ oz	?	1	?	?	?	53
w/whole milk	1 oz	?	1	?	?	?	32
mixed cereal							
dry	½ oz	?	1	?	?	?	54
w/whole milk	1 oz	?	1	?	?	?	32
mixed cereal w/applesauce & bananas							
strained	about 4.8 oz	?	1	?	?	?	111
junior	about 7.8 oz	?	1	?	?	?	183
mixed cereal w/bananas							
dry	½ oz	?	1	?	?	?	56
w/whole milk	1 oz	?	1	?	?	?	33
mixed cereal w/honey							
dry	½ oz	?	1	?	?	?	55
w/whole milk	1 oz	?	1	?	?	?	33
oatmeal							
dry	½ oz	?	1	?	?	?	56
w/whole milk	1 oz	?	1	?	?	?	33
oatmeal w/applesauce & bananas							
strained	about 4.8 oz	?	1	?	?	?	99
junior	about 7.8 oz	?	2	?	?	?	165
junior	1 oz	?	tr	?	?	?	21
oatmeal w/bananas							
dry	½ oz	?	1	?	?	?	56
w/whole milk	1 oz	?	1	?	?	?	33

	Portion	Chol (mg)	Total Fat(g)	Satur'd Fat(g)	Mono Fat(g)	Poly Fat(g)	Total Calor
oatmeal w/honey							
dry	1/2 oz	?	1	?	?	?	55
w/whole milk	1 oz	?	1	?	?	?	33
rice							
dry	1/2 oz	?	1	?	?	?	56
w/whole milk	1 oz	?	1	?	?	?	33
rice w/applesauce & bananas, strained	about 4.8 oz	?	1	?	?	?	107
rice w/bananas							
dry	1/2 oz	?	1	?	?	?	57
w/whole milk	1 oz	?	1	?	?	?	33
rice, w/honey							
dry	1/2 oz	?	tr	?	?	?	56
w/whole milk	1 oz	?	1	?	?	?	33
rice w/mixed fruit, junior	about 7.8 oz	?	1	?	?	?	186

Desserts

	Portion	Chol (mg)	Total Fat(g)	Satur'd Fat(g)	Mono Fat(g)	Poly Fat(g)	Total Calor
apple Betty							
strained	about 4.8 oz	?	0	?	?	?	97
junior	about 7.8 oz	?	0	?	?	?	153
caramel pudding							
strained	about 4.8 oz	?	1	?	?	?	104
junior	about 7 1/2 oz	?	2	?	?	?	167
cherry vanilla pudding							
strained	about 4.8 oz	?	tr	?	?	?	91
junior	about 7.8 oz	?	tr	?	?	?	152
chocolate custard pudding							
strained	about 4 1/2 oz	?	2	?	?	?	107
junior	about 7.8 oz	?	4	?	?	?	195
cottage cheese w/pineapple							
strained	about 4.8 oz	?	1	?	?	?	94
junior	about 7.8 oz	?	2	?	?	?	172
Dutch apple							
strained	about 4.8 oz	?	1	1	?	?	92
junior	about 7.8 oz	?	2	1	?	?	151

	Portion	Chol (mg)	Total Fat(g)	Satur'd Fat(g)	Mono Fat(g)	Poly Fat(g)	Total Calor
fruit dessert strained	about 4.8 oz	?	0	?	?	?	79
junior	about 7.8 oz	?	0	?	?	?	138
peach cobbler strained	about 4.8 oz	?	0	?	?	?	88
junior	about 7.8 oz	?	0	?	?	?	147
peach melba strained	about 4.8 oz	?	0	?	?	?	81
junior	about 7.8 oz	?	0	?	?	?	132
pineapple orange, strained	about 4½ oz	?	0	?	?	?	89
pineapple pudding strained	about 4½ oz	?	tr	?	?	?	104
junior	about 7.8 oz	?	1	?	?	?	192
tropical fruit, junior	about 7.8 oz	?	0	?	?	?	131
vanilla custard pudding strained	about 4½ oz	?	3	1	?	?	109
junior	about 7.8 oz	?	5	3	?	?	196

Dinners

REGULAR

	Portion	Chol (mg)	Total Fat(g)	Satur'd Fat(g)	Mono Fat(g)	Poly Fat(g)	Total Calor
beef & egg noodles strained	about 4½ oz	?	2	?	?	?	68
junior	about 7½ oz	?	4	?	?	?	122
beef & rice, toddler	about 6.2 oz	?	5	?	?	?	146
beef lasagna, toddler	about 6.2 oz	?	4	?	?	?	137
beef stew, toddler	about 6.2 oz	22	2	1	?	?	90
chicken & noodles strained	about 4½ oz	?	2	?	?	?	67
junior	about 7½ oz	?	3	?	?	?	109
chicken soup, cream of, strained	about 4½ oz	?	2	?	?	?	74
chicken soup, strained	about 4½ oz	?	2	?	?	?	64

	Portion	Chol (mg)	Total Fat(g)	Satur'd Fat(g)	Mono Fat(g)	Poly Fat(g)	Total Calor
chicken stew, toddler	about 6 oz	49	6	2	?	?	132
lamb & noodles, junior	about 1½ oz	?	5	?	?	?	138
macaroni & bacon, toddler	about 7½ oz	?	7	?	?	?	160
macaroni & cheese strained	about 4½ oz	?	3	?	?	?	76
junior	about 7½ oz	?	4	?	?	?	130
macaroni & ham, junior	about 7½ oz	?	3	?	?	?	127
macaroni, tomato, & beef strained	about 4½ oz	?	1	?	?	?	71
junior	about 7½ oz	?	2	?	?	?	125
mixed vegetables strained	about 4½ oz	?	tr	?	?	?	52
junior	about 7½ oz	?	tr	?	?	?	71
spaghetti, tomato, & meat junior	about 7½ oz	?	3	?	?	?	135
toddler	about 6.2 oz	?	2	?	?	?	133
split peas & ham, junior	about 7½ oz	?	3	?	?	?	152
turkey & rice strained	about 4½ oz	13	2	1	?	?	63
junior	about 7½ oz	?	3	1	?	?	104
vegetables & bacon strained	about 4½ oz	4	4	2	?	?	88
junior	about 7½ oz	?	8	3	?	?	150
vegetables & beef strained	about 4½ oz	?	3	?	?	?	67
junior	about 7½ oz	?	4	?	?	?	113
vegetables & chicken strained	about 4½ oz	?	1	?	?	?	55
junior	about 7½ oz	?	2	?	?	?	106

	Portion	Chol (mg)	Total Fat(g)	Satur'd Fat(g)	Mono Fat(g)	Poly Fat(g)	Total Calor
vegetables & ham							
strained	about 4½ oz	?	2	?	?	?	62
junior	about 7½ oz	?	4	?	?	?	110
toddler	about 6.2 oz	14	5	2	?	?	128
vegetables & lamb							
strained	about 4½ oz	?	3	?	?	?	67
junior	about 7½ oz	?	4	?	?	?	108
vegetables & liver							
strained	about 4½ oz	?	1	?	?	?	50
junior	about 7½ oz	?	1	?	?	?	93
vegetables & turkey							
strained	about 4½ oz	?	2	?	?	?	54
junior	about 7½ oz	?	3	?	?	?	101
toddler	about 6.2 oz	?	6	?	?	?	141
vegetables, dumplings, & beef							
strained	about 4½ oz	?	1	?	?	?	61
junior	about 7½ oz	?	2	?	?	?	103
vegetables, noodles, & chicken							
strained	about 4½ oz	?	3	?	?	?	81
junior	about 7½ oz	?	5	?	?	?	137
vegetables, noodles, & turkey							
strained	about 4½ oz	?	2	?	?	?	56
junior	about 7½ oz	?	3	?	?	?	110
HIGH IN MEAT OR CHEESE							
beef w/vegetables							
strained	about 4½ oz	?	5	?	?	?	96
junior	about 4½ oz	?	6	?	?	?	108
chicken w/vegetables							
strained	about 4½ oz	?	5	?	?	?	100

	Portion	Chol (mg)	Total Fat(g)	Satur'd Fat(g)	Mono Fat(g)	Poly Fat(g)	Total Calor
junior	about 4½ oz	?	7	?	?	?	117
cottage cheese w/pineapple, strained	about 4.8 oz	?	3	?	?	?	157
ham w/vegetables							
strained	about 4½ oz	?	4	2	?	?	97
junior	about 4½ oz	23	4	1	?	?	98
turkey w/vegetables							
strained	about 4½ oz	?	6	?	?	?	111
junior	about 4½ oz	?	6	?	?	?	115
veal w/vegetables							
strained	about 4½ oz	?	3	?	?	?	89
junior	about 4½ oz	?	4	?	?	?	93

Fruits

See also DESSERTS, above

all types		?	0 or tr	?	?	?	var

Fruit Juices

all types		?	0 or tr	?	?	?	var

Meats & Egg Yolks

	Portion	Chol (mg)	Total Fat(g)	Satur'd Fat(g)	Mono Fat(g)	Poly Fat(g)	Total Calor
beef							
strained	about 3½ oz	?	5	3	?	?	106
junior	about 3½ oz	?	5	3	?	?	105
beef w/beef heart, strained	about 3½ oz	?	4	2	?	?	93
chicken							
strained	about 3½ oz	?	8	2	?	?	128
junior	about 3½ oz	?	10	2	?	?	148
chicken sticks, junior	1 stick = .35 g	?	1	?	?	?	19
egg yolks, strained	about 3.3 oz	739	16	5	?	?	191
ham							
strained	about 3½ oz	?	6	2	?	?	110

	Portion	Chol (mg)	Total Fat(g)	Satur'd Fat(g)	Mono Fat(g)	Poly Fat(g)	Total Calor
junior	about 3½ oz	?	7	2	?	?	123
lamb							
strained	about 3½ oz	?	5	2	?	?	102
junior	about 3½ oz	?	5	3	?	?	111
liver, strained	about 3½ oz	182	4	1	?	?	100
meat sticks, junior	1 stick = .35 g	?	2	1	?	?	18
pork, strained	about 3½ oz	?	7	2	?	?	123
turkey							
strained	about 3½ oz	?	6	2	?	?	113
junior	about 3½ oz	?	7	2	?	?	128
turkey sticks, junior	1 stick = .35 g	?	1	?	?	?	18
veal							
strained	about 3½ oz	?	5	2	?	?	100
junior	about 3½ oz	?	5	2	?	?	109

Vegetables

	Portion	Chol (mg)	Total Fat(g)	Satur'd Fat(g)	Mono Fat(g)	Poly Fat(g)	Total Calor
beans, green							
plain							
strained	about 4½ oz	?	tr	?	?	?	32
junior	about 7.3 oz	?	tr	?	?	?	51
buttered							
strained	about 4½ oz	?	1	?	?	?	42
junior	about 7.3 oz	?	2	?	?	?	67
creamed, junior	about 7½ oz	?	1	?	?	?	68
beets, strained	about 4½ oz	?	tr	?	?	?	43
carrots							
plain							
strained	about 4½ oz	?	tr	?	?	?	34
junior	about 7½ oz	?	tr	?	?	?	67
buttered							
strained	about 4½ oz	?	1	?	?	?	46

	Portion	Chol (mg)	Total Fat(g)	Satur'd Fat(g)	Mono Fat(g)	Poly Fat(g)	Total Calor
junior	about 7½ oz	?	1	?	?	?	70
corn, creamed							
strained	about 4½ oz	?	1	?	?	?	73
junior	about 7½ oz	?	1	?	?	?	138
garden vegetables, strained	about 4½ oz	?	tr	?	?	?	48
mixed vegetables							
strained	about 4½ oz	?	1	?	?	?	52
junior	about 7½ oz	?	1	?	?	?	88
peas							
plain							
strained	about 4½ oz	?	tr	?	?	?	52
buttered							
strained	about 4½ oz	?	1	?	?	?	72
junior	about 7.3 oz	?	3	?	?	?	123
creamed, strained	about 4½ oz	?	2	?	?	?	68
spinach, creamed							
strained	about 4½ oz	?	2	?	?	?	48
junior	about 7½ oz	?	3	?	?	?	90
squash							
plain							
strained	about 4½ oz	?	tr	?	?	?	30
junior	about 7½ oz	?	tr	?	?	?	51
buttered							
strained	about 4½ oz	?	tr	?	?	?	37
junior	about 7½ oz	?	1	?	?	?	63
sweet potatoes							
plain							
strained	about 4.8 oz	?	tr	?	?	?	77
junior	about 7.8 oz	?	tr	?	?	?	133
buttered							
strained	about 4.8 oz	?	1	?	?	?	76

	Portion	Chol (mg)	Total Fat(g)	Satur'd Fat(g)	Mono Fat(g)	Poly Fat(g)	Total Calor
junior	about 7.8 oz	?	2	?	?	?	126

■ BRAND NAME

Beech-Nut
STAGE 1
Cereal
barley	½ oz dry	?	0	?	?	?	60
barley	½ oz dry + 2.4 fl oz formula	?	4	?	?	?	120
oatmeal	½ oz dry	?	2	?	?	?	70
oatmeal	½ oz dry + 2.4 fl oz formula	?	5	?	?	?	120
rice	2 oz dry	?	0	?	?	?	60
rice	2 oz dry + 2.4 fl oz formula	?	4	?	?	?	120

Fruit & Fruit Dishes
applesauce, golden delicious	4½ oz	?	0	?	?	?	70
bananas, chiquita	4½ oz	?	0	?	?	?	120
pears, bartlett	4½ oz	?	0	?	?	?	70

Fruit Juices
| apple | 4 fl oz | ? | 0 | ? | ? | ? | 60 |
| pear | 4 fl oz | 0 | ? | ? | ? | 70 | |

Meat
beef	3½ oz	?	8	?	?	?	120
chicken	3½ oz	?	6	?	?	?	110
turkey	3½ oz	?	7	?	?	?	120
veal	3½ oz	?	7	?	?	?	120

Vegetables
green beans	4½ oz	?	0	?	?	?	40
peas, tender sweet	4½ oz	?	0	?	?	?	70
squash, butternut	4½ oz	?	0	?	?	?	60
sweet potatoes	4½ oz	?	0	?	?	?	90

STAGE 2
Cereals
| mixed | ½ oz dry | ? | 0 | ? | ? | ? | 60 |
| mixed | ½ oz dry + 2.4 fl oz formula | ? | 4 | ? | ? | ? | 120 |

	Portion	Chol (mg)	Total Fat(g)	Satur'd Fat(g)	Mono Fat(g)	Poly Fat(g)	Total Calor
w/applesauce & bananas	4½ oz	?	0	?	?	?	90
oatmeal							
w/applesauce & bananas	4½ oz	?	1	?	?	?	90
w/bananas	½ oz dry	?	1	?	?	?	70
w/bananas	½ oz dry + 2.4 fl oz formula	?	4	?	?	?	120
rice							
w/applesauce & bananas	4½ oz	?	0	?	?	?	90
w/bananas	½ oz dry	?	0	?	?	?	70
w/bananas	½ oz dry + 2.4 fl oz formula	?	4	?	?	?	120
Desserts							
applesauce & apricots	4½ oz	?	0	?	?	?	80
applesauce & bananas	4½ oz	?	0	?	?	?	80
apples, pears, & bananas	4½ oz	?	0	?	?	?	90
bananas w/pears & applesauce	4½ oz	?	0	?	?	?	100
bartlett pears & pineapple	4½ oz	?	0	?	?	?	90
fruit dessert	4½ oz	?	0	?	?	?	80
Juice							
Juice Plus	4 fl oz	?	0	?	?	?	90
Main Courses							
beef & egg noodles	4½ oz	?	4	?	?	?	90
beef dinner supreme	4½ oz	?	7	?	?	?	130
chicken & rice	4½ oz	?	3	?	?	?	80
macaroni & beef	4½ oz	?	4	?	?	?	100
turkey dinner supreme	4½ oz	?	6	?	?	?	110
turkey rice	4½ oz	?	2	?	?	?	70
vegetable beef	4½ oz	?	4	?	?	?	80
vegetable chicken	4½ oz	?	3	?	?	?	90
vegetable ham	4½ oz	?	3	?	?	?	90
Vegetables							
creamed corn	4½ oz	?	0	?	?	?	100
garden vegetables	4½ oz	?	0	?	?	?	60
mixed vegetables	4½ oz	?	0	?	?	?	60
peas & carrots	4½ oz	?	0	?	?	?	50

	Portion	Chol (mg)	Total Fat(g)	Satur'd Fat(g)	Mono Fat(g)	Poly Fat(g)	Total Calor
STAGE 3							
FRUITS							
applesauce	6 oz	?	0	?	?	?	90
apples & bananas	6 oz	?	0	?	?	?	100
apricots w/pears & apples	6 oz	?	0	?	?	?	120
bananas w/pears & apples	6 oz	?	0	?	?	?	130
bartlett pears	7½ oz	?	0	?	?	?	110
fruit dessert	6 oz	?	0	?	?	?	120
peaches	6	?	0	?	?	?	90
Main Courses & Dinners							
beef & egg noodles	6 oz	?	5	?	?	?	120
chicken noodles	6 oz	?	3	?	?	?	100
macaroni & beef	6 oz	?	6	?	?	?	130
spaghetti & beef	6 oz	?	6	?	?	?	130
turkey rice	6 oz	?	3	?	?	?	100
vegetable beef	6 oz	?	5	?	?	?	120
vegetable chicken	6 oz	?	4	?	?	?	110
Desserts							
cottage cheese w/pineapple	6 oz	?	2	?	?	?	170
mixed fruit yogurt	6 oz	?	2	?	?	?	160
vanilla custard	6 oz	?	5	?	?	?	180
Juice							
orange	4 oz	?	0	?	?	?	70
Special Harvest							
single foods							
oatmeal	½ oz dry	?	1	?	?	?	70
oatmeal	½ oz dry + 2.4 oz formula	?	4	?	?	?	110
applesauce	4.5 oz	?	0	?	?	?	70
bananas	4.5 oz	?	0	?	?	?	100
peaches	4.5 oz	?	0	?	?	?	70
carrots	4.5 oz	?	0	?	?	?	40
green beans	4.25 oz	?	0	?	?	?	35
peas	4.5 oz	?	?	?	?	?	60
squash	4.5 oz	?	0	?	?	?	50
sweet potatoes	4.5 oz	?	0	?	?	?	90
combination foods							
mixed grain cereal	½ oz dry	?	1	?	?	?	70
mixed grain cereal	½ oz dry + 2.4 oz formula	?	4	?	?	?	110
apples & apricots	4.5 oz	?	0	?	?	?	60

	Portion	Chol (mg)	Total Fat (g)	Satur'd Fat (g)	Mono Fat (g)	Poly Fat (g)	Total Calor
apples & bananas	4.5 oz	?	0	?	?	?	60
peaches & bananas	4.5 oz	?	0	?	?	?	70
chicken rice dinner	4.5 oz	?	3	?	?	?	80
spaghetti beef dinner	4.5 oz	?	3	?	?	?	90
vegetable beef dinner	4.5 oz	?	4	?	?	?	110
vegetable chicken dinner	4.5 oz	?	3	?	?	?	90
vegetable turkey dinner	4.5 oz	?	2	?	?	?	70
mixed fruit juice	4.2 oz	?	0	?	?	?	60
Vegetables							
carrots	6 oz	?	0	?	?	?	60
green beans	5¾ oz	?	0	?	?	?	60
sweet potatoes	6 oz	?	0	?	?	?	110
UNSTAGED							
Juices							
apple	4 fl oz	?	0	?	?	?	60
apple banana	4.2 fl oz	?	0	?	?	?	60
apple cherry	4.2 fl oz	?	0	?	?	?	50
apple grape	4.2 fl oz	?	0	?	?	?	60
mixed fruit	4.2 fl oz	?	0	?	?	?	60
orange	4.2 fl oz	?	0	?	?	?	60
pear	4 fl oz	?	0	?	?	?	60
tropical blend	4 fl oz	?	0	?	?	?	70
TABLE TIME							
Main Courses							
beef stew	6 oz	?	4	?	?	?	140
pasta squares in meat sauce	6 oz	?	4	?	?	?	140
vegetable stew w/chicken	6 oz	?	8	?	?	?	190
Soups							
hearty chicken w/stars	6 oz	?	9	?	?	?	180
hearty vegetable	6 oz	?	0	?	?	?	70
Gerber							
BAKED GOODS							
animal crackers	4	?	2	?	?	?	50
animal shaped cookies	2	tr	2	?	?	?	60
arrowroot cookies	2	tr	2	?	?	?	50
pretzels	2	0	0	?	?	?	45
zwieback toast	2	tr	2	?	?	?	70
CHUNKY PRODUCTS							
homestyle noodles & beef	6 oz	14	6	?	?	?	150
macaroni alphabets w/beef & tomato sauce	6¼ oz	13	4	?	?	?	140

	Portion	Chol (mg)	Total Fat (g)	Satur'd Fat (g)	Mono Fat (g)	Poly Fat (g)	Total Calor
noodles & chicken w/carrots & peas	6 oz	20	3	?	?	?	110
saucy rice w/chicken	6 oz	18	3	?	?	?	120
spaghetti-tomato sauce & beef	6¼ oz	10	4	?	?	?	150
vegetables & beef	6¼ oz	10	5	?	?	?	130
vegetables & chicken	6¼ oz	16	5	?	?	?	140
vegetables & ham	6¼ oz	10	5	?	?	?	130
vegetables & turkey	6¼ oz	20	3	?	?	?	110

READY-TO-SERVE DRY CEREALS

	Portion	Chol (mg)	Total Fat (g)	Satur'd Fat (g)	Mono Fat (g)	Poly Fat (g)	Total Calor
barley	½ oz dry	?	1	?	?	?	60
barley	½ oz dry + 2.4 fl oz milk	?	4	?	?	?	110
high protein	½ oz dry	?	1	?	?	?	50
high protein	½ oz dry + 2.4 fl oz milk	?	4	?	?	?	100
mixed	½ oz dry	?	1	?	?	?	60
mixed	½ oz dry + 2.4 fl oz milk	?	4	?	?	?	100
w/banana	½ oz dry	?	1	?	?	?	60
w/banana	½ oz dry + 2.4 fl oz milk	?	4	?	?	?	100
oatmeal	½ oz dry	?	1	?	?	?	60
oatmeal	½ oz dry + 2.4 fl oz milk	?	4	?	?	?	100
w/banana	½ oz dry	?	1	?	?	?	60
w/banana	½ oz dry + 2.4 fl oz milk	?	4	?	?	?	100
rice	/2 oz dry	?	1	?	?	?	60
rice	½ oz dry + 2.4 fl oz milk	?	4	?	?	?	100
w/banana	½ oz dry	?	1	?	?	?	60
w/banana	½ oz dry + 2.4 fl oz milk	?	4	?	?	?	100

FIRST FOODS

Fruit

	Portion	Chol (mg)	Total Fat (g)	Satur'd Fat (g)	Mono Fat (g)	Poly Fat (g)	Total Calor
applesauce	2½ oz	?	0	?	?	?	35
bananas	2½ oz	?	0	?	?	?	70
peaches	2½ oz	?	0	?	?	?	40
pears	2½ oz	?	0	?	?	?	45
prunes	2½ oz	?	0	?	?	?	70

	Portion	Chol (mg)	Total Fat(g)	Satur'd Fat(g)	Mono Fat(g)	Poly Fat(g)	Total Calor
SECOND FOODS							
Cereals w/Fruit							
mixed w/applesauce & bananas	4 oz	?	1	?	?	?	90
oatmeal w/applesauce & bananas	4 oz	?	1	?	?	?	90
rice w/applesauce & bananas	4 oz	?	0	?	?	?	90
Desserts							
banana apple	4 oz	0	0	?	?	?	80
cherry vanilla pudding	4 oz	3	0	?	?	?	80
Dutch apple	4 oz	4	0	?	?	?	80
fruit	4 oz	0	0	?	?	?	90
Hawaiian delight	4 oz	2	0	?	?	?	100
vanilla custard pudding	4 oz	14	1	?	?	?	100
Dinners, Regular							
beef egg noodle	4 oz	6	3	?	?	?	80
chicken noodle	4 oz	10	2	?	?	?	70
macaroni cheese	4 oz	3	2	?	?	?	70
macaroni tomato beef	4 oz	3	2	?	?	?	70
turkey rice	4 oz	13	3	?	?	?	70
vegetable beef	4 oz	4	3	?	?	?	70
vegetable chicken	4 oz	6	2	?	?	?	70
vegetable ham	4 oz	4	3	?	?	?	70
vegetable turkey	4 oz	11	2	?	?	?	60
Dinners, Lean Meat							
beef w/vegetables	4 oz	10	3	?	?	?	80
chicken w/vegetables	4 oz	16	2	?	?	?	70
ham w/vegetables	4 oz	16	2	?	?	?	100
turkey w/vegetables	4 oz	15	3	?	?	?	80
Fruits & Tropical Fruits							
apple blueberry	4 oz	?	1	?	?	?	50
applesauce	4 oz	?	0	?	?	?	50
applesauce apricot	4 oz	?	1	?	?	?	50
apricots w/tapioca	4 oz	?	1	?	?	?	70
bananas w/pineapple & tapioca	4 oz	?	1	?	?	?	60
bananas w/tapioca	4 oz	?	0	?	?	?	80
mango w/tapioca	4 oz	?	0	?	?	?	80
papaya w/tapioca	4 oz	?	0	?	?	?	70
peaches	4 oz	?	0	?	?	?	80
peaches mango w/tapioca	4 oz	?	0	?	?	?	80
pears	4 oz	?	0	?	?	?	60

	Portion	Chol (mg)	Total Fat(g)	Satur'd Fat(g)	Mono Fat(g)	Poly Fat(g)	Total Calor
pear pineapple	4 oz	?	0	?	?	?	80
tropical fruits w/tapioca	4 oz	?	0	?	?	?	70
Meats & Egg Yolks							
beef	2½ oz	21	4	?	?	?	80
chicken	2½ oz	44	6	?	?	?	90
egg yolks	2¼ oz	398	11	?	?	?	130
ham	2½ oz	17	6	?	?	?	90
lamb	2½ oz	27	4	?	?	?	80
turkey	2½ oz	42	5	?	?	?	80
veal	2½ oz	18	4	?	?	?	70
Strained Vegetables							
beets	4 oz	?	0	?	?	?	45
carrots	4 oz	?	0	?	?	?	30
creamed corn	4 oz	?	1	?	?	?	80
creamed spinach	4 oz	?	1	?	?	?	50
garden vegetables	4 oz	?	1	?	?	?	50
green beans	4 oz	?	0	?	?	?	35
mixed vegetables	4 oz	?	1	?	?	?	50
peas	4 oz	?	1	?	?	?	60
squash	4 oz	?	0	?	?	?	30
sweet potatoes	4 oz	?	0	?	?	?	70
Vegetables							
carrots	2½ oz	?	0	?	?	?	30
green beans	2½ oz	?	0	?	?	?	25
peas	2½ oz	?	0	?	?	?	30
squash	2½ oz	?	0	?	?	?	25
sweet potatoes	2½ oz	?	0	?	?	?	50
THIRD FOODS							
Cereals w/Fruit							
mixed w/applesauce & bananas	6 oz	?	1	?	?	?	140
oatmeal w/applesauce & bananas	6 oz	?	1	?	?	?	140
rice w/mixed fruit	6 oz	?	0	?	?	?	130
Desserts							
Dutch apple	6 oz	7	2	?	?	?	130
fruit	6 oz	0	0	?	?	?	120
Hawaiian delight	6 oz	3	1	?	?	?	150
peach cobbler	6 oz	0	0	?	?	?	120
vanilla custard pudding	6 oz	24	2	?	?	?	150
Dinners							
beef egg noodle	6 oz	10	4	?	?	?	110
chicken noodle	6 oz	14	3	?	?	?	100
macaroni tomato beef	6 oz	6	2	?	?	?	110

	Portion	Chol (mg)	Total Fat(g)	Satur'd Fat(g)	Mono Fat(g)	Poly Fat(g)	Total Calor
spaghetti tomato sauce beef	6 oz	7	3	?	?	?	120
turkey rice	6 oz	19	3	?	?	?	100
vegetable bacon	6 oz	6	6	?	?	?	130
vegetable beef	6 oz	7	4	?	?	?	120
vegetable chicken	6 oz	13	3	?	?	?	100
vegetable ham	6 oz	7	4	?	?	?	110
vegetable turkey	6 oz	20	3	?	?	?	100
Dinners Lean in Meat							
beef w/vegetables	4 oz	12	3	?	?	?	90
chicken w/vegetables	4 oz	19	2	?	?	?	70
ham w/vegetables	4 oz	11	4	?	?	?	100
turkey w/vegetables	4 oz	16	3	?	?	?	90
Fruits							
applesauce	6 oz	?	1	?	?	?	90
apricots w/tapioca	6 oz	?	0	?	?	?	110
bananas w/pineapple & tapioca	6 oz	?	0	?	?	?	130
bananas w/tapioca	6 oz	?	0	?	?	?	80
peaches	6 oz	?	0	?	?	?	110
pears	6 oz	?	1	?	?	?	100
Meats							
beef	2½ oz	20	4	?	?	?	80
chicken	2½ oz	42	6	?	?	?	90
ham	2½ oz	21	5	?	?	?	90
turkey	2½ oz	38	6	?	?	?	90
veal	2½ oz	19	4	?	?	?	80
Vegetables							
broccoli carrots cheese	6 oz	?	2	?	?	?	80
carrots	6 oz	?	0	?	?	?	45
creamed green beans	6 oz	?	1	?	?	?	80
mixed vegetables	6 oz	?	1	?	?	?	70
peas	6 oz	?	1	?	?	?	90
squash	6 oz	?	1	?	?	?	60
sweet potatoes	6 oz	?	0	?	?	?	100
TODDLER FOODS							
Juice w/Lowfat Yogurt							
apple	4 oz	?	1	?	?	?	100
banana	4 oz	?	1	?	?	?	110
mixed fruit	4 oz	?	1	?	?	?	100
Juices, 8 oz							
apple	4 oz	?	0	?	?	?	60
apple cherry	4 oz	?	0	?	?	?	60
apple grape	4 oz	?	0	?	?	?	60
grape	4 oz	?	0	?	?	?	80

	Portion	Chol (mg)	Total Fat(g)	Satur'd Fat(g)	Mono Fat(g)	Poly Fat(g)	Total Calor
Cereals							
Toasted Oat Rings	½ oz dry	?	1	?	?	?	60
Toasted Oat Rings	½ oz dry + 2.7 fl oz milk	?	4	?	?	?	110
Juices							
all	4 oz	?	0	0	?	?	60
Meat & Poultry Sticks							
chicken	2½ oz	65	8	?	?	?	120
meat	2½ oz	33	7	?	?	?	110
turkey	2½ oz	61	9	?	?	?	120

❏ **JAMS & JELLIES** *See* **FRUIT SPREADS**

❏ **JUICE, FROZEN** *See* **DESSERTS, FROZEN**

❏ **JUICES & JUICE DRINKS** *See* **BEVERAGES**

❏ **LAMB, VEAL, & MISCELLANEOUS MEATS**

Lamb, Cooked

LAMB CHOPS (3/LB W/BONE)

Lean & Fat							
arm, braised	2.2 oz	77	15	7	?	?	220
loin, broiled	2.8 oz	78	16	7	?	?	235
rib	3½ oz	70	37	?	?	?	423
arm, braised	1.7 oz	59	7	3	?	?	135
loin, broiled	2.3 oz	60	6	3	?	?	140
Lean Only							
LEG OF LAMB, ROASTED							
lean & fat	3 oz	78	13	6	?	?	205
lean only	2.6 oz	65	6	2	?	?	140
RIB, ROASTED							
lean & fat	3 oz	77	26	12	?	?	315
lean only	2 oz	50	7	3	?	?	130

Veal, Cooked

| arm steak, lean & fat | 3½ oz | 90 | 19 | ? | ? | ? | 298 |

	Portion	Chol (mg)	Total Fat(g)	Satur'd Fat(g)	Mono Fat(g)	Poly Fat(g)	Total Calor
blade, lean & fat	3½ oz	90	17	?	?	?	276
breast, stewed w/gravy	2.6 oz	?	19	?	?	?	256
cutlet, medium fat, bone removed							
braised or broiled	3 oz	109	9	4	?	?	185
breaded	3½ oz	?	15	?	?	?	319
flank, medium fat, stewed	3½ oz	90	32	?	?	?	390
foreshank, medium fat, stewed	3½ oz	90	10	?	?	?	216
loin chop, lean & fat	3½ oz	90	36	?	?	?	421
plate, medium fat, stewed	3½ oz	90	21	?	?	?	303
rib, roasted	3 oz	109	14	6	?	?	230

Other Meats

	Portion	Chol (mg)	Total Fat(g)	Satur'd Fat(g)	Mono Fat(g)	Poly Fat(g)	Total Calor
frog legs							
raw	4 large	50	tr	?	?	?	73
flour coated & fried	6 large	?	29	?	?	?	418
goat, raw	3½ oz	?	9	?	?	?	165
hare, raw	3½ oz	?	5	?	?	?	135
rabbit, stewed	3½ oz	?	10	?	?	?	216
venison, roasted	3½ oz	?	2	?	?	?	146

❑ LEGUMES & LEGUME PRODUCTS

Beans

	Portion	Chol (mg)	Total Fat(g)	Satur'd Fat(g)	Mono Fat(g)	Poly Fat(g)	Total Calor
adzuki							
boiled	½ c	0	tr	?	?	?	147
canned, sweetened	½ c	0	tr	?	?	?	351
yokan (sugar & bean confection)	1½ oz	0	tr	tr	?	?	36
black, boiled	½ c	0	tr	tr	?	?	113
black turtle soup							
boiled	1 c	0	1	tr	?	?	241
canned	½ c	0	tr	tr	?	?	109
broad							
raw	1 bean-0.3 oz	0	tr	tr	?	?	6
raw	1 c	0	1	tr	?	?	79
canned (solids & liquids)	½ c	0	tr	tr	?	?	91
dry, boiled	½ c	0	tr	tr	?	?	93
fresh, boiled, drained	3½ oz	0	1	tr	?	?	56
cannellini See KIDNEY, below							
cranberry							
boiled	½ c	0	tr	tr	?	?	120

	Portion	Chol (mg)	Total Fat (g)	Satur'd Fat (g)	Mono Fat (g)	Poly Fat (g)	Total Calor
canned, solids & liquids	½ c	0	tr	tr	?	?	108
fava *See* BROAD, above							
French, boiled	½ c	0	1	tr	?	?	111
garbanzo *See* CHICKPEAS, under PEAS & LENTILS, below							
great northern							
boiled	½ c	0	tr	tr	?	?	104
canned, solids & liquids	½ c	0	1	tr	?	?	150
green gram *See* MUNG, below							
kidney							
all types							
boiled	½ c	0	tr	tr	?	?	112
canned, solids & liquids	½ c	0	tr	tr	?	?	104
California red, boiled	½ c	0	tr	tr	?	?	109
red							
boiled	½ c	0	tr	tr	?	?	112
canned (solids & liquid)	½ c	0	tr	tr	?	?	108
royal red, boiled	½ c	0	tr	tr	?	?	108
lima							
regular							
fresh, boiled, drained	½ c	0	tr	tr	?	?	104
frozen, boiled, drained	10 oz pkg	0	1	tr	?	?	312
frozen, boiled, drained	½ c	0	tr	tr	?	?	85
baby							
fresh, boiled	½ c	0	tr	tr	?	?	115
frozen, boiled, drained	10 oz pkg	0	1	tr	?	?	326
frozen, boiled, drained	½ c	0	tr	tr	?	?	94
large							
canned (solids & liquid)	½ c	0	tr	tr	?	?	95
dry, boiled	½ c	0	tr	tr	?	?	108
long rice *See* MUNG, below							
miso *See* SOYBEANS & SOYBEAN PRODUCTS							
mung							
boiled	½ c	0	tr	tr	?	?	107
mature seeds, sprouted							
raw	½ c	0	tr	tr	?	?	16
raw	12 oz pkg	0	1	tr	?	?	102
boiled, drained	½ c	0	tr	tr	?	?	13
canned, drained	½ c	0	tr	tr	?	?	8
stir-fried	½ c	0	tr	tr	?	?	31
long rice, dehydrated, prepared from mung bean starch	½ c	0	tr	tr	?	?	246
natto *See* SOYBEANS & SOYBEAN PRODUCTS							
navy, canned, solids & liquids	½ c	0	1	tr	?	?	148
okara *See* TOFU, OKARA, under SOYBEANS & SOYBEAN PRODUCTS							
pink, boiled	½ c	0	tr	tr	?	?	125

	Portion	Chol (mg)	Total Fat(g)	Satur'd Fat(g)	Mono Fat(g)	Poly Fat(g)	Total Calor
pinto							
boiled	½ c	0	tr	tr	?	?	117
canned, solids & liquids	½ c	0	tr	tr	?	?	93
frozen, boiled, drained	10 oz pkg	0	1	tr	?	?	460
Roman *See* CRANBERRY, above							
shellie *See* VEGETABLES, PLAIN & PREPARED							
snap *See* VEGETABLES, PLAIN & PREPARED							
soybeans *See* SOYBEANS & SOYBEAN PRODUCTS							
white							
boiled	½ c	0	tr	tr	?	?	125
canned, solids & liquids	½ c	0	tr	tr	?	?	153
small, boiled	½ c	0	1	tr	?	?	127
winged							
raw, fresh	1 pod = 0.6 oz	0	tr	tr	?	?	8
dry, boiled	½ c	0	5	1	?	?	126
fresh, boiled, drained	½ c	0	tr	tr	?	?	12
yellow, boiled	½ c	0	1	tr	?	?	126
yokan *See* adzuki, above							

Peas & Lentils

	Portion	Chol (mg)	Total Fat(g)	Satur'd Fat(g)	Mono Fat(g)	Poly Fat(g)	Total Calor
Bengal gram *See* chickpeas, below							
black-eyed *See* COWPEAS, COMMON, below							
chickpeas							
boiled	½ c	0	2	tr	?	?	134
canned, solids & liquids	½ c	0	1	tr	?	?	143
cowpeas, catjang, boiled	½ c	0	1	tr	?	?	100
cowpeas, common							
boiled	½ c	0	tr	tr	?	?	100
canned, plain, solids & liquids	½ c	0	1	tr	?	?	92
frozen, boiled, drained	½ c	0	1	tr	?	?	112
leafy tips							
raw	1 c	0	tr	tr	?	?	10
boiled, drained	½ c	0	tr	tr	?	?	6
young pods w/seeds							
raw	1 pod	0	tr	tr	?	?	5
boiled, drained	½ c	0	tr	tr	?	?	16
crowder peas *See* COWPEAS, COMMON, above							
golden gram *See* CHICKPEAS, above							
lentils							
boiled	½ c	0	tr	tr	?	?	115
sprouted							
raw	½ c	0	tr	tr	?	?	40
stir-fried	3½ oz	0	tr	tr	?	?	101
southern peas *See* COWPEAS, COMMON, above							
split peas, boiled	½ c	0	tr	tr	?	?	116

	Portion	Chol (mg)	Total Fat(g)	Satur'd Fat(g)	Mono Fat(g)	Poly Fat(g)	Total Calor
Prepared Bean Dishes							
baked beans							
canned							
plain or vegetarian	½ c	0	1	tr	?	?	118
w/beef	½ c	29	5	2	?	?	161
w/franks	½ c	8	8	3	?	?	182
w/pork	½ c	9	2	1	?	?	133
w/pork & tomato sauce	½ c	9	1	tr	?	?	123
homemade	½ c	6	7	2	?	?	190
chili w/beans, canned	½ c	22	7	3	?	?	144
falafel	0.6 oz	0	3	tr	?	?	57
falafel	1.8 oz	0	9	1	?	?	170
hummus	1 c	0	21	3	?	?	420
refried beans, canned	½ c	?	1	1	?	?	134
▪ BRAND NAME							
Arrowhead Mills							
adzuki beans	2 oz	0	1	?	?	?	190
anasazi beans	2 oz	0	1	?	?	?	200
black turtle beans	2 oz	0	1	?	?	?	190
chickpeas	2 oz	0	3	?	?	?	200
kidney beans	2 oz	0	1	?	?	?	190
lentils							
green	2 oz	0	1	?	?	?	190
red	2 oz	0	1	?	?	?	195
mung beans							
dry, raw	2 oz	0	?	?	?	?	?
sprouted	1 c	0	0	0	?	?	50
pinto beans	2 oz	0	1	?	?	?	200
split peas, green	2 oz	0	1	?	?	?	200
B & M							
brick oven baked beans							
barbeque	8 oz	5	6	?	?	?	260
honey	8 oz	0	2	?	?	?	240
hot 'n spicy	8 oz	3	3	1	?	1	240
maple	8 oz	<5	2	1	?	1	240
small red	8 oz	5	5	2	?	1	223
tomato	8 oz	1	3	1	?	1	230
vegetarian	8 oz	0	3	?	?	?	230
vegetarian, 50% less sodium	8 oz	0	3	?	?	?	230
Campbell's							
Barbecue Beans	7⅞ oz	?	4	?	?	?	210
Home Style Beans	8 oz	?	4	?	?	?	220
hot chili beans	7¾ oz	?	4	?	?	?	180
Old Fashioned Beans in Molasses & Brown Sugar	8 oz	?	3	?	?	?	230
Pork & Beans in Tomato Sauce	8 oz	?	3	?	?	?	200

	Portion	Chol (mg)	Total Fat(g)	Satur'd Fat(g)	Mono Fat(g)	Poly Fat(g)	Total Calor
vegetarian beans	7¾ oz	?	1	?	?	?	170
Friends							
maple baked beans	8 oz	<5	2	1	?	1	240
red kidney beans	8 oz	4	4	2	?	1	340
small pea beans	8 oz	6	4	3	?	1	360
Health Valley							
BEANS							
fat-free baked beans							
regular or no salt	7.5 oz	0	<1	?	?	?	190
w/miso	7.5 oz	0	<1	?	?	?	180
fat-free chilis							
mild vegetarian w/black beans	5 oz	0	<1	?	?	?	290
spicy vegetarian w/black beans	5 oz	0	<1	?	?	?	290
mild vegetarian w/3 beans	5 oz	0	<1	?	?	?	180
Old El Paso							
garbanzo beans	½ c	?	<1	?	?	?	190
mexe-beans	½ c	0	1	0	0	?	163
pinto beans	½ c	0	0	0	0	?	100
refried beans	¼ c	1	<1	?	?	?	55
spicy refried beans	¼ c	1	1	0	0	?	35
vegetarian refried beans	¼ c	0	1	?	?	?	70
Progresso							
red kidney beans	½ c	0	<1	?	?	?	100
cannellini beans	½ c	0	<1	?	?	?	80
chick beans	½ c	0	1	?	?	?	110
pinto beans	½ c	0	<1	?	?	?	110
black beans	½ c	0	1	?	?	?	90
Van Camp's							
baked beans	1 c	?	2	?	?	?	260
baked beans, deluxe	1 c	?	4	?	?	?	320
beanie weenie	1 c	15	15	5	6	2	326
brown sugar beans	1 c	?	5	?	?	?	290
butter beans	1 c	?	1	?	?	?	162
chili w/beans	1 c	?	23	?	?	?	352
chili w/out beans	1 c	?	34	?	?	?	412
dark red kidney beans	1 c	?	1	?	?	?	182
light red kidney beans	1 c	?	1	?	?	?	184
Mexican style chili beans	1 c	?	2	?	?	?	210
New Orleans style red kidney beans	1 c	?	1	?	?	?	178
pork & beans	1 c	0	2	1	1	1	216
red beans	1 c	?	1	?	?	?	194
vegetarian style beans	1 c	?	1	?	?	?	206
Wolf							
chili w/beans	<1 c	?	22	?	?	?	345
chili w/out beans							
regular	1 c	?	27	?	?	?	387
extra spicy	scant c	?	25	?	?	?	363

	Portion	Chol (mg)	Total Fat(g)	Satur'd Fat(g)	Mono Fat(g)	Poly Fat(g)	Total Calor

❑ **LUNCHEON MEATS** *See* PROCESSED
MEAT & POULTRY PRODUCTS

❑ **MAIN COURSES** *See* ENTREES & MAIN
COURSES, CANNED & BOXED; ENTREES &
MAIN COURSES, FROZEN

❑ **MARGARINES** *See* BUTTER & MARGARINE
SPREADS

❑ **MARMALADES** *See* FRUIT SPREADS

❑ **MAYONNAISE** *See* SALAD DRESSINGS,
MAYONNAISE, VINEGAR, & DIPS

❑ **MEAT** *See* BEEF, FRESH & CURED;
LAMB, VEAL, & MISCELLANEOUS MEATS;
PORK, FRESH & CURED; PROCESSED
MEAT & POULTRY PRODUCTS

❑ **MEAT PRODUCTS, SIMULATED** *See*
LEGUMES & LEGUME PRODUCTS; NUTS
& NUT-BASED BUTTERS, FLOURS, MEALS,
MILKS, PASTES, & POWDERS; SOYBEANS
& SOYBEAN PRODUCTS

❑ **MEAT SPREADS** *See* PROCESSED MEAT
& POULTRY PRODUCTS

❑ **MILK, MILK SUBSTITUTES, & MILK
PRODUCTS: CREAM, SOUR CREAM,
CREAM SUBSTITUTES, MILK, MILK
SUBSTITUTES, WHEY, & YOGURT**
See also CHEESE & CHEESE FOODS
See also DESSERT SAUCES, SYRUPS, & TOPPINGS
See also FLAVORED MILK BEVERAGES under
Beverages

	Portion	Chol (mg)	Total Fat(g)	Satur'd Fat(g)	Mono Fat(g)	Poly Fat(g)	Total Calor
Cream & Sour Cream							
CREAM							
half & half	1 T	6	2	1	?	?	20
light	1 T	10	3	2	?	?	29
medium, 25% fat	1 T	13	4	2	?	?	37
whipping							
light	1 T	17	5	3	?	?	44
heavy	1 oz	21	6	3	?	?	52
SOUR CREAM							
half & half, cultured	1 T	6	2	1	?	?	20
Cream & Sour Cream Substitutes							
coffee whitener, nondairy							
liquid, frozen	½ fl oz	0	2	tr	(.29)	?	20
liquid, frozen, containing lauric acid oil & sodium caseinate	½ fl oz	0	2	1	?	?	20
powdered, containing lauric acid oil & sodium caseinate	1 t	0	1	1	?	?	11
imitation sour cream, nondairy, cultured, containing lauric acid oil & sodium caseinate	1 oz	0	6	5	?	?	59
sour dressing, nonbutterfat, cultured (made by combining oils or fats other than milk fat w/milk solids)	1 T	1	2	2	?	?	21
Cow's Milk							
FRESH							
whole							
3.7% fat, pasteurized or raw	1 c	35	9	6	?	?	157
low-sodium	1 c	33	8	5	?	?	149
low-fat							
2% fat	1 c	18	5	3	?	?	121
2% fat, nonfat milk solids added	1 c	18	5	3	?	?	125
2% fat, protein-fortified	1 c	19	5	3	?	?	137
1% fat	1 c	10	2	3	?	?	102
1% fat, nonfat milk solids added	1 c	10	2	1	?	?	104
1% fat, protein-fortified	1 c	10	3	2	?	?	119

	Portion	Chol (mg)	Total Fat(g)	Satur'd Fat(g)	Mono Fat(g)	Poly Fat(g)	Total Calor
skim	1 c	4	tr	tr	?	?	86
skim, nonfat milk solids added	1 c	5	1	tr	?	?	90
skim, protein-fortified	1 c	5	1	tr	?	?	100
buttermilk, cultured	1 c	9	2	1	?	?	99

CONDENSED & EVAPORATED

	Portion	Chol (mg)	Total Fat(g)	Satur'd Fat(g)	Mono Fat(g)	Poly Fat(g)	Total Calor
condensed, sweetened, canned	1 oz	13	3	2	?	?	123
evaporated, canned							
whole	1 oz	9	2	1	?	?	42
skim	1 fl oz	1	tr	tr	?	?	25

DRY

	Portion	Chol (mg)	Total Fat(g)	Satur'd Fat(g)	Mono Fat(g)	Poly Fat(g)	Total Calor
whole	¼ c	31	9	5	?	?	159
nonfat							
regular	¼ c	6	tr	tr	?	?	109
calcium-reduced	1 oz	1	tr	tr	?	?	100
instant	3.2 oz	17	1	tr	?	?	326
instant	1 c	12	tr	tr	?	?	244
buttermilk, sweet cream	1 T	5	tr	tr	?	?	25
buttermilk, sweet cream	1 c	83	7	4	?	?	464

Milk of Other Animals

	Portion	Chol (mg)	Total Fat(g)	Satur'd Fat(g)	Mono Fat(g)	Poly Fat(g)	Total Calor
goat	1 c	28	10	7	?	?	168
human	1 oz	4	1	1	?	?	21

Milk Substitutes

	Portion	Chol (mg)	Total Fat(g)	Satur'd Fat(g)	Mono Fat(g)	Poly Fat(g)	Total Calor
filled (made by blending hydrogenated vegetable oils w/milk solids)	1 c	4	8	2	?	?	154
filled, w/lauric acid oil (made by combining milk solids w/fats or oils other than milk fat)	1 c	4	8	8	?	?	153
imitation, containing blend of hydrogenated vegetable oils	1 c	tr	8	2	?	?	150
imitation, containing lauric acid	1 c	tr	8	7	?	?	150

Whey

	Portion	Chol (mg)	Total Fat(g)	Satur'd Fat(g)	Mono Fat(g)	Poly Fat(g)	Total Calor
acid							
dry	1 T	?	tr	tr	?	?	10
fluid	1 c	?	tr	tr	?	?	59
sweet							
dry	1 T	tr	tr	tr	?	?	26
fluid	1 c	5	1	1	?	?	66

	Portion	Chol (mg)	Total Fat(g)	Satur'd Fat(g)	Mono Fat(g)	Poly Fat(g)	Total Calor
Yogurt							
plain							
8 g protein	1 c	29	7	5	?	?	139
low-fat, 12 g protein	1 c	14	4	2	?	?	144
skim milk, 13 g protein	1 c	4	tr	tr	?	?	127
coffee & vanilla varieties, low-fat, 11 g protein	1 c	11	3	2	?	?	194
fruit varieties, low-fat							
9 g protein	1 c	10	3	2	?	?	225
10 g protein	1 c	10	2	2	?	?	231
11 g protein	1 c	12	3	2	?	?	239
▪ BRAND NAME							
Carnation							
instant nonfat dry milk	5 T	5	0	0	0	0	80
evaporated milk	½ c	37	10	6	3	<1	170
evaporated lowfat milk	½ c	10	3	2	1	<1	110
evaporated skim milk	½ c	5	0	0	0	0	100
sweetened condensed milk	about ⅓ c	24	8	5	2	0	320
Coffee-mate non-dairy creamer	1 t	0	<1	0	0	0	10
liquid	1 T	0	1	0	0	0	16
lite	1 t	0	<1	0	0	0	8
Colombo Yogurt							
nonfat							
lite plain	8 oz	5	<1	?	?	?	110
lite vanilla	8 oz	5	<1	?	?	?	160
fruit on bottom	8 oz	5	<1	?	?	?	190
lite mini-pack	4.4 oz	?	0	?	?	?	100
whole milk							
plain	8 oz	?	8	?	?	?	160
French vanilla	8 oz	?	7	?	?	?	215
strawberry	8 oz	?	7	?	?	?	210
fruit on bottom	8 oz	?	6	?	?	?	230
Dannon							
lowfat yogurt							
plain	8 oz	15	4	?	?	?	140
flavored	8 oz	10	3	?	?	?	200
fruit on bottom	8 oz	10	3	?	?	?	240
fruit on bottom, mini-pack	4.4 oz	5	2	?	?	?	130
nonfat yogurt, plain	8 oz	5	0	?	?	?	110
yogurt w/fruit on bottom	8 oz	10	3	?	?	?	240
Friendship							
buttermilk, low-fat (1½% milk fat)	1 c	14	4	?	?	?	120
lite delite low-fat sour cream	2 T	8	2	?	?	?	35

	Portion	Chol (mg)	Total Fat(g)	Satur'd Fat(g)	Mono Fat(g)	Poly Fat(g)	Total Calor
sour cream	2 T	42	5	?	?	?	55
yogurt							
plain, lowfat	1 c	14	3	?	?	?	150
low-fat vanilla & coffee (1½% milk fat)	1 c	14	3	?	?	?	210
low-fat w/fruit (1½% milk fat)	1 c	14	3	?	?	?	230
Pet/Dairymate							
evaporated milk	½ c	36	10	?	?	?	170
evaporated skimmed milk	½ c	10	<1	?	?	?	100
evaporated filled milk	½ c	5	8	1	?	3	150
imitation sour cream	1 T	<1	2	?	?	?	25
Rich's nondairy creamers							
Coffee Rich	½ oz	0	2	?	?	?	20
Poly Rich	½ oz	0	1	?	?	?	20
Weight Watchers							
skim milk	1 c	?	<1	?	?	?	90
light sour cream	2 T	?	2	?	?	?	35
yogurt							
Ultimate 90	1 c	5	?	?	?	?	90
plain nonfat	1 c	5	?	?	?	?	90
Dairy Creamer instant, nonfat dry milk	1 packet	?	?	?	?	?	10
Whitney's yogurt							
apples & raisins	6 oz	20	5	?	?	?	190
blueberry	6 oz	20	5	?	?	?	190
cherry	6 oz	20	5	?	?	?	190
lemon	6 oz	?	5	?	?	?	190
peach	6 oz	20	5	?	?	?	190
raspberry	6 oz	20	5	?	?	?	190
strawberry	6 oz	20	5	?	?	?	190
tropical fruit	6 oz	20	6	?	?	?	190
vanilla	6 oz	?	5	?	?	?	190
wild berries	6 oz	20	5	?	?	?	190
Yoplait Yogurt							
fat free, fruit flavors	6 oz	5	0	?	?	?	150
light, fruit flavors	6 oz	<5	0	?	?	?	80
original							
fruit flavors	6 oz	10	3	?	?	?	190
vanilla	6 oz	10	3	?	?	?	180
plain	6 oz	15	3	?	?	?	130
custard style							
fruit flavors	6 oz	20	4	?	?	?	190
cherry & mixed berry	6 oz	20	4	?	?	?	180
vanilla	6 oz	20	4	?	?	?	180
nonfat							
plain	8 oz	5	0	?	?	?	120
vanilla	8 oz	5	0	?	?	?	180

	Portion	Chol (mg)	Total Fat(g)	Satur'd Fat(g)	Mono Fat(g)	Poly Fat(g)	Total Calor

❑ MOLASSES *See* SUGARS & SWEETENERS

❑ MUFFINS *See* BREADS, ROLLS, BISCUITS, & MUFFINS

❑ NOODLES & PASTA, PLAIN

Noodles

	Portion	Chol (mg)	Total Fat(g)	Satur'd Fat(g)	Mono Fat(g)	Poly Fat(g)	Total Calor
chow funn, dry (oriental wheat noodles)	1 oz	0	tr	?	?	?	102
chow mein, canned	1 c	5	11	2	?	?	220
egg, enriched, cooked	1 c	50	2	1	?	?	200
Japanese-style, seasoned *See* SOUPS, PREPARED							
rice, dry	1 oz	0	1	?	?	?	130
saimin, dry (oriental wheat noodles)	1 oz	0	0	?	?	?	95
suba, dry (oriental buckwheat noodles)	1 oz	0	1	?	?	?	99

Pasta

	Portion	Chol (mg)	Total Fat(g)	Satur'd Fat(g)	Mono Fat(g)	Poly Fat(g)	Total Calor
macaroni, enriched, cooked (cut lengths, elbows, shells)							
firm stage, hot	1 c	0	1	tr	?	?	190
tender stage							
cold	1 c	0	tr	tr	?	?	115
hot	1 c	0	1	tr	?	?	155
prepared & seasoned pasta dishes *See* ENTREES & MAIN COURSES, CANNED & BOXED; ENTREES & MAIN COURSES, FROZEN							
spaghetti, enriched, cooked							
firm stage, hot	1 c	0	1	tr	?	?	190
tender stage, hot	1 c	0	1	tr	?	?	155

▪ BRAND NAME

Contadina

	Portion	Chol (mg)	Total Fat(g)	Satur'd Fat(g)	Mono Fat(g)	Poly Fat(g)	Total Calor
fresh pasta & cheese							
fettucini, linguini & angel's hair	3 oz	75	4	1	?	<1	260
spinach linguini & spinach fettucini	3 oz	85	4	2	?	<1	260

Health Valley

	Portion	Chol (mg)	Total Fat(g)	Satur'd Fat(g)	Mono Fat(g)	Poly Fat(g)	Total Calor
lasagna, whole-wheat	2 oz	0	1	?	?	?	200
spaghetti whole-wheat	2 oz	0	1	?	?	?	200

	Portion	Chol (mg)	Total Fat(g)	Satur'd Fat(g)	Mono Fat(g)	Poly Fat(g)	Total Calor
whole-wheat amaranth	2 oz	0	1	?	?	?	200
Mueller's							
egg noodles	2 oz dry	55	3	?	?	?	220
golden rich egg noodles	2 oz dry	70	3	?	?	?	220
lasagna	2 oz dry	0	1	?	?	?	210
noodle trio	2 oz dry	0	1	?	?	?	210
spaghetti & macaroni	2 oz dry	0	1	?	?	?	210
super shapes	2 oz dry	55	2	?	?	?	220
tricolor twists	2 oz dry	0	1	?	?	?	210

❏ NUTS & NUT-BASED BUTTERS, FLOURS, MEALS, MILKS, PASTES, & POWDERS

	Portion	Chol (mg)	Total Fat(g)	Satur'd Fat(g)	Mono Fat(g)	Poly Fat(g)	Total Calor
almond butter							
plain	1 T	0	9	1	?	?	101
honey & cinnamon	1 T	0	8	1	?	?	96
almond meal, partially defatted	1 oz	0	5	tr	?	?	116
almond paste	1 oz	0	8	1	?	?	127
almond powder							
full-fat	1 oz	0	15	1	?	?	168
partially defatted	1 oz	0	5	tr	?	?	112
almonds							
dried							
blanched	1 oz	0	15	1	?	?	166
unblanched	1 oz	0	15	1	?	?	167
dry roasted, unblanched	1 oz	0	15	1	?	?	167
oil roasted							
blanched	1 oz	0	16	2	?	?	174
unblanched	1 oz	0	16	2	?	?	176
toasted, unblanched	1 oz	0	14	1	?	?	167
brazil nuts, dried, unblanched	1 oz	0	19	5	?	?	186
butternuts, dried	1 oz	0	16	tr	?	?	174
cashew butter, plain	1 T	0	8	2	?	?	94
cashew nuts							
dry roasted	1 oz	0	13	3	?	?	163
oil roasted	1 oz	0	14	3	?	?	163
chestnuts, Chinese							
raw	1 oz	0	tr	tr	?	?	64
boiled & steamed	1 oz	0	tr	tr	?	?	44
dried	1 oz	0	1	tr	?	?	103
roasted	1 oz	0	tr	tr	?	?	68
chestnuts, European							
raw							
peeled	1 oz	0	tr	tr	?	?	56
unpeeled	1 oz	0	1	tr	?	?	60

	Portion	Chol (mg)	Total Fat (g)	Satur'd Fat (g)	Mono Fat (g)	Poly Fat (g)	Total Calor
boiled & steamed	1 oz	0	tr	tr	?	?	37
dried, peeled	1 oz	0	1	tr	?	?	105
dried, unpeeled	1 oz	0	1	tr	?	?	106
roasted	1 oz	0	1	tr	?	?	70
chestnuts, Japanese							
raw	1 oz	0	tr	tr	?	?	44
boiled & steamed	1 oz	0	tr	tr	?	?	16
dried	1 oz	0	tr	tr	?	?	102
roasted	1 oz	0	tr	tr	?	?	57
coconut cream							
raw	1 T	0	5	5	?	?	49
canned	1 T	0	3	3	?	?	36
coconut meat							
raw	1.6 oz	0	15	13	?	?	159
dried (desiccated)							
creamed	1 oz	0	20	17	?	?	194
sweetened, flaked, canned	4 oz	0	36	32	?	?	505
sweetened, flaked, packaged	7 oz pkg	0	64	57	?	?	944
sweetened, shredded	7 oz pkg	0	71	63	?	?	997
toasted	1 oz	0	13	12	?	?	168
unsweetened	1 oz	0	18	16	?	?	187
coconut milk							
raw	1 T	0	4	3	?	?	35
canned	1 T	0	3	3	?	?	30
frozen	1 T	0	3	3	?	?	30
coconut water	1 T	0	tr	tr	?	?	3
filberts or hazelnuts							
dried							
blanched	1 oz	0	19	1	?	?	191
unblanched	1 oz	0	18	1	?	?	179
dry roasted, unblanched	1 oz	0	19	1	?	?	188
oil roasted, unblanched	1 oz	0	18	1	?	?	187
formulated nuts, wheat-based							
unflavored (mixture of hydrogenated soybean oil, wheat germ, fructose, wheat starch, sodium caseinate, soy protein, & salt)	1 oz	0	16	2	?	?	177
macadamia flavored (mixture of hydro-genated soybean oil, wheat germ, sugar, wheat starch, so-dium caseinate, soy protein, & natural & artificial flavor)	1 oz	0	16	2	?	?	176

	Portion	Chol (mg)	Total Fat(g)	Satur'd Fat(g)	Mono Fat(g)	Poly Fat(g)	Total Calor
all other flavors (mixture of hydrogenated soybean oil, wheat germ, sugar, sodium caseinate, soy protein, natural & artificial flavors, & artificial color)	1 oz	0	18	3	?	?	184
hazlenuts *See* FILBERTS, above							
hickory nuts, dried	1 oz	0	18	2	?	?	187
macadamia nuts							
dried	1 oz	0	21	3	?	?	199
oil roasted	1 oz	0	22	3	?	?	204
mixed nuts (cashew nuts, almonds, filberts, & pecans)							
dry roasted, w/peanuts	1 oz	0	15	2	?	?	169
oil roasted							
w/peanuts	1 oz	0	16	2	?	?	175
w/out peanuts	1 oz	0	16	3	?	?	175
peanut butter, w/added fat, sugar, & salt							
chunk style	2 T	0	16	3	?	?	188
smooth style	2 T	0	16	3	?	?	188
peanuts (all types)							
raw	1 oz	0	14	2	?	?	159
boiled	½ c	0	7	1	?	?	102
dried	1 oz	0	14	2	?	?	161
dry roasted	1 oz	0	14	2	?	?	164
oil roasted	1 oz	0	14	2	?	?	163
Spanish, oil roasted	1 oz	0	14	2	?	?	162
Valencia, oil roasted	1 oz	0	14	2	?	?	165
Virginia, oil roasted	1 oz	0	14	2	?	?	161
pecan flour	1 oz	0	tr	tr	?	?	93
pecans							
dried	1 oz	0	19	2	?	?	190
dry roasted	1 oz	0	18	1	?	?	187
oil roasted	1 oz	0	20	2	?	?	195
pignolias *See* PINE NUTS, PIGNOLIA, below							
pili nuts, dried	1 oz	0	23	9	?	?	204
pine nuts							
pignolia, dried	1 oz	0	14	2	?	?	146
piñon, dried	1 oz	0	17	3	?	?	161
pistachio nuts							
dried	1 oz	0	14	2	?	?	164
dry roasted	1 oz	0	15	2	?	?	172
sweet chestnuts *See* CHESTNUTS, EUROPEAN, above							
walnuts							
black, dried	1 oz	0	16	1	?	?	172

	Portion	Chol (mg)	Total Fat(g)	Satur'd Fat(g)	Mono Fat(g)	Poly Fat(g)	Total Calor
English or Persian, dried	1 oz	0	18	2	?	?	182

■ BRAND NAME

Arrowhead Mills
peanut butter, creamy or chunky	2 T	0	16	?	?	?	190

Blue Diamond
almonds
smokehouse	1 oz	0	14	1	9	4	150
lightly salted	1 oz	0	13	1	9	3	150
honey roasted	1 oz	0	12	1	8	3	140
barbeque	1 oz	0	16	1	11	4	160
toasted, no salt	1 oz	0	13	1	9	3	150
natural	1 oz	0	13	1	9	3	150
no salt, dry roasted	1 oz	0	13	1	9	3	150
pistachios, dry roasted	½ oz	0	12	2	6	4	140
macadamias							
lightly salted	1 oz	0	18	2	15	1	190
whole	1 oz	0	13	1	9	3	150
whole, blanched	1 oz	0	13	1	9	3	150
slivered	1 oz	0	13	1	9	3	150

Erewhon
almond butter	1 T	0	8	?	?	?	90
peanut butter							
chunky or creamy, salted	2 T	0	14	?	?	?	190
chunky or creamy, unsalted	2 T	0	14	?	?	?	190
sesame butter	2 T	?	17	?	?	?	190
sunflower butter	2 T	?	18	?	?	?	200
sesame tahini	2 T	?	18	?	?	?	200

Hain
natural raw almond butter	2 T	0	18	2	?	4	190
raw cashew butter	2 T	0	15	3	?	4	190
toasted blanched almond butter	2 T	0	19	2	?	4	220
raw unsalted cashew butter	2 T	0	19	3	?	7	210

Peter Pan Peanut Butter
creamy or crunchy	2 T	0	16	2	?	5	180
sodium-free or sodium-free crunchy	2 T	0	17	2	?	5	180

Skippy Peanut Butter
creamy or superchunk	2 T	0	17	3	8	5	190

Smucker's
natural peanut butter, regular, no salt added	2 T	0	16	3	8	5	200

	Portion	Chol (mg)	Total Fat(g)	Satur'd Fat(g)	Mono Fat(g)	Poly Fat(g)	Total Calor
honey sweetened peanut butter	2 T	0	10	2	5	3	180
Goober grape	2 T	0	10	2	5	3	180
Weight Watchers							
roasted peanuts	1 pouch	?	7	?	?	?	100

❏ OILS *See* FATS, OILS, & SHORTENINGS

❏ OLIVES *See* PICKLES, OLIVES, RELISHES, & CHUTNEYS

❏ PASTA *See* NOODLES & PASTA, PLAIN

❏ PASTRIES *See* DESSERTS: CAKES, PASTRIES, & PIES

❏ PATÉS *See* PROCESSED MEAT & POULTRY

❏ PEANUT BUTTER *See* NUTS & NUT-BASED BUTTERS, FLOURS, MEALS, MILKS, PASTES, & POWDERS

❏ PICKLES, OLIVES, RELISHES, & CHUTNEYS
See also PEPPERS, UNDER VEGETABLES, PLAIN & PREPARED

CHUTNEYS

apple	1 T	0	tr	?	?	?	41
tomato	1 T	0	?	n/a	?	?	31

Olives Canned

green	4 medium	0	2	tr	?	?	15
ripe, mission, pitted	3 small	0	2	tr	?	?	15

Pickles, Cucumber

bread & butter	4 slices	0	tr	?	?	?	18
dill, medium, whole	1 pickle, about 2¼ oz	0	tr	tr	?	?	5

	Portion	Chol (mg)	Total Fat(g)	Satur'd Fat(g)	Mono Fat(g)	Poly Fat(g)	Total Calor
fresh-pack slices	2 slices, about 1/2 oz	0	tr	tr	?	?	10
kosher	1	0	tr	tr	?	?	7
sour	1 large	0	tr	tr	?	?	10
sweet	1 large	0	tr	tr	?	?	146
sweet & sour, sliced	1 slice	0	tr	tr	?	?	3
sweet gherkin, small, whole	1, about 1/2 oz	0	tr	tr	?	?	20

Relishes

cranberry-orange	1 T	0	tr	?	?	?	27
cranberry-orange, canned	1/2 c	0	tr	?	?	?	246
strawberry	1 T	0	0	0	?	?	53
strawberry-pineapple	1 T	0	0	0	?	?	54
tomato	1 T	0	tr	?	?	?	53
pickle							
chow chow							
sour	1 oz	0	tr	tr	?	?	8
sweet	1 oz	0	tr	?	?	?	32
sour	1 T	0	tr	?	?	?	3
sweet, finely chopped	1 T	0	tr	tr	?	?	20

■ BRAND NAME

Claussen
kosher tomatoes	1	0	tr	tr	?	?	5
pickled cucumbers	1	0	0 or tr	0 or tr	?	?	?
sauerkraut	1/2 c	?	tr	tr	?	?	17

Dromedary
pimientos, all types, drained	1 oz	?	0	?	?	?	10

Progresso
olive condite	1/2 c	0	14	2	?	3	130
olive appetizer	1/2 c	0	21	3	?	5	180
salan olives	1/2 c	0	15	2	?	<1	120

Vlasic
relishes, hamburger & hotdog		?0	0	0	?	?	?

❏ PIE FILLINGS *See* DESSERTS: CUSTARDS, GELATINS, PUDDINGS, & PIE FILLINGS

	Portion	Chol (mg)	Total Fat(g)	Satur'd Fat(g)	Mono Fat(g)	Poly Fat(g)	Total Calor

❏ **PIES** *See* **DESSERTS: CAKES, PASTRIES, & PIES**

❏ **PIZZA**

pizza, cheese	⅛ pizza 15″ diam	56	9	4	?	?	290

■ **BRAND NAME**

Banquet
zap

cheese French bread pizza	1	35	10	?	?	?	310
pepperoni French bread pizza	1	40	16	?	?	?	350
deluxe French bread pizza	1	25	13	?	?	?	330

Celentano

thick crust	4.3 oz	15	11	?	?	?	290
9-slice	2.7 oz	8	4	?	?	?	150

Celeste Frozen Pizza
pizza-for-one

cheese	1 pizza	40	24.5	11	5	2	497
deluxe	1 pizza	20	31.8	10	9	3	582
pepperoni	1 pizza	20	29.6	9	7	2	546
sausage	1 pizza	20	31.7	10	7	3	571
sausage & mushroom	1 pizza	20	32.3	11	10	3	592
suprema	1 pizza	20	39.3	12	11	4	678
cheese	¼ pizza	20	16.6	7	3	1	317
deluxe	¼ pizza	20	22.1	7	7	2	378
pepperoni	¼ pizza	15	21.3	7	7	2	368
sausage	¼ pizza	15	21.7	7	6	2	376
suprema	¼ pizza	15	24.1	7	6	2	381

Contadina Fresh

pizza	⅛ pizza	20	7	3	2	<1	180
toppings							
pepperoni	.19 oz	5	2	<1	1	<1	25
Italian sausage	.21 oz	5	2	<1	<1	0	20
three-cheese	.35 oz	10	3	2	<1	0	35

Jeno's
pizza packets

supreme	1	20	19	7	?	4	370
sausage & pepperoni	1	20	20	7	?	4	360
pepperoni	1	25	20	6	?	4	370
sausage	1	15	19	7	?	4	360

	Portion	Chol (mg)	Total Fat(g)	Satur'd Fat(g)	Mono Fat(g)	Poly Fat(g)	Total Calor
pizza rolls							
cheese	3 oz	20	5	2	?	1	200
combination	3 oz	15	9	3	?	1	220
hamburger	3 oz	20	8	3	?	1	220
pepperoni	3 oz	20	9	3	?	1	220
sausage	3 oz	15	7	2	?	1	210
CNT							
sausage	½ pizza	15	16	4	?	2	290
combination	½ pizza	15	16	4	?	2	290
pepperoni	½ pizza	15	15	4	?	2	280
Canadian style bacon	½ pizza	10	10	2	?	2	240
Mr. P's							
pepperoni	½ pizza	15	13	3	?	2	250
golden topping	½ pizza	10	10	2	?	2	220
sausage	½ pizza	10	13	3	?	2	250
combination	½ pizza	10	13	3	?	2	250
hamburger	½ pizza	10	9	2	?	2	230
Pappalo's Traditional Crust Pizza							
pepperoni	¼ pizza	45	11	5	?	1	350
sausage	¼ pizza	40	12	6	?	1	350
sausage pepperoni	¼ pizza	45	12	6	?	1	360
supreme	¼ pizza	45	12	6	?	1	350
Pepperidge Farm Croissant Pastry Pizza							
cheese	1 pizza	?	23	?	?	?	430
deluxe	1 pizza	?	23	?	?	?	440
pepperoni	1 pizza	?	22	?	?	?	420
Pillsbury							
oven lovin' microwave pizza							
cheese	½ pizza	10	12	4	?	2	240
pepperoni	½ pizza	25	17	6	?	2	310
sausage	½ pizza	20	18	6	?	3	310
microwave French bread pizza							
cheese	1 pizza	15	14	5	?	2	350
combination	1 pizza	30	21	10	?	3	420
pepperoni	1 pizza	35	21	8	?	3	410
sausage	1 pizza	25	20	10	?	3	400
Stouffer's							
FRENCH BREAD PIZZA							
Canadian style bacon	½ pkg	?	14	?	?	?	360
cheese	½ pkg	?	13	?	?	?	340
double cheese	½ pkg	?	18	?	?	?	410
deluxe	½ pkg	?	21	?	?	?	430
hamburger	½ pkg	?	19	?	?	?	410
pepperoni	½ pkg	?	17	?	?	?	410
pepperoni & mushroom	½ pkg	?	22	?	?	?	430
sausage	½ pkg	?	20	?	?	?	420
sausage & pepperoni	½ pkg	?	23	?	?	?	450
vegetable deluxe	½ pkg	?	20	?	?	?	420

	Portion	Chol (mg)	Total Fat (g)	Satur'd Fat (g)	Mono Fat (g)	Poly Fat (g)	Total Calor
LEAN CUISINE							
French bread pizza							
cheese	1 pkg	15	9	3	?	<1	300
deluxe	1 pkg	40	8	3	?	<1	320
pepperoni	1 pkg	25	11	3	?	1	330
sausage	1 pkg	40	9	3	?	<1	330
TRADITIONAL PIZZA							
cheese	½ pkg	?	15	?	?	?	320
deluxe	½ pkg	?	19	?	?	?	370
pepperoni	½ pkg	?	18	?	?	?	350
sausage	½ pkg	?	18	?	?	?	360
Totinos							
PARTY PIZZA							
Canadian bacon	½ pizza	10	10	2	?	2	290
cheese	½ pizza	15	10	3	?	2	280
combination	½ pizza	15	15	4	?	3	340
hamburger	½ pizza	15	13	3	?	2	320
pepperoni	½ pizza	20	14	3	?	3	330
sausage	½ pizza	15	15	3	?	3	340
MICROWAVE PIZZA							
cheese	1 pizza	15	10	4	?	2	250
combination	1 pizza	15	13	3	?	2	290
pepperoni	1 pizza	15	13	3	?	2	270
sausage	1 pizza	10	13	3	?	2	280
PAN PIZZA							
3 cheese	⅙ pizza	?	10	?	?	?	290
sausage	⅙ pizza	?	13	?	?	?	320
pepperoni	⅙ pizza	?	14	?	?	?	330
sausage & pepperoni combination	⅙ pizza	?	15	?	?	?	340
Weight Watchers							
cheese	6 oz	35	7	3	3	1	300
deluxe combination	7 oz	25	10	3	5	2	330
pepperoni	6 oz	35	10	3	5	2	320
bread pizza							
pepperoni	5 oz	30	11	3	6	2	320
deluxe	6 oz	30	12	3	7	2	330
sausage	6¼ oz	35	10	2	6	2	320

❏ **PORK, FRESH & CURED**
See also PROCESSED MEAT & POULTRY PRODUCTS

Pork, fresh

	Portion	Chol (mg)	Total Fat (g)	Satur'd Fat (g)	Mono Fat (g)	Poly Fat (g)	Total Calor
retail cuts, separable fat, cooked	1 oz	26	21	8	?	?	200

	Portion	Chol (mg)	Total Fat(g)	Satur'd Fat(g)	Mono Fat(g)	Poly Fat(g)	Total Calor
LEG (HAM)							
Lean & Fat							
whole, roasted	3 oz	79	18	6	?	?	250
rump half, roasted	3 oz	81	15	5	?	?	233
shank half, roasted	3 oz	78	19	7	?	?	258
Lean Only							
whole, roasted	3 oz	80	9	3	?	?	187
rump half, roasted	3 oz	81	9	3	?	?	187
shank half, roasted	3 oz	78	9	3	?	?	183
LOIN, WHOLE							
Lean & Fat							
braised	3 oz	87	24	9	?	?	312
braised	1 chop (3 chops/lb as pur- chased)	73	20	7	?	?	261
broiled	3 oz	80	23	8	?	?	294
broiled	1 chop (3 chops/lb as pur- chased)	77	22	8	?	?	284
roasted	3 oz	77	21	7	?	?	271
roasted	1 chop (3 chops/lb as pur- chased)	74	20	7	?	?	262
Lean Only							
braised	3 oz	90	12	4	?	?	232
braised	1 chop (3 chops/lb as pur- chased)	58	8	3	?	?	150
broiled	3 oz	81	13	4	?	?	218
broiled	1 chop (3 chops/lb as pur- chased)	63	10	3	?	?	169
roasted	3 oz	77	12	4	?	?	204
roasted	1 chop (3 chops/lb as pur- chased)	62	10	3	?	?	166
LOIN, BLADE							
Lean & Fat							
braised	3 oz	92	29	10	?	?	348

	Portion	Chol (mg)	Total Fat(g)	Satur'd Fat(g)	Mono Fat(g)	Poly Fat(g)	Total Calor
braised	1 chop (3 chops/lb as purchased)	72	23	8	?	?	275
broiled	3 oz	83	29	10	?	?	334
broiled	1 chop (3 chops/lb as purchased)	75	26	9	?	?	303
pan-fried	3 oz	81	31	11	?	?	352
pan-fried	1 chop (3 chops/lb as purchased)	85	33	12	?	?	368
roasted	3 oz	76	26	9	?	?	310
roasted	1 chop (3 chops/lb as purchased)	79	27	10	?	?	321
Lean Only							
braised	3 oz	96	18	6	?	?	266
braised	1 chop (3 chops/lb as purchased)	57	10	4	?	?	156
broiled	3 oz	85	18	6	?	?	255
broiled	1 chop (3 chops/lb as purchased)	59	13	4	?	?	177
pan-fried	3 oz	82	17	6	?	?	240
pan-fried	1 chop (3 chops/lb as purchased)	60	12	4	?	?	175
roasted	3 oz	76	16	6	?	?	238
roasted	1 chop (3 chops/lb as purchased)	63	14	5	?	?	198

LOIN, CENTER
Lean & Fat

	Portion	Chol (mg)	Total Fat(g)	Satur'd Fat(g)	Mono Fat(g)	Poly Fat(g)	Total Calor
braised	3 oz	91	22	8	?	?	301
braised	1 chop (3 chops/lb as purchased)	81	19	7	?	?	266

	Portion	Chol (mg)	Total Fat(g)	Satur'd Fat(g)	Mono Fat(g)	Poly Fat(g)	Total Calor
broiled	3 oz	82	19	7	?	?	269
broiled	1 chop (3 chops/lb as pur- chased)	84	19	7	?	?	275
pan-fried	3 oz	87	26	9	?	?	318
pan-fried	1 chop (3 chops/lb as pur- chased)	92	27	10	?	?	333
roasted	3 oz	78	18	7	?	?	259
roasted	1 chop (3 chops/lb as pur- chased)	80	19	7	?	?	268
Lean Only							
braised	3 oz	95	12	4	?	?	231
braised	1 chop (3 chops/lb as pur- chased)	68	8	3	?	?	166
broiled	3 oz	83	9	3	?	?	196
broiled	1 chop (3 chops/lb as pur- chased)	71	8	3	?	?	166
pan-fried	3 oz	91	14	5	?	?	226
pan-fried	1 chop (3 chops/lb as pur- chased)	71	11	4	?	?	178
roasted	3 oz	78	11	4	?	?	204
roasted	1 chop (3 chops/lb as pur- chased)	68	10	3	?	?	180
LOIN, CENTER RIB							
Lean & Fat							
braised	3 oz	81	23	8	?	?	312
braised	1 chop (3 chops/lb as pur- chased)	64	18	7	?	?	246
broiled	3 oz	79	22	8	?	?	291
broiled	1 chop (3 chops/lb as pur- chased)	72	20	7	?	?	264

	Portion	Chol (mg)	Total Fat(g)	Satur'd Fat(g)	Mono Fat(g)	Poly Fat(g)	Total Calor
pan-fried	3 oz	71	28	10	?	?	331
pan-fried	1 chop (3 chops/lb as purchased)	74	29	10	?	?	343
roasted	3 oz	69	20	7	?	?	271
roasted	1 chop (3 chops/lb as purchased)	64	19	7	?	?	252
Lean Only							
braised	3 oz	82	12	4	?	?	236
braised	1 chop (3 chops/lb as purchased)	51	8	3	?	?	147
broiled	3 oz	80	13	4	?	?	219
broiled	1 chop (3 chops/lb as purchased)	59	9	3	?	?	162
pan-fried	3 oz	69	13	4	?	?	219
pan-fried	1 chop (3 chops/lb as purchased)	50	9	3	?	?	160
roasted	3 oz	67	12	4	?	?	208
roasted	1 chop (3 chops/lb as purchased)	52	9	3	?	?	162
LOIN, SIRLOIN							
Lean & Fat							
braised	3 oz	90	22	8	?	?	299
braised	1 chop (3 chops/lb as purchased)	75	18	7	?	?	250
broiled	3 oz	82	21	8	?	?	281
broiled	1 chop (3 chops/lb as purchased)	81	21	8	?	?	278
roasted	3 oz	77	17	6	?	?	247
roasted	1 chop (3 chops/lb as purchased)	76	17	6	?	?	244

	Portion	Chol (mg)	Total Fat(g)	Satur'd Fat(g)	Mono Fat(g)	Poly Fat(g)	Total Calor
Lean Only							
braised	3 oz	94	11	4	?	?	221
braised	1 chop (3 chops/lb as purchased)	63	7	3	?	?	149
broiled	3 oz	83	12	4	?	?	207
broiled	1 chop (3 chops/lb as purchased)	67	9	3	?	?	165
roasted	3 oz	77	11	4	?	?	201
roasted	1 chop (3 chops/lb as purchased)	67	10	3	?	?	175
LOIN, TENDERLOIN							
lean							
roasted	3 oz	79	4	1	?	?	141
LOIN, TOP							
Lean & Fat							
braised	3 oz	81	25	9	?	?	324
braised	1 chop (3 chops/lb as purchased)	67	20	7	?	?	267
broiled	3 oz	79	24	9	?	?	306
broiled	1 chop (3 chops/lb as purchased)	76	23	8	?	?	295
pan-fried	3 oz	71	28	10	?	?	333
pan-fried	1 chop (3 chops/lb as purchased)	72	29	10	?	?	337
roasted	3 oz	69	21	8	?	?	280
roasted	1 chop (3 chops/lb as purchased)	68	21	8	?	?	274
Lean Only							
braised	3 oz	82	12	4	?	?	236

	Portion	Chol (mg)	Total Fat(g)	Satur'd Fat(g)	Mono Fat(g)	Poly Fat(g)	Total Calor
braised	1 chop (3 chops/lb as pur- chased)	51	8	3	?	?	147
broiled	3 oz	80	13	4	?	?	219
broiled	1 chop (3 chops/lb as pur- chased)	60	10	3	?	?	165
pan-fried	3 oz	69	13	4	?	?	219
pan-fried	1 chop (3 chops/lb as pur- chased)	49	9	3	?	?	157
roasted	3 oz	67	12	4	?	?	208
roasted	1 chop (3 chops/lb as pur- chased)	54	9	3	?	?	167

SHOULDER, WHOLE

Lean & Fat

roasted	3 oz	81	22	8	?	?	277

Lean Only

roasted	3 oz	82	13	4	?	?	207

SHOULDER, ARM, PICNIC

Lean & Fat

braised	3 oz	93	22	8	?	?	293
roasted	3 oz	80	22	8	?	?	281

Lean Only

braised	3 oz	97	10	4	?	?	211
roasted	3 oz	81	11	4	?	?	194

SHOULDER, BLADE, BOSTON

Lean & Fat

braised	3 oz	95	24	9	?	?	316
braised	1 steak	178	46	17	?	?	594
broiled	3 oz	87	24	9	?	?	297
broiled	1 steak	190	53	19	?	?	647
roasted	3 oz	82	21	8	?	?	273
roasted	1 steak	179	47	17	?	?	594

Lean Only

braised	3 oz	99	15	5	?	?	250
braised	1 steak	151	23	8	?	?	382
broiled	3 oz	89	16	5	?	?	233

	Portion	Chol (mg)	Total Fat(g)	Satur'd Fat(g)	Mono Fat(g)	Poly Fat(g)	Total Calor
broiled	1 steak	159	28	10	?	?	413
roasted	3 oz	83	14	5	?	?	218
roasted	1 steak	155	27	9	?	?	404

SPARERIBS

Lean & Fat

	Portion	Chol (mg)	Total Fat(g)	Satur'd Fat(g)	Mono Fat(g)	Poly Fat(g)	Total Calor
braised	3 oz	103	26	10	?	?	338
braised	6¼ oz (yield from 1 lb as pur- chased)	214	54	21	?	?	703

Pork, Fresh, Variety Meats

	Portion	Chol (mg)	Total Fat(g)	Satur'd Fat(g)	Mono Fat(g)	Poly Fat(g)	Total Calor
brains, braised	3 oz	2169	8	2	?	?	117
chitterlings, simmered	3 oz	122	24	9	?	?	258
ears, simmered	1	99	12	?	?	?	183
feet, simmered	2½ oz	71	9	3	?	?	138
heart, braised	1	285	7	2	?	?	191
kidneys, braised	1 c	673	7	2	?	?	211
liver, braised	3 oz	302	4	1	?	?	141
lungs, braised	3 oz	329	3	1	?	?	84
tail, simmered	3 oz	110	30	11	?	?	336
tongue, braised	3 oz	124	16	5	?	?	230

Pork, Cured

	Portion	Chol (mg)	Total Fat(g)	Satur'd Fat(g)	Mono Fat(g)	Poly Fat(g)	Total Calor
bacon, pan-fried or roasted	3 slices (20 slices/lb)	16	9	3	?	?	109
breakfast strips, cooked	3 slices (15 slices/ 12 oz)	36	12	4	?	?	156
breakfast strips, cooked	6 oz	179	62	22	?	?	780
Canadian-style bacon, unheated, fully cooked as purchased	2 oz	28	4	1	?	?	89
feet, pickled	1 oz	26	5	2	?	?	58
ham, boneless extra lean (about 5% fat)							
unheated	1 oz	13	1	tr	?	?	37
roasted	3 oz	45	5	2	?	?	123
regular (about 11% fat)							
unheated	1 oz	16	3	1	?	?	52
roasted	3 oz	50	8	3	?	?	151

	Portion	Chol (mg)	Total Fat(g)	Satur'd Fat(g)	Mono Fat(g)	Poly Fat(g)	Total Calor
ham, canned							
extra lean (about 4% fat)							
unheated	1 oz	11	1	tr	?	?	34
roasted	3 oz	25	4	1	?	?	116
regular (about 13% fat)							
unheated	1 oz	11	4	1	?	?	54
roasted	3 oz	52	13	4	?	?	192
ham, center slice							
country-style, lean only, raw	4 oz	?	9	3	?	?	220
lean & fat, unheated, fully cooked as purchased	4 oz	61	15	5	?	?	229
ham patties							
unheated, fully cooked as purchased	1	46	18	7	?	?	206
grilled	1	43	18	7	?	?	203
ham steak, boneless, extra lean, unheated, fully cooked as purchased	2 oz	26	2	1	?	?	69
ham, whole							
lean & fat							
unheated, fully cooked as purchased	1 oz	16	5	2	?	?	70
roasted	3 oz	52	14	5	?	?	207
lean only							
unheated, fully cooked as purchased	1 oz	15	2	1	?	?	42
roasted	3 oz	47	5	2	?	?	133
salt, pork, raw	1 oz	25	23	8	?	?	212
separable fat (from ham & arm picnic)							
unheated, fully cooked as purchased	1 oz	19	17	6	?	?	164
roasted	1 oz	24	18	6	?	?	167
shoulder							
arm picnic, roasted							
lean & fat	3 oz	49	18	7	?	?	238
lean only	3 oz	41	6	2	?	?	145
blade roll, lean & fat							
unheated, fully cooked as purchased	1 oz	15	6	2	?	?	76
roasted	3 oz	57	20	7	?	?	244

	Portion	Chol (mg)	Total Fat(g)	Satur'd Fat(g)	Mono Fat(g)	Poly Fat(g)	Total Calor

■ **BRAND NAME**

Oscar Mayer

BACON

regular	1 slice	5	3	?	?	?	35
⅛ thick slice	1 slice	10	5	?	?	?	55
center cut	1 slice	5	2	?	?	?	25
lower salt	1 slice	5	3	?	?	?	35
bits	1 T	5	1	?	?	?	20

HAM

breakfast honey	1 slice	20	2	?	?	?	45
boneless jubilee	1 slice	15	2	?	?	?	45
chopped & formed jubilee	1 slice	15	2	?	?	?	40
canned	1 slice	15	1	?	?	?	30
ham slice	1 slice	15	1	?	?	?	30
ham steaks	1 slice	30	2	?	?	?	55

❏ **POULTRY, FRESH & PROCESSED**
See also PROCESSED MEAT & POULTRY PRODUCTS

NOTE: Values are based on the following weights as purchased w/giblets & neck.

chicken	
broilers or fryers	3.33 lbs
roasting	4.56 lbs
stewing	2.93 lbs
capons	6½ lbs

duck	
domesticated	4.42 lbs
wild	2.26 lbs
goose	8.25 lbs
guinea	1.92 lbs
pheasant	2.15 lbs
quail	0.27 lbs
squab	0.67 lbs

turkey	
all classes	15.47 lbs
fryer-roasters	7.05 lbs
young hens	12.56 lbs
young toms	23.06 lbs

	Portion	Chol (mg)	Total Fat(g)	Satur'd Fat(g)	Mono Fat(g)	Poly Fat(g)	Total Calor

Chicken, Fresh

CHICKEN, BROILERS OR FRYERS

flesh, skin, giblets &
   neck
   fried

	Portion	Chol (mg)	Total Fat(g)	Satur'd Fat(g)	Mono Fat(g)	Poly Fat(g)	Total Calor
batter-dipped	1 chicken	1,054	180	48	?	?	2,987
flour-coated	1 chicken	795	108	29	?	?	1,928
roasted	1 chicken	730	90	25	?	?	1,598
stewed	1 chicken	726	93	26	?	?	1,625
flesh & skin							
fried							
batter-dipped	½ chicken	404	81	22	?	?	1,347
flour-coated	½ chicken	283	47	13	?	?	844
roasted	½ chicken	263	41	11	?	?	715
stewed	½ chicken	262	42	12	?	?	730
flesh only							
fried							
roasted	1 c	125	10	3	?	?	266
fried	1 c	131	13	3	?	?	307
stewed	1 c	116	9	3	?	?	248
skin only							
fried							
batter-dipped	½ chicken	140	55	14	?	?	748
flour-coated	½ chicken	41	24	7	?	?	281
roasted	½ chicken	46	23	6	?	?	254
stewed	½ chicken	45	24	7	?	?	261
giblets							
fried, flour-coated	1 c	647	20	6	?	?	402
simmered	1 c	570	7	2	?	?	228
gizzard, simmered	1 c	281	5	2	?	?	222
heart, simmered	1 c	350	11	3	?	?	268
liver, simmered	1 c	883	8	3	?	?	219
fried							
batter-dipped	½ chicken	157	29	8	?	?	520
flour-coated	½ chicken	113	16	4	?	?	320
roasted	½ chicken	111	14	4	?	?	293
stewed	½ chicken	111	15	4	?	?	302
dark meat w/skin							
fried							
batter-dipped	½ chicken	247	52	14	?	?	828
flour-coated	½ chicken	169	31	8	?	?	523
roasted	½ chicken	152	26	7	?	?	423
stewed	½ chicken	151	27	7	?	?	428
light meat w/out skin							
fried	1 c	125	8	2	?	?	268
roasted	1 c	118	6	2	?	?	242
stewed	1 c	107	6	2	?	?	223
dark meat w/out skin							
fried	1 c	135	16	4	?	?	334
roasted	1 c	130	14	4	?	?	286

	Portion	Chol (mg)	Total Fat(g)	Satur'd Fat(g)	Mono Fat(g)	Poly Fat(g)	Total Calor
stewed	1 c	123	13	3	?	?	269
back, meat & skin							
fried							
batter-dipped	½ back	105	26	7	?	?	397
flour-coated	½ back	64	15	4	?	?	238
roasted	½ back	46	11	3	?	?	159
stewed	½ back	48	11	3	?	?	158
back, meat only							
fried	½ back	54	9	2	?	?	167
roasted	½ back	36	5	1	?	?	96
stewed	½ back	36	5	1	?	?	88
breast, meat & skin							
fried							
batter-dipped	½ breast	119	18	5	?	?	364
flour-coated	½ breast	88	9	2	?	?	218
roasted	½ breast	83	8	2	?	?	193
stewed	½ breast	83	8	2	?	?	202
breast, meat only							
fried	½ breast	78	4	1	?	?	161
roasted	½ breast	73	3	1	?	?	142
stewed	½ breast	73	3	1	?	?	144
drumstick, meat & skin							
fried							
batter-dipped	1	62	11	3	?	?	193
flour-coated	1	44	7	2	?	?	120
roasted	1	48	6	2	?	?	112
stewed	1	48	6	2	?	?	116
drumstick, meat only							
fried	1	40	3	1	?	?	82
roasted	1	41	2	1	?	?	76
stewed	1	40	3	1	?	?	78
leg (drumstick & thigh) meat & skin							
fried							
batter-dipped	1	142	26	7	?	?	431
flour-coated	1	105	16	4	?	?	285
roasted	1	105	15	4	?	?	265
stewed	1	105	16	4	?	?	275
leg (drumstick & thigh) meat only							
fried	1	93	9	2	?	?	195
roasted	1	89	8	2	?	?	182
stewed	1	90	8	2	?	?	187
neck, meat & skin							
fried							
batter-dipped	1	47	12	3	?	?	172
flour-coated	1	34	9	2	?	?	119
simmered	1	27	7	2	?	?	94
neck, meat only							
fried	1	23	3	1	?	?	50
simmered	1	14	1	tr	?	?	32

	Portion	Chol (mg)	Total Fat(g)	Satur'd Fat(g)	Mono Fat(g)	Poly Fat(g)	Total Calor
thigh, meat & skin							
fried							
batter-dipped	1	80	14	4	?	?	238
flour-coated	1	60	9	3	?	?	162
roasted	1	58	10	3	?	?	153
stewed	1	57	10	3	?	?	158
thigh, meat only							
fried	1	53	5	1	?	?	113
roasted	1	49	6	2	?	?	109
stewed	1	49	5	1	?	?	107
wing, meat & skin							
fried							
batter-dipped	1	39	11	3	?	?	159
flour-coated	1	26	7	2	?	?	103
roasted	1	29	7	2	?	?	99
stewed	1	28	7	2	?	?	100
wing, meat only							
fried	1	17	2	1	?	?	42
roasted	1	18	2	tr	?	?	43
stewed	1	18	2	tr	?	?	43
CHICKEN, ROASTING							
flesh & skin, roasted	½ chicken	365	64	18	?	?	1,071
flesh only, roasted	1 c	104	9	3	?	?	233
giblets, simmered	1 c	517	7	2	?	?	239
light meat w/out skin, roasted	1 c	105	6	2	?	?	214
dark meat w/out skin, roasted	1 c	104	12	3	?	?	250
CHICKEN, STEWING							
flesh, skin, giblets, & neck, stewed	1 chicken	603	107	29	?	?	1,636
flesh & skin, stewed	½ chicken	205	49	13	?	?	744
flesh only, stewed	1 c	117	17	4	?	?	332
giblets, simmered	1 c	515	13	4	?	?	281
light meat w/out skin, stewed	1 c	98	11	3	?	?	298
dark meat w/out skin, stewed	1 c	132	21	6	?	?	361
CHICKEN, CAPONS							
flesh, skin, giblets & neck, roasted	1 chicken	1,458	165	46	?	?	3,211
flesh & skin, roasted	½ chicken	549	74	21	?	?	1,457
giblets, simmered	1 c	629	8	3	?	?	238
Duck, Fresh							
DOMESTICATED							
flesh & skin, roasted	½ duck	320	108	37	?	?	1,287

	Portion	Chol (mg)	Total Fat(g)	Satur'd Fat(g)	Mono Fat(g)	Poly Fat(g)	Total Calor
flesh only, roasted	½ duck	198	25	9	?	?	445
WILD							
flesh & skin, raw	1 lb of ready-to-cook bird	191	36	12	?	?	505
breast, meat only, raw	½ breast	?	4	1	?	?	102

Goose, Fresh, Domesticated

	Portion	Chol (mg)	Total Fat(g)	Satur'd Fat(g)	Mono Fat(g)	Poly Fat(g)	Total Calor
flesh & skin, roasted	½ goose	708	170	53	?	?	2,362
flesh only, roasted	½ goose	569	75	27	?	?	1,406
liver, raw	1	?	4	1	?	?	125

Guinea, Fresh

	Portion	Chol (mg)	Total Fat(g)	Satur'd Fat(g)	Mono Fat(g)	Poly Fat(g)	Total Calor
flesh & skin, raw	1 lb of ready-to-cook bird	?	23	?	?	?	568
flesh only, raw	1 lb of ready-to-cook bird	?	7	?	?	?	304

Pheasant, Fresh

	Portion	Chol (mg)	Total Fat(g)	Satur'd Fat(g)	Mono Fat(g)	Poly Fat(g)	Total Calor
flesh & skin, raw	1 lb of ready-to-cook bird	?	34	10	?	?	670
flesh only, raw	1 lb of ready-to-cook bird	?	12	4	?	?	435
breast, meat only, raw	½ breast	?	6	2	?	?	243
leg, meat only, raw	1	?	5	2	?	?	143

Quail, Fresh

	Portion	Chol (mg)	Total Fat(g)	Satur'd Fat(g)	Mono Fat(g)	Poly Fat(g)	Total Calor
flesh & skin, raw	1 quail	?	13	4	?	?	210
flesh only, raw	1 quail	?	4	1	?	?	123
breast, meat only, raw	1	?	2	tr	?	?	69

Squab (Pigeon), Fresh

	Portion	Chol (mg)	Total Fat(g)	Satur'd Fat(g)	Mono Fat(g)	Poly Fat(g)	Total Calor
flesh only, raw	1 squab	?	13	3	?	?	239
breast, meat only, raw	1	91	5	1	?	?	135

Turkey, Fresh

TURKEY, ALL CLASSES

	Portion	Chol (mg)	Total Fat(g)	Satur'd Fat(g)	Mono Fat(g)	Poly Fat(g)	Total Calor
flesh, skin, giblets, & neck, roasted	1 lb of ready-to-cook bird	248	25	7	?	?	533

	Portion	Chol (mg)	Total Fat(g)	Satur'd Fat(g)	Mono Fat(g)	Poly Fat(g)	Total Calor
flesh, skin, giblets, & neck, roasted	1 turkey	3,839	380	111	?	?	8,245
flesh & skin, roasted	1 lb of ready-to-cook bird	196	23	7	?	?	498
flesh & skin, roasted	½ turkey	1,514	180	53	?	?	3,857
flesh only, roasted	1 c	107	7	2	?	?	238
skin only, roasted	½ turkey	281	98	26	?	?	1,096
giblets, simmered	1 c	606	7	2	?	?	243
gizzard, simmered	1 c	336	6	2	?	?	236
heart, simmered	1 c	327	9	3	?	?	257
liver, simmered	1 c	876	8	3	?	?	237
light meat w/skin, roasted	½ turkey	794	87	25	?	?	2,069
dark meat w/skin, roasted	½ turkey	720	93	28	?	?	1,789
light meat w/out skin, roasted	1 c	97	5	1	?	?	219
dark meat w/out skin, roasted	1 c	119	10	3	?	?	262
back, meat & skin, roasted	½ back	238	38	11	?	?	637
breast, meat & skin, roasted	½ breast	643	64	18	?	?	1,637
leg, meat & skin, roasted	1	466	54	17	?	?	1,133
neck, meat only, simmered	1	186	11	4	?	?	274
wing, meat & skin, roasted	1	150	23	6	?	?	426

TURKEY, FRYER ROASTERS

	Portion	Chol (mg)	Total Fat(g)	Satur'd Fat(g)	Mono Fat(g)	Poly Fat(g)	Total Calor
flesh, skin, giblets, & neck, roasted	1 lb of ready-to-cook bird	297	14	4	?	?	429
flesh, skin, giblets & neck, roasted	1 turkey	2093	100	29	?	?	3,029
flesh & skin, roasted	1 lb of ready-to-cook bird	241	13	4	?	?	395
flesh & skin, roasted	½ turkey	849	46	13	?	?	1,392
flesh only, roasted	1 lb ready to cook bird	192	5	2	?	?	292
flesh only, roasted	1 c	138	4	1	?	?	210
skin only, roasted	½ turkey	175	28	7	?	?	362
light meat w/skin, roasted	½ turkey	413	20	5	?	?	711
dark meat w/skin, roasted	½ turkey	436	26	8	?	?	680

	Portion	Chol (mg)	Total Fat(g)	Satur'd Fat(g)	Mono Fat(g)	Poly Fat(g)	Total Calor
light meat w/out skin, roasted	1 c	121	2	1	?	?	195
dark meat w/out skin, roasted	1 c	157	6	2	?	?	227
back							
meat & skin, roasted	½ back	140	11	4	?	?	265
meat only, roasted	½ back	91	5	2	?	?	164
breast							
meat & skin, roasted	½ breast	310	11	3	?	?	526
meat only, roasted	½ breast	255	2	1	?	?	413
leg							
meat & skin, roasted	1	171	13	4	?	?	418
meat only, roasted	1	267	8	3	?	?	355
wing							
meat & skin, roasted	1	104	9	2	?	?	186
meat only, roasted	1	61	2	1	?	?	98

TURKEY, YOUNG HENS

	Portion	Chol (mg)	Total Fat(g)	Satur'd Fat(g)	Mono Fat(g)	Poly Fat(g)	Total Calor
flesh, skin, giblets, & neck, roasted	1 lb of ready-to-cook bird	246	28	8	?	?	565
flesh, skin, giblets, & neck, roasted	1 turkey	3,092	348	102	?	?	7,094
flesh & skin, roasted	½ turkey	1,190	166	48	?	?	3,323
flesh only, roasted	1 c	102	8	3	?	?	244
skin only, roasted	½ turkey	207	87	23	?	?	945
light meat w/skin, roasted	½ turkey	633	81	23	?	?	1,778
dark meat w/skin, roasted	½ bird	557	85	26	?	?	1,544
light meat w/out skin, roasted	1 c	95	5	2	?	?	226
dark meat w/out skin, roasted	1 c	111	11	4	?	?	268
back, meat & skin, roasted	½ back	185	34	10	?	?	551
breast, meat & skin, roasted	½ breast	492	54	15	?	?	1,330
leg, meat & skin, roasted	1	365	47	15	?	?	955
wing, meat & skin, roasted	1	134	23	6	?	?	414

TURKEY, YOUNG TOMS

	Portion	Chol (mg)	Total Fat(g)	Satur'd Fat(g)	Mono Fat(g)	Poly Fat(g)	Total Calor
flesh, skin, giblets, & neck, roasted	1 lb of ready-to-cook bird	249	23	7	?	?	514
flesh, skin, giblets, & neck, roasted	1 turkey	5,745	525	154	?	?	11,873

	Portion	Chol (mg)	Total Fat(g)	Satur'd Fat(g)	Mono Fat(g)	Poly Fat(g)	Total Calor
flesh & skin, roasted	1 lb of ready-to-cook bird	197	22	6	?	?	482
flesh & skin, roasted	½ turkey	2,265	249	73	?	?	5,545
flesh only, roasted	1 c	108	7	2	?	?	235
skin only, roasted	½ turkey	436	139	36	?	?	1,578
light meat w/skin, roasted	½ turkey	1,182	121	34	?	?	2,992
dark meat w/skin, roasted	½ turkey	1,081	128	39	?	?	2,553
light meat w/out skin, roasted	1 c	97	4	1	?	?	215
dark meat w/out skin, roasted	1 c	123	10	3	?	?	260
back, meat & skin							
raw	½ back	416	58	16	?	?	940
roasted	½ back	358	52	15	?	?	903
breast, meat & skin, roasted	½ breast	1,002	98	28	?	?	2,510
leg, meat & skin, roasted	1	727	78	24	?	?	1,660
wing, meat & skin, roasted	1	192	27	7	?	?	524

Poultry, Processed

TURKEY

	Portion	Chol (mg)	Total Fat(g)	Satur'd Fat(g)	Mono Fat(g)	Poly Fat(g)	Total Calor
gravy & turkey, frozen	5 oz	?	4	1	?	?	95
prebasted breast, meat & skin, roasted	½ breast	359	30	8	?	?	1,087
thigh, meat & skin, roasted	1	194	27	8	?	?	494
patties, breaded, battered, fried	2¼ oz	?	12	?	?	?	181
patties, breaded, battered, fried	3.33 oz	?	17	?	?	?	266
roasts, boneless, frozen, seasoned, light & dark meat, roasted	0.43 lb	103	11	?	?	?	304
roasts, boneless, frozen, seasoned, light & dark meat, roasted	1.72 lb	413	45	?	?	?	1,213
breaded, battered, fried	1 stick = 2¼ oz	?	11	?	?	?	178

MECHANICALLY DEBONED POULTRY

	Portion	Chol (mg)	Total Fat(g)	Satur'd Fat(g)	Mono Fat(g)	Poly Fat(g)	Total Calor
from broiler backs & necks							
w/skin, raw	½ lb	?	56	17	?	?	616
w/out skin, raw	½ lb	?	35	11	?	?	450

	Portion	Chol (mg)	Total Fat(g)	Satur'd Fat(g)	Mono Fat(g)	Poly Fat(g)	Total Calor
from mature hens, raw	½ lb	324	45	11	?	?	551

■ BRAND NAME

Poultry

Louis Rich
BREADED ITEMS

turkey nuggets (80% fat free)	1 oz	10	4	?	?	?	60
turkey sticks (80% fat free)	1 oz	10	5	?	?	?	80
turkey patties (80% fat free)	1 oz	30	12	?	?	?	210

BREAST OF TURKEY (FULLY COOKED, SKINLESS)

hickory smoked (98% fat free)	1 oz	10	<1	?	?	?	30
honey roasted (98% fat free)	1 oz	10	<1	?	?	?	30
oven roasted (98% fat free)	1 oz	10	<1	?	?	?	25

FRESH TURKEY CUTS

breast	1 oz	20	2	?	?	?	45
breast roast	1 oz	20	<1	?	?	?	40
breast steaks	1 oz	20	<1	?	?	?	40
breast tenderloins/ tenderloin steaks	1 oz	20	<1	?	?	?	40
drumsticks	1 oz	30	3	?	?	?	55
thighs	1 oz	30	4	?	?	?	65
wings	1 oz	30	3	?	?	?	55

FRESH WHOLE TURKEY (EXCLUDING GIBLETS)

regular	1 oz	25	2	?	?	?	50

GROUND ITEMS

fresh ground turkey w/natural flavorings (90% fat free)	1 oz	25	2	?	?	?	50
ground turkey (85% fat free)	1 oz	30	3	?	?	?	60
ground turkey (90% fat free)	1 oz	25	3	?	?	?	50
turkey breakfast sausage (85% fat free)	1 oz	25	3	?	?	?	55

Tyson/Holly Farms
FULLY COOKED ROASTED CHICKEN

wings	1 oz	45	5	?	?	?	70
drumsticks	1 oz	40	3	?	?	?	50

	Portion	Chol (mg)	Total Fat(g)	Satur'd Fat(g)	Mono Fat(g)	Poly Fat(g)	Total Calor
thighs	1 oz	40	5	?	?	?	70
breast	1 oz	15	3	?	?	?	50
breast fillet	1 oz	15	2	?	?	?	50
whole bird	1 oz	30	4	?	?	?	60
CORNISH HENS							
regular	3.5 oz	155	15	?	?	?	250
FULLY COOKED WINGS							
barbeque	3.5 oz	?	14	?	?	?	220
hot & spicy	3.5 oz	?	14	?	?	?	220
Italian	3.5 oz	?	14	?	?	?	220
teriyaki	3.5 oz	?	14	?	?	?	220
READY-TO-COOK BREAST FILLETS							
lemon pepper	3.75 oz	?	2	?	?	?	130
barbeque	3.75 oz	?	1	?	?	?	120
teriyaki	3.75 oz	?	2	?	?	?	120
Italian	3.75 oz	?	2	?	?	?	130
FROZEN BONELESS ITEMS							
breast chunks	3 oz	30	17	?	?	?	240
chick 'n cheddar	2.6 oz	40	15	?	?	?	220
southern fried breast fillets	3 oz	25	11	?	?	?	220
breast patties	2.6 oz	35	15	?	?	?	220
southern fried breast patties	2.6 oz	35	15	?	?	?	220
breast fillets	3 oz	25	9	?	?	?	190
diced meat	3 oz	70	3	?	?	?	130
southern fried chick 'n chunks	2.6 oz	35	15	?	?	?	220
grilled chicken sandwich	per sandwich	32	9	?	?	?	230
breast tenders	3 oz	?	13	?	?	?	220
microwave breast sandwich	per sandwich	?	12	?	?	?	275
BBQ beef	per sandwich	30	3	?	?	?	200
tenders	3.5 oz	?	11	?	?	?	230
chunk	3.5 oz	?	15	?	?	?	220
BBQ chicken sandwich	per sandwich	50	4	?	?	?	208

	Portion	Chol (mg)	Total Fat(g)	Satur'd Fat(g)	Mono Fat(g)	Poly Fat(g)	Total Calor

❏ **POULTRY SPREADS** *See* PROCESSED MEAT & POULTRY PRODUCTS

❏ **PRESERVES** *See* FRUIT SPREADS

❏ **PROCESSED MEAT & POULTRY PRODUCTS: SAUSAGES, FRANKFURTERS, COLD CUTS, PÂTÉS, & SPREADS**
See also BEEF, FRESH & CURED
See also PORK, FRESH & CURED
See also POULTRY, FRESH & PROCESSED

	Portion	Chol (mg)	Total Fat(g)	Satur'd Fat(g)	Mono Fat(g)	Poly Fat(g)	Total Calor
bacon & Canadian style bacon *See* PORK, FRESH & CURED							
barbecue loaf, pork, beef	1 oz	11	3	1	?	?	49
beef sausage, smoked	1 oz	19	8	3	?	?	89
beerwurst, beer salami							
beef	0.8 oz	13	7	3	?	?	75
pork	0.8 oz	13	4	1	?	?	55
blood sausage	1 oz	34	10	4	?	?	107
bockwurst, raw (pork, veal)	2½ oz	?	18	7	?	?	200
bockwurst, raw (pork, veal)	1 oz	?	8	3	?	?	87
bologna							
beef	1 oz	16	8	3	?	?	89
beef & pork	1 oz	16	8	3	?	?	89
pork	1 oz	17	6	2	?	?	70
turkey	1 oz	28	4	?	?	?	57
bratwurst, cooked, pork	1 oz	17	7	3	?	?	85
braunschweiger (a liver sausage), pork	1 oz	44	9	3	?	?	102
breakfast strips *See* BEEF, FRESH & CURED; PORK, FRESH & CURED							
brotwurst, pork, beef	1 oz	18	8	3	?	?	92
chicken, canned, boned, w/broth	5 oz	?	11	3	?	?	234
chicken roll, light meat	2 oz	28	4	1	?	?	90
chicken spread, canned	1 T	?	2	?	?	?	25
chorizo, pork & beef	1 oz	?	11	4	?	?	?
corned beef, braised *See* BEEF, FRESH & CURED							
corned beef, canned	1 oz	24	4	2	?	?	71
corned beef loaf, jellied	1 oz	12	2	1	?	?	46
dried beef	1 oz	?	1	tr	?	?	47
Dutch brand loaf, pork, beef	1 oz	13	5	2	?	?	68

	Portion	Chol (mg)	Total Fat(g)	Satur'd Fat(g)	Mono Fat(g)	Poly Fat(g)	Total Calor
frankfurter							
beef	2 oz	27	17	7	?	?	184
beef & pork	2 oz	29	17	6	?	?	183
chicken	1.6 oz	45	9	2	?	?	116
turkey	1.6 oz	48	8	?	?	?	102
ham, chopped	1 oz	15	5	2	?	?	65
ham, chopped, canned	1 oz	14	5	2	?	?	68
ham, minced	1 oz	20	6	2	?	?	75
ham & cheese loaf or roll	1 oz	16	6	2	?	?	73
ham & cheese spread	1 T	9	3	1	?	?	37
ham & cheese spread	1 oz	17	5	2	?	?	69
ham salad spread	1 T	6	2	1	?	?	32
ham salad spread	1 oz	10	4	1	?	?	61
head cheese, pork	1 oz	23	4	1	?	?	60
honey loaf, pork, beef	1 oz	10	1	tr	?	?	36
honey roll sausage, beef	1 oz	14	3	1	?	?	52
Italian sausage, pork							
raw	4 oz	86	35	13	?	?	391
cooked	2.9 oz	65	21	8	?	?	268
kielbasa, pork, beef	1 oz	19	8	3	?	?	88
knockwurst, pork, beef	1 oz	16	8	3	?	?	87
lebanon bologna, beef	1 oz	19	4	2	?	?	64
liver cheese, pork	1 oz	49	7	3	?	?	86
liver sausage (liverwurst), pork	1 oz	45	8	3	?	?	93
luncheon meat							
beef, jellied	1 oz	?	1	tr	?	?	31
beef, loaved	1 oz	18	7	3	?	?	87
beef, thin-sliced	1 oz	12	1	tr	?	?	35
pork, beef	1 oz	15	9	3	?	?	100
pork, canned	1 oz	18	9	3	?	?	95
luncheon sausage, pork & beef	1 oz	18	6	2	?	?	74
mortadella, beef, pork	about ½ oz (15 per 8 oz pkg)	8	4	1	?	?	47
mortadella, beef, pork	1 oz	16	7	3	?	?	88
New England brand sausage, pork, beef	0.8 oz	11	2	1	?	?	37
New England brand sausage, pork, beef	1 oz	14	2	1	?	?	46
olive loaf, pork	1 oz	11	5	2	?	?	67
pastrami, beef See BEEF, FRESH & CURED							
pastrami, turkey	2 oz	?	4	1	?	?	80
paté							
chicken liver, canned	1 T	?	2	?	?	?	26
goose liver, smoked, canned	1 T	20	6	?	?	?	60

	Portion	Chol (mg)	Total Fat(g)	Satur'd Fat(g)	Mono Fat(g)	Poly Fat(g)	Total Calor
liver (not specified), canned	1 T	?	4	?	?	?	41
peppered loaf, pork, beef	1 oz	13	2	1	?	?	42
pepperoni, pork, beef	8.8 oz	?110		40	?	?	1,248
pickle & pimento loaf, pork	1 oz	10	6	2	?	?	74
picnic loaf, pork, beef	1 oz	11	5	2	?	?	66
Polish sausage, pork	1 oz	20	8	3	?	?	92
pork & beef sausage, fresh, cooked	about 1 oz	?	10	4	?	?	107
pork & beef sausage, fresh, cooked	about ½ oz	?	5	2	?	?	52
pork sausage, country-style, fresh, cooked	about 1 oz	22	8	3	?	?	100
pork sausage, country-style, fresh, cooked	about ½ oz	11	4	1	?	?	48
salami							
cooked							
beef	1 oz	17	6	2	?	?	72
beef & pork	1 oz	18	6	2	?	?	71
turkey	2 slices = 2 oz	46	8	?	?	?	111
dry or hard							
pork	4 oz	?	38	13	?	?	460
pork, beef	4 oz	89	39	14	?	?	472
sandwich spread							
pork, beef	1 T	6	3	1	?	?	35
poultry salad	1 T	4	2	tr	?	?	26
smoked chopped beef	1 oz	13	1	1	?	?	38
smoked link sausage							
pork, grilled	2.4 oz	46	22	8	?	?	265
pork, grilled	about ½ oz	11	5	2	?	?	62
pork & beef	2.4 oz	48	21	7	?	?	229
pork & beef	about ½ oz	11	5	2	?	?	54
flour & nonfat dry milk added	2.4 oz	59	15	5	?	?	182
flour & nonfat dry milk added	about ½ oz	14	3	1	?	?	43
nonfat dry milk added	2.4 oz	44	19	7	?	?	213
nonfat dry milk added	about ½ oz	10	4	2	?	?	50
Thuringer, cervelat, summer sausage: beef, pork	1 oz	19	8	3	?	?	98
turkey							
canned, boned, w/broth	5 oz	?	10	3	?	?	231

	Portion	Chol (mg)	Total Fat(g)	Satur'd Fat(g)	Mono Fat(g)	Poly Fat(g)	Total Calor
diced, light & dark, seasoned	1 oz	?	2	1	?	?	39
turkey breast meat	0.7 oz	9	tr	tr	?	?	23
turkey ham (cured, turkey thigh meat)	2 oz	?	3	1	?	?	73
turkey loaf, breast meat	1½ oz	17	1	tr	?	?	47
turkey pastrami *See* PASTRAMI, TURKEY, ABOVE							
turkey roll, light meat	1 oz	12	2	1	?	?	42
turkey roll, light & dark meat	1 oz	16	2	1	?	?	42
Vienna sausage, canned, beef & pork	about 0.6 oz	8	4	1	?	?	45

▪ BRAND NAME

Carl Buddig Luncheon Meats
LUNCHEON MEATS

beef	1 oz	20	2	1	?	<1	40
corned beef	1 oz	20	2	1	?	<1	40
chicken	1 oz	20	4	2	?	1	60
ham	1 oz	20	3	1	?	<1	50
pastrami	1 oz	20	2	1	?	<1	40
turkey	1 oz	15	3	1	?	1	50
turkey ham	1 oz	15	2	1	?	1	40
honey ham	1 oz	20	3	1	?	<1	50

Louis Rich
COLD CUTS

chopped turkey ham, water added (92% fat free)	1 slice	25	2	?	?	?	45
deluxe oven roasted chicken breast (96% fat free)	1 slice	15	1	?	?	?	30
honey cured turkey ham (96% fat free)	1 slice	15	<1	?	?	?	25
honey roasted turkey breast (95% fat free)	1 slice	10	1	?	?	?	35
mild turkey bologna (82% fat free)	1 slice	20	5	?	?	?	60
oven roasted turkey breast (97% fat free)	1 slice	10	<1	?	?	?	30
oven roasted white chicken (93% fat free)	1 slice	15	1	?	?	?	35
smoked turkey (96% fat free)	1 slice	15	1	?	?	?	30
turkey bologna (82% fat free)	1 slice	25	5	?	?	?	60

	Portion	Chol (mg)	Total Fat(g)	Satur'd Fat(g)	Mono Fat(g)	Poly Fat(g)	Total Calor
turkey cotto salami (85% fat free)	1 slice	25	4	?	?	?	55
turkey ham, water added (round) (95% fat free)	1 slice	20	1	?	?	?	30
turkey luncheon loaf (89% fat free)	1 slice	15	3	?	?	?	45
turkey pastrami (square) (96% fat free)	1 slice	15	<1	?	?	?	25
turkey summer sausage (85% fat free)	1 slice	25	4	?	?	?	55

DELI, THIN BRAND (THIN SLICED COLD CUTS)

	Portion	Chol (mg)	Total Fat(g)	Satur'd Fat(g)	Mono Fat(g)	Poly Fat(g)	Total Calor
oven roasted chicken breast (96% fat free)	1 slice	5	<1	?	?	?	10
oven roasted turkey breast (97% fat free)	1 slice	5	<1	?	?	?	10
smoked turkey breast (98% fat free)	1 slice	5	<1	?	?	?	10
turkey ham (96% fat free)	1 slice	5	<1	?	?	?	15
turkey pastrami (96% fat free)	1 slice	5	<1	?	?	?	10

LUNCH BREAKS

	Portion	Chol (mg)	Total Fat(g)	Satur'd Fat(g)	Mono Fat(g)	Poly Fat(g)	Total Calor
oven roasted turkey breast & cheddar	1 pkg	70	26	?	?	?	410
turkey ham & Swiss	1 pkg	75	22	?	?	?	380
turkey salami & cheddar	1 pkg	85	29	?	?	?	430

TURKEY BACON

	Portion	Chol (mg)	Total Fat(g)	Satur'd Fat(g)	Mono Fat(g)	Poly Fat(g)	Total Calor
80% fat free	1 slice	10	2	?	?	?	35

TURKEY FRANKS

	Portion	Chol (mg)	Total Fat(g)	Satur'd Fat(g)	Mono Fat(g)	Poly Fat(g)	Total Calor
bun-length franks (80% fat free)	1 frank	55	10	?	?	?	130
cheese franks (80% fat free)	1 frank	45	9	?	?	?	110
regular (80% fat free)	1 frank	40	8	?	?	?	100

TURKEY HAM & CHUNK SPECIALTIES

	Portion	Chol (mg)	Total Fat(g)	Satur'd Fat(g)	Mono Fat(g)	Poly Fat(g)	Total Calor
oven roasted turkey breast (97% fat free)	1 oz	10	1	?	?	?	30
smoked turkey breast (96% fat free)	1 oz	10	1	?	?	?	35
turkey bologna (82% fat free)	1 oz	25	5	?	?	?	60
turkey ham (95% fat free)	1 oz	20	1	?	?	?	35
turkey pastrami (96% fat free)	1 oz	20	1	?	?	?	35

	Portion	Chol (mg)	Total Fat (g)	Satur'd Fat (g)	Mono Fat (g)	Poly Fat (g)	Total Calor
turkey salami (85% fat free)	1 oz	20	4	?	?	?	55

TURKEY SMOKED SAUSAGE

	Portion	Chol (mg)	Total Fat (g)	Satur'd Fat (g)	Mono Fat (g)	Poly Fat (g)	Total Calor
turkey & cheddar smoked sausage (90% fat free)	1 oz	20	3	?	?	?	45
turkey polska kielbasa (90% fat free)	1 oz	20	2	?	?	?	40
turkey smoked sausage (90% fat free)	1 oz	20	2	?	?	?	40

Oscar Mayer

CLASSIC COLD CUTS

	Portion	Chol (mg)	Total Fat (g)	Satur'd Fat (g)	Mono Fat (g)	Poly Fat (g)	Total Calor
braunschweiger, liver sausage	1 slice	50	9	?	?	?	95
chopped ham w/natural juices (87% fat free)	1 slice	15	4	?	?	?	55
corned beef loaf, jellied (93% fat free)	1 slice	15	2	?	?	?	40
cotto salami	1 slice	20	4	?	?	?	55
cotto salami, beef	1 slice	20	3	?	?	?	45
Genoa salami	1 slice	10	3	?	?	?	35
ham, chopped, prepared w/natural juices (87% fat free)	1 slice	15	4	?	?	?	55
ham & cheese loaf	1 slice	20	5	?	?	?	70
head cheese	1 slice	25	4	?	?	?	55
liver cheese, pork fat wrapped	1 slice	80	10	?	?	?	115
luncheon loaf	1 slice	20	6	?	?	?	75
New England brand sausage (94% fat free)	1 slice	15	1	?	?	?	30
old fashioned loaf	1 slice	15	5	?	?	?	65
salami for beer, beef	1 slice	15	6	?	?	?	65
salami, hard	1 slice	10	3	?	?	?	35
summer sausage (Thuringer Cervelat)	1 slice	20	6	?	?	?	70
summer sausage, beef (Thuringer Cervelat)	1 slice	20	6	?	?	?	70

"OUR LEANEST CUTS" COLD CUTS

	Portion	Chol (mg)	Total Fat (g)	Satur'd Fat (g)	Mono Fat (g)	Poly Fat (g)	Total Calor
beef, smoked (97% fat free)	1 slice	5	<1	?	?	?	15
Canadian style bacon (95% fat free)	1 slice	10	<1	?	?	?	25
chicken breast, oven roasted (98% fat free)	1 slice	10	<1	?	?	?	25
chicken breast, smoked (98% fat free)	1 slice	10	<1	?	?	?	25

	Portion	Chol (mg)	Total Fat(g)	Satur'd Fat(g)	Mono Fat(g)	Poly Fat(g)	Total Calor
corned beef (98% fat free)	1 slice	10	<1	?	?	?	15
ham, baked w/natural juices (97% fat free)	1 slice	10	<1	?	?	?	20
ham, boiled w/natural juices (96% fat free)	1 slice	10	<1	?	?	?	25
ham, cracked black pepper w/natural juices (96% fat free)	1 slice	10	<1	?	?	?	20
ham, honey w/natural juices (96% fat free)	1 slice	10	<1	?	?	?	25
ham, lower salt, water added (95% fat free)	1 slice	10	<1	?	?	?	20
honey loaf (96% fat free)	1 slice	15	<1	?	?	?	35
pastrami (98% fat free)	1 slice	5	<1	?	?	?	15
turkey breast, oven roasted (97% fat free)	1 slice	5	<1	?	?	?	20
PORK SAUSAGE							
pork sausage link	1 cooked link	20	7	?	?	?	85
SMOKIES							
smokies link sausage	1 link	30	11	?	?	?	125
smokies, beef	1 link	25	11	?	?	?	125
SPREADS							
branschweiger, German brand	28 gr	45	9	?	?	?	95
branschweiger, liver sausage	28 gr	45	9	?	?	?	95
sandwich spread	28 gr	10	5	?	?	?	65
weiners, lite (80% fat free)	1 link	30	11	?	?	?	130
weiners, little	1 link	5	3	?	?	?	30
BOLOGNA							
regular	1 slice	20	8	?	?	?	90
regular w/cheese	1 slice	15	7	?	?	?	75
beef	1 slice	20	8	?	?	?	90
beef Lebanon	1 slice	15	3	?	?	?	45
beef light (80% fat free)	1 slice	15	5	?	?	?	65
garlic	1 slice	25	12	?	?	?	130
light (80% fat free)	1 slice	15	6	?	?	?	65
THIN SLICED							
beef, roast (96% fat free)	1 slice	5	<1	?	?	?	15
chicken, roast (96% fat free)	1 slice	5	<1	?	?	?	15

	Portion	Chol (mg)	Total Fat(g)	Satur'd Fat(g)	Mono Fat(g)	Poly Fat(g)	Total Calor
ham, honey w/natural juices (96% fat free)	1 slice	5	<1	?	?	?	15
ham, smoked cooked w/natural juices (96% fat free)	1 slice	5	<1	?	?	?	15
turkey, roast (96% fat free)	1 slice	5	<1	?	?	?	15
turkey, smoked (98% fat free)	1 slice	5	<1	?	?	?	10
WEINERS & FRANKS							
bacon & cheese hot dogs	1 link	30	13	?	?	?	145
franks, beef	1 link	30	13	?	?	?	130
franks, beef w/cheddar	1 link	30	11	?	?	?	130
franks, beef little	1 link	5	3	?	?	?	30
franks, beef light (80% fat free)	1 link	25	11	?	?	?	135
franks, bun-length, 1/4 lb	1 link	65	34	?	?	?	360
weiners	1 link	30	13	?	?	?	145
Swanson							
white chicken	2 1/2 oz	?	4	?	?	?	100
white turkey	2 1/2 oz	?	1	?	?	?	80
white & dark chicken	2 1/4 oz	?	4	?	?	?	100
Tyson							
SLICED MEATS							
chicken bologna	1 slice	?	.5	?	?	?	44
chicken roll	1 slice	?	.5	?	?	?	26
hickory smoked breast	1 slice	?	.5	?	?	?	26
oven roasted breast	1 slice	?	.5	?	?	?	25
turkey breast	1 slice	?	.4	?	?	?	20
turkey ham	1 slice	?	.2	?	?	?	23
Underwood							
MEAT SPREADS							
chunky chicken	2 1/8 oz	40	9	3	?	2	150
deviled ham	2 1/8 oz	50	19	6	?	2	220
liverwurst	2 1/8 oz	90	15	?	?	?	180
mesquite smoked roast beef	2 1/8 oz	45	11	5	?	<1	126
roast beef	2 1/8 oz	45	11	5	?	<1	140
smoky flavored chicken	2 1/8 oz	40	8	2	?	1	150
LIGHT MEAT SPREADS							
chunky chicken	2 1/8 oz	30	3	1	?	1	80
deviled ham	2 1/8 oz	35	8	1	?	3	120
roast beef	2 1/8 oz	30	6	2	?	<1	90
chunky turkey	2 1/8 oz	25	2	<1	?	<1	75

	Portion	Chol (mg)	Total Fat(g)	Satur'd Fat(g)	Mono Fat(g)	Poly Fat(g)	Total Calor

❏ **PUDDING DESSERTS, FROZEN**
See DESSERTS, FROZEN

❏ **PUDDINGS & PIE FILLINGS**
See DESSERTS: CUSTARDS, GELATINS, PUDDINGS, & PIE FILLINGS

❏ **RELISHES** *See* PICKLES, OLIVES, RELISHES, & CHUTNEYS

❏ **RICE & GRAINS, PLAIN & PREPARED**
See also VEGETABLES, PLAIN & PREPARED

	Portion	Chol (mg)	Total Fat(g)	Satur'd Fat(g)	Mono Fat(g)	Poly Fat(g)	Total Calor
barley, pearled, light, uncooked	1 c	0	2	tr	?	?	700
bulgur, uncooked	1 c	0	3	1	?	?	600
popcorn *See* SNACKS							
rice							
brown cooked, hot	1 c	0	1	tr	?	?	230
white enriched							
raw	1 c	0	1	tr	?	?	670
cooked, hot	1 c	6	tr	tr	?	?	225
instant, ready-to-serve, hot	1 c	0	0	tr	?	?	180
parboiled, raw	1 c	0	1	tr	?	?	685
parboiled, cooked, hot	1 c	0	tr	tr	?	?	185

■ **BRAND NAMES**

Arrowhead Mills
PLAIN RICE & GRAINS

	Portion	Chol (mg)	Total Fat(g)	Satur'd Fat(g)	Mono Fat(g)	Poly Fat(g)	Total Calor
barley, pearled	2 oz	0	1	?	?	?	200
barley flakes	2 oz	0	1	?	?	?	200
buckwheat groats							
brown	2 oz	0	1	?	?	?	190
white	2 oz	0	1	?	?	?	190
bulgur wheat	2 oz	0	1	?	?	?	200
corn							
blue	2 oz	0	3	?	?	?	210
yellow	2 oz	0	2	?	?	?	210
millet	2 oz	0	1	?	?	?	90
oat flakes	2 oz	0	4	?	?	?	220
oat groats	2 oz	0	4	?	?	?	220
quinoa	2 oz	0	3	?	?	?	200

	Portion	Chol (mg)	Total Fat (g)	Satur'd Fat (g)	Mono Fat (g)	Poly Fat (g)	Total Calor
rice							
brown							
long	2 oz	0	1	?	?	?	200
long basmati	2 oz	0	1	?	?	?	200
medium	2 oz	0	1	?	?	?	200
short	2 oz	0	1	?	?	?	200
rye	2 oz	0	1	?	?	?	190
rye flakes	2 oz	0	1	?	?	?	190
wheat, hard, red, winter	2 oz	0	1	?	?	?	190
wheat, soft pastry	2 oz	0	1	?	?	?	190
wheat flakes	2 oz	0	1	?	?	?	210

PREPARED RICE & GRAINS

	Portion	Chol (mg)	Total Fat (g)	Satur'd Fat (g)	Mono Fat (g)	Poly Fat (g)	Total Calor
quick brown rice	2 oz	0	1	?	?	?	200
Spanish style quick brown rice	¼ of 5.65 oz pkg	0	1	?	?	?	150
vegetable herb quick brown rice	¼ of 5.6 oz pkg	0	1	?	?	?	150
wild rice & herbs quick brown rice	¼ of 5.35 oz pkg	0	1	?	?	?	140

Birds Eye International Rice Recipes

	Portion	Chol (mg)	Total Fat (g)	Satur'd Fat (g)	Mono Fat (g)	Poly Fat (g)	Total Calor
country style	3.3 oz	0	0	?	?	?	90
French style	3.3 oz	0	0	0	?	?	110
Spanish style	3.3 oz	0	0	?	?	?	110

Carolina Rice

	Portion	Chol (mg)	Total Fat (g)	Satur'd Fat (g)	Mono Fat (g)	Poly Fat (g)	Total Calor
extra long grain, enriched	about ½ c cooked	0	0	0	?	?	100
long grain, enriched, precooked instant	about ½ c cooked	0	0	0	?	?	110

Fearn

	Portion	Chol (mg)	Total Fat (g)	Satur'd Fat (g)	Mono Fat (g)	Poly Fat (g)	Total Calor
naturfresh corn germ	¼ c or ¹⁄₁₀ of 10 oz bag	0	7	1	?	?	130
naturfresh raw wheat germ	¼ c or ¹⁄₁₀ of 10 oz bag	0	3	tr	?	?	100

Hain

3-GRAIN SIDE DISHES

	Portion	Chol (mg)	Total Fat (g)	Satur'd Fat (g)	Mono Fat (g)	Poly Fat (g)	Total Calor
rice almondine	½ c	0	5	?	?	?	130
chicken meatless style	½ c	0	1	?	?	?	100
herb	½ c	0	1	?	?	?	80
rice oriental 3-grain goodness	½ c	?	5	?	?	?	120

Mahatma

RICE MIXES

	Portion	Chol (mg)	Total Fat (g)	Satur'd Fat (g)	Mono Fat (g)	Poly Fat (g)	Total Calor
almond beef	½ c	?	0	?	?	?	100
classic pilaf	½ c	?	0	?	?	?	100
wild	½ c	?	0	?	?	?	100
sesame chicken	½ c	?	0	?	?	?	100

	Portion	Chol (mg)	Total Fat(g)	Satur'd Fat(g)	Mono Fat(g)	Poly Fat(g)	Total Calor
saffron yellow	½ c	?	0	?	?	?	100
authentic Spanish	½ c	?	0	?	?	?	100
red beans & rice	½ c	?	0	?	?	?	200
long grain rice, enriched	about ½ c cooked	0	0	0	?	?	100
long grain, enriched, precooked instant	about ½ c cooked	0	0	0	?	?	110
natural long grain rice, brown	about ½ c cooked	0	0	0	?	?	110
Minute Rice							
boil-in-a-bag rice w/o salt or butter	½ c	0	0	?	?	?	90
premium long grain rice w/o salt or butter	⅔ c	0	0	?	?	?	120
rice mix							
drumstick, w/butter (salted)	½	10	4	?	?	?	150
fried rice, w/oil	½ c	0	5	?	?	?	160
long grain & wild rice w/butter (salted)	½ c	10	4	?	?	?	150
rib roast w/butter (salted)	½ c	10	4	?	?	?	150
microwave dishes							
beef flavored rice, family size, w/butter (salted)	½ c	10	3	?	?	?	160
cheddar cheese, broccoli & rice, family size, w/butter (salted)	½ c	10	5	?	?	?	160
chicken flavored rice, family size, w/butter (salted)	½ c	10	4	?	?	?	160
French style rice pilaf, family size, w/butter (salted)	½ c	10	3	?	?	?	130
Quaker Oats							
Scotch brand medium pearled barley	¼ c	?	1	?	?	?	172
Scotch brand quick pearled barley	⅓ c	?	1	?	?	?	172
Rice-A-Roni							
SAVORY CLASSICS							
broccoli au gratin	1.12 oz dry mix	4	3	1	1	<1	129
chicken Florentine	1.12 oz dry mix	1	1	<1	<1	<1	108
creamy parmesan & herbs	1.22 oz dry mix	7	4	1	1	<1	145

	Portion	Chol (mg)	Total Fat(g)	Satur'd Fat(g)	Mono Fat(g)	Poly Fat(g)	Total Calor
garden pilaf	1.12 oz dry mix	1	1	<1	<1	<1	113
green bean almondine	1.25 oz dry mix	6	5	1	1	<1	152
spring vegetables & cheese	1.22 oz dry mix	6	4	1	1	<1	141
zesty cheddar	1.30 oz dry mix	6	4	1	1	<1	151

RICE & PASTA MIXES

	Portion	Chol (mg)	Total Fat(g)	Satur'd Fat(g)	Mono Fat(g)	Poly Fat(g)	Total Calor
beef flavor	1.33 oz dry mix	1	1	<1	<1	0	135
chicken flavor	1.33 oz dry mix	1	1	<1	<1	<1	136
chicken & mushroom	1.25 oz dry mix	1	1	<1	<1	<1	129
chicken & vegetables	1.2 oz dry mix	?	1	<1	<1	<1	124
fried rice w/almonds	1 oz dry mix	<1	1	<1	<1	<1	106
herb & butter	1 oz dry mix	1	1	<1	<1	<1	105
rice pilaf	1.45 oz dry mix	1	1	<1	<1	<1	147
risotto	1.5 oz dry mix	2	1	<1	<1	<1	157
Spanish rice	1 oz dry mix	1	1	<1	<1	<1	107
yellow rice	2 oz dry mix	1	1	<1	<1	<1	196

River

	Portion	Chol (mg)	Total Fat(g)	Satur'd Fat(g)	Mono Fat(g)	Poly Fat(g)	Total Calor
enriched rice	about ½ c cooked	0	0	0	?	?	100
natural long grain rice, brown	about ½ c cooked	0	0	0	?	?	110

Success

	Portion	Chol (mg)	Total Fat(g)	Satur'd Fat(g)	Mono Fat(g)	Poly Fat(g)	Total Calor
enriched, precooked, natural long grain rice	about ½ c cooked	0	0	0	?	?	90
10-minute brown	about ½ c	0	0	?	?	?	103
flavored rice mixes							
au gratin herb	½ c	?	0	?	?	?	100
broccoli & cheese	½ c	?	0	<1	?	?	120
brown & wild	½ c	?	0	?	?	?	120
beef oriental	½ c	?	0	?	?	?	100
classic chicken	½ c	?	0	?	?	?	100
chicken almondine	½ c	?	2	?	?	?	110
pilaf	½ c	?	0	?	?	?	120
saffron yellow	½ c	?	0	?	?	?	100
Spanish	½ c	?	0	?	?	?	110

	Portion	Chol (mg)	Total Fat(g)	Satur'd Fat(g)	Mono Fat(g)	Poly Fat(g)	Total Calor
Water Maid							
enriched rice	about ½ c cooked	0	0	0	?	?	100

❏ ROLLS *See* BREADS, ROLLS, BISCUITS, & MUFFINS

❏ SALAD DRESSINGS, MAYONNAISE, VINEGAR, & DIPS

Mayonnaise Commercial

	Portion	Chol (mg)	Total Fat(g)	Satur'd Fat(g)	Mono Fat(g)	Poly Fat(g)	Total Calor
mayonnaise							
safflower & soybean	1 T	?	11	1	?	?	99
soybean	1 T	8	11	2	?	?	99
mayonnaise, imitation							
milk, cream	1 T	6	1	tr	?	?	15
soybean	1 T	4	3	1	?	?	35
soybean w/out cholesterol	1 T	0	7	1	?	?	68
mayonnaise-type dressing	1 T	4	5	1	?	?	57
low-cal	1 T	?	2	?	?	?	19
bleu cheese commercial							
regular	1 T	?	8	2	?	?	77
low-cal	1 T	?	9	?	?	?	11
Caesar, commercial	1 T	?	7	?	?	?	70
cole slaw, commercial low cal	1 T	?	3	?	?	?	31
cooked, homemade	1 T	?	2	1	?	?	25
French commercial							
regular	1 T	?	6	2	?	?	67
creamy	1 T	?	7	?	?	?	70
low-cal	1 T	1	1	tr	?	?	22
homemade	1 T	?	10	2	?	?	88
Green Goddess, commercial	1 T	?	7	?	?	?	68
low-cal	1 T	?	2	?	?	?	27
Italian, commercial							
regular	1 T	?	7	1	?	?	69
creamy	1 T	?	5	?	?	?	52
low-cal	1 T	1	2	tr	?	?	16
Russian							
regular	1 T	?	8	1	?	?	76
low-cal	1 T	1	1	tr	?	?	23
poppy seed	1 oz	?	11	?	?	?	121

	Portion	Chol (mg)	Total Fat(g)	Satur'd Fat(g)	Mono Fat(g)	Poly Fat(g)	Total Calor
sesame seed, commercial	1 T	0	7	1	?	?	68
sweet & sour, commercial	1 T	?	tr	?	?	?	29
Thousand Island, commercial							
regular	1 T	?	6	1	?	?	59
low-cal	1 T	2	2	tr	?	?	24
vinegar & oil, homemade	1 T	?	8	2	?	?	72
vinegar (redwine) & oil, commercial	1 oz	?	9	?	?	?	103

Vinegar

cider	1 T	0	0	0	?	?	tr
distilled	1 T	0	0	0	?	?	2

▪ BRAND NAME

Frito-Lay
dips

cheese	1 oz	5	3	?	?	?	45
jalapeño bean	1 oz	0	1	?	?	?	30
French onion	1 oz	10	5	?	?	?	60
picante	1 oz	0	0	?	?	?	10

Good Seasons Salad Dressing Mixes

bleu cheese & herbs w/vinegar, water, & salad oil	1 T	0	8	?	?	?	70
buttermilk farm style w/whole milk & mayonnaise	1 T	5	6	?	?	?	60
cheese garlic w/vinegar, water, & salad oil	1 T	0	8	?	?	?	70
cheese Italian w/vinegar, water, & salad oil	1 T	0	8	?	?	?	70
classic herb w/vinegar, water, & salad oil	1 T	0	8	?	?	?	70
garlic & herbs w/vinegar, water, & salad oil	1 T	0	8	?	?	?	70
Italian w/vinegar, water & salad oil	1 T	0	8	?	?	?	70
lemon & herbs w/vinegar, water & salad oil	1 T	0	8	?	?	?	70
lite cheese Italian w/vinegar, water & salad oil	1 T	0	3	?	?	?	25
lite Italian w/vinegar, water & salad oil	1 T	0	3	?	?	?	25

	Portion	Chol (mg)	Total Fat(g)	Satur'd Fat(g)	Mono Fat(g)	Poly Fat(g)	Total Calor
lite Ranch, prepared w/whole milk & mayonnaise	1 T	5	2	?	?	?	30
lite zesty Italian, prepared w/vinegar, water & salad oil	1 T	0	3	?	?	?	25
mild Italian, prepared w/vinegar, water & salad oil	1 T	0	8	?	?	?	70
no oil Italian w/vinegar & water	1 T	0	0	0	?	?	6
Ranch, prepared w/vinegar, whole milk & mayonnaise	1 T	0	0	?	?	?	2
zesty Italian, prepared w/vinegar, water, & salad oil	1 T	0	8	?	?	?	70
Hain							
mayonnaise							
cold processed	1 T	5	12	2	?	7	110
eggless, no salt added	1 T	0	12	2	?	7	110
light, low sodium	1 T	10	6	1	?	4	60
real, no salt added	1 T	5	12	2	?	7	110
safflower	1 T	5	12	1	?	9	110
canola	1 T	5	11	1	?	3	100
reduced calorie canola	1 T	0	5	0	?	2	60
pourable dressings							
creamy Caesar	1 T	<5	6	?	?	?	60
creamy Caesar, low salt	1 T	<5	6	?	?	?	60
creamy French	1 T	0	6	?	?	?	60
creamy Italian	1 T	0	8	?	?	?	80
creamy Italian, no salt added	1 T	0	8	?	?	?	80
cucumber dill	1 T	5	8	?	?	?	80
Dijon vinaigrette	1 T	<5	5	?	?	?	50
garlic & sour cream	1 T	0	7	?	?	?	70
honey & sesame	1 T	0	5	?	?	?	60
Italian & cheese vinaigrette	1 T	<5	6	?	?	?	55
old fashioned buttermilk	1 T	0	7	?	?	?	70
poppy seed rancher's	1 T	<5	7	?	?	?	60
savory herb, no salt added	1 T	0	10	?	?	?	90
Swiss cheese vinaigrette	1 T	<5	7	?	?	?	60
1000 island	1 T	0	5	?	?	?	50
traditional Italian	1 T	0	8	?	?	?	80
traditional Italian, no salt added	1 T	0	6	?	?	?	60

	Portion	Chol (mg)	Total Fat(g)	Satur'd Fat(g)	Mono Fat(g)	Poly Fat(g)	Total Calor
canola oil dressings							
garden tomato vinaigrette	1 T	0	6	?	?	?	60
Italian	1 T	0	5	?	?	?	50
spicy French mustard	1 T	5	5	?	?	?	50
tangy citrus	1 T	0	5	?	?	?	50
no oil dry mixes							
bleu cheese	1 T	<5	1	?	?	?	14
buttermilk	1 T	0	<1	?	?	?	11
Caesar	1 T	0	<1	?	?	?	6
French	1 T	0	0	?	?	?	12
garlic & cheese	1 T	0	<1	?	?	?	6
herb	1 T	0	0	?	?	?	2
Italian	1 T	0	0	?	?	?	2
1000 island	1 T	<1	0	?	?	?	12
Hellman's							
cholesterol-free reduced calorie mayonnaise	1 T	0	5	1	2	2	50
light reduced calorie mayonnaise	1 T	5	5	1	2	2	50
real mayonnaise	1 T	5	11	2	3	5	100
reduced calorie mayonnaise							
cholesterol free	1 T	0	5	<1	?	?	50
light	1 T	5	5	1	?	?	50
sandwich spread	1 T	5	5	1	2	2	50
tartar sauce	1 T	5	8	5	3	1	70
Hollywood							
pourable dressings							
Caesar	1 T	0	7	1	?	3	70
creamy French	1 T	0	7	1	?	3	70
creamy Italian	1 T	0	9	1	?	4	90
Dijon vinaigrette	1 T	0	6	1	?	2	60
Italian	1 T	0	9	1	?	4	90
Italian cheese	1 T	0	8	1	?	3	80
old fashioned buttermilk	1 T	0	8	1	?	3	75
poppy seed rancher's	1 T	?	8	1	?	3	75
thousand island	1 T	5	6	1	?	2	60
mayonnaise							
canola	1 T	5	11	1	?	3	100
regular	1 T	5	12	1	?	8	110
safflower	1 T	5	12	1	?	8	100
Kraft							
dips							
avocado (guacamole)	2 T	0	4	2	?	1	50
bacon & horseradish	2 T	0	5	3	?	1	60
clam	2 T	10	4	1	?	3	60
French onion	2 T	0	4	2	?	1	60
green onion	2 T	0	4	2	?	1	60
jalapeño pepper	2 T	0	4	2	?	1	50

	Portion	Chol (mg)	Total Fat(g)	Satur'd Fat(g)	Mono Fat(g)	Poly Fat(g)	Total Calor
premium bacon & onion	2 T	15	5	3	?	0	60
premium blue cheese	2 T	10	4	2	?	0	50
premium creamy cucmber	2 T	10	4	3	?	0	50
premium creamy onion	2 T	10	4	2	?	0	45
premium creamy French onion	2 T	10	4	2	?	0	45
premium creamy nacho cheese	2 T	10	4	2	?	0	55
viscous dressings							
real mayonnaise	1 T	5	12	2	?	7	100
sandwich spread	1 T	5	5	1	?	3	50
light reduced calorie mayonnaise	1 T	0	5	1	?	3	50
nonfat mayonnaise dressing	1 T	0	0	0	?	0	12
miracle whip							
coleslaw dressing	1 T	5	6	1	?	4	70
salad dressing	1 T	5	7	1	?	4	70
light reduced calorie salad dressing	1 T	0	4	1	?	2	45
free nonfat dressing	1 T	0	0	0	?	0	20
pourable							
Catalina French	1 T	0	5	1	?	3	60
buttermilk creamy	1 T	<5	8	1	?	5	80
chunky blue cheese	1 T	<5	6	3	?	3	60
coleslaw	1 T	10	6	1	?	3	70
creamy cucumber	1 T	0	8	1	?	4	70
creamy Italian w/real sour cream	1 T	0	5	1	?	3	50
French	1 T	5	6	1	?	3	60
golden Caesar	1 T	0	7	1	?	4	70
creamy garlic	1 T	0	5	1	?	3	50
house Italian	1 T	0	6	1	?	3	60
miracle French	1 T	0	6	1	?	3	70
oil & vinegar	1 T	0	8	1	?	4	70
presto Italian	1 T	0	7	1	?	4	70
red wine vinegar & oil	1 T	0	4	1	?	2	60
thousand island	1 T	5	5	1	?	3	60
zesty Italian	1 T	0	5	1	?	3	50
rancher's choice creamy	1 T	5	10	1	?	6	90
roka blue cheese	1 T	10	6	1	?	3	60
thousand island & bacon	1 T	0	6	1	?	3	60
reduced calorie pourable							
Catalina	1 T	0	1	0	?	0	18
bacon & tomato	1 T	0	2	0	?	1	30
buttermilk creamy	1 T	<5	3	0	?	1	30

	Portion	Chol (mg)	Total Fat(g)	Satur'd Fat(g)	Mono Fat(g)	Poly Fat(g)	Total Calor
chunky blue cheese	1 T	<5	2	1	?	1	30
creamy bacon	1 T	0	2	0	?	1	30
creamy Italian	1 T	0	2	0	?	1	25
French	1 T	0	1	0	?	1	20
house Italian	1 T	0	2	0	?	1	30
oil-free Italian	1 T	0	0	0	?	0	4
Russian	1 T	0	1	0	?	1	30
thousand island	1 T	0	1	0	?	1	30
zesty Italian	1 T	0	2	0	?	1	20
rancher's choice creamy	1 T	5	3	0	?	1	30
roka blue cheese	1 T	5	1	1	?	0	16
nonfat pourable							
free Catalina	1 T	0	0	0	?	0	16
free French	1 T	0	0	0	?	0	20
free Italian	1 T	0	0	0	?	0	6
free ranch	1 T	0	0	0	?	0	16
free thousand island	1 T	0	0	0	?	0	20
Regina							
wine vinegars, all flavors	1 fl oz	?	0	?	?	?	4
Seven Seas							
buttermilk	1 T	5	8	1	?	5	80
creamy French	1 T	0	6	1	?	3	60
thousand island creamy	1 T	5	5	1	?	3	50
viva herb & spice	1 T	0	6	1	?	4	60
viva Italian	1 T	0	5	1	?	3	50
viva ranch	1 T	5	8	1	?	5	80
viva red wine vinegar & oil	1 T	0	7	1	?	4	70
creamy Italian	1 T	0	7	1	?	4	70
reduced calorie							
buttermilk recipe ranch! light	1 T	0	5	1	?	3	50
thousand island! light	1 T	5	2	0	?	1	30
viva creamy Italian! light	1 T	0	4	1	?	2	45
French! light	1 T	0	3	0	?	1	35
viva herb & spices! light	1 T	0	3	0	?	1	30
viva Italian! light	1 T	0	3	0	?	2	30
viva ranch! light	1 T	5	5	1	?	2	50
viva red wine! vinegar & oil light	1 T	0	4	1	?	3	45
nonfat							
free ranch	1 T	0	0	0	?	0	16
free red wine vinegar	1 T	0	0	0	?	0	6
free viva	1 T	0	0	0	?	0	4
Weight Watchers							
mayonnaise							
regular	1 T	5	5	1	?	3	50
cholesterol free	1 T	0	5	1	?	3	50

	Portion	Chol (mg)	Total Fat(g)	Satur'd Fat(g)	Mono Fat(g)	Poly Fat(g)	Total Calor
low sodium	1 T	5	5	1	?	3	50
whipped dressing	1 T	0	4	1	?	2	45
creamy Italian	1 T	5	5	1	?	3	50
thousand island/Russian	1 T	5	5	1	?	3	50
mixes							
creamy ranch	1 T	?	?	?	?	?	25
Italian style	1 T	?	?	?	?	?	6
creamy Italian	1 T	?	?	?	?	?	12
Caesar salad	1 T	?	?	?	?	?	4
tomato vinaigrette	1 T	?	?	?	?	?	8
French style	1 T	?	?	?	?	?	10
creamy cucumber	1 T	?	?	?	?	?	18
creamy peppercorn	1 T	?	?	?	?	?	8

❏ **SALADS, COMMERCIALLY PREPARED**
See FAST FOODS; FRUIT, FRESH
& PROCESSED; VEGETABLES, PLAIN
& PREPARED

❏ **SAUCES, DESSERT** *See* DESSERT
SAUCES, SYRUPS, & TOPPINGS

❏ **SAUCES, GRAVIES, & CONDIMENTS**
See also FRUIT, FRESH & PROCESSED
See also PICKLES, OLIVES, RELISHES, & CHUTNEYS

Condiments

	Portion	Chol (mg)	Total Fat(g)	Satur'd Fat(g)	Mono Fat(g)	Poly Fat(g)	Total Calor
catsup	1 c	0	1	tr	?	?	290
mustard, prepared, yellow	1 t	0	tr	tr	?	?	5

Gravies

	Portion	Chol (mg)	Total Fat(g)	Satur'd Fat(g)	Mono Fat(g)	Poly Fat(g)	Total Calor
au jus							
canned	1 c	1	tr	tr	?	?	38
dehydrated, prepared w/water	1 c	1	1	tr	?	?	19
beef, canned	1 c	7	5	3	?	?	124
brown, dehydrated, prepared w/water	1 c	tr	tr	tr	?	?	9
chicken							
canned	1 c	5	14	3	?	?	189
dehydrated, prepared w/water	1 c	3	2	1	?	?	83
mushroom							
canned	1 c	0	6	1	?	?	120

	Portion	Chol (mg)	Total Fat(g)	Satur'd Fat(g)	Mono Fat(g)	Poly Fat(g)	Total Calor
dehydrated, prepared w/water	1 c	1	1	1	?	?	70
turkey							
canned	1 c	5	5	1	?	?	122
dehydrated, prepared w/water	1 c	3	2	1	?	?	87

Sauces

	Portion	Chol (mg)	Total Fat(g)	Satur'd Fat(g)	Mono Fat(g)	Poly Fat(g)	Total Calor
barbecue, ready to serve	1 c	0	5	1	?	?	188
bearnaise							
dehydrated	0.9 oz	tr	2	tr	?	?	90
dehydrated, prepared w/milk & butter	1 c	189	68	42	?	?	701
dehydrated, prepared w/milk & butter	13½ oz	283	102	63	?	?	1,052
cheese							
dehydrated	1.2 oz	18	9	4	?	?	158
dehydrated, prepared w/whole milk	1 c	53	17	9	?	?	307
curry							
dehydrated	1.2 oz	tr	8	1	?	?	151
dehydrated, prepared w/whole milk	1 c	35	15	6	?	?	270
dehydrated, prepared w/whole milk	12 oz	44	18	8	?	?	337
hollandaise, dehydrated							
w/butterfat	1.2 oz	40	16	9	?	?	187
w/butterfat, prepared w/water	1 c	51	20	12	?	?	237
w/butterfat, prepared w/water	7.2 oz	40	16	9	?	?	187
w/vegetable oil	1 oz	tr	2	tr	?	?	93
w/vegetable oil, prepared w/milk & butter	1 c	189	68	42	?	?	703
w/vegetable oil, prepared w/milk & butter	13½ oz	283	102	63	?	?	1,055
marinara, canned	1 c	0	8	1	?	?	171
marinara, canned	15½ oz	0	15	2	?	?	300
mushroom, dehydrated	1 oz	0	3	tr	?	?	99
dehydrated, prepared w/whole milk	1 c	34	10	5	?	?	228
dehydrated, prepared w/whole milk	11.7 oz	43	13	7	?	?	285
sour cream							
dehydrated	1.2 oz	28	11	6	?	?	180
dehydrated, prepared w/whole milk	1 c	91	30	16	?	?	509

	Portion	Chol (mg)	Total Fat(g)	Satur'd Fat(g)	Mono Fat(g)	Poly Fat(g)	Total Calor
dehydrated, prepared w/whole milk	5½ oz	46	15	8	?	?	255
soy *See* SOYBEANS & SOYBEAN PRODUCTS							
spaghetti							
canned	1 c	0	12	2	?	?	272
canned	15½ oz	0	21	3	?	?	479
dehydrated	0.35 oz = 10 g	0	tr	tr	?	?	28
dehydrated	1½ oz = 42 g	0	tr	tr	?	?	118
dehydrated, w/mushrooms	0.35 oz	3	1	1	?	?	30
dehydrated, w/mushrooms	1.4 oz	11	4	2	?	?	118
stroganoff							
dehydrated	1.6 oz	12	4	3	?	?	161
dehydrated, prepared w/whole milk & water	1 c	38	11	7	?	?	271
dehydrated, prepared w/whole milk & water	11.2 oz	41	12	7	?	?	292
sweet & sour							
dehydrated	2 oz	0	tr	tr	?	?	220
dehydrated, prepared w/water & vinegar	1 c	0	tr	tr	?	?	294
dehydrated, prepared w/water & vinegar	8.3 oz	0	tr	tr	?	?	220
tamari *See* SOY BEANS & SOY BEAN PRODUCTS							
teriyaki *See* SOY BEANS & SOY BEAN PRODUCTS							
tomato paste & puree *See* VEGETABLES, PLAIN & PREPARED							
tomato, canned	½ c	0	tr	tr	?	?	37
Spanish style	½ c	0	tr	tr	?	?	40
w/herbs & cheese	½ c	?	2	1	?	?	72
w/mushrooms	½ c	0	tr	tr	?	?	42
w/onions	½ c	0	tr	tr	?	?	52
w/onions, green peppers, & celery	½ c	0	1	tr	?	?	50
w/tomato tidbits	½ c	0	tr	tr	?	?	39
white							
dehydrated	1.7 oz	tr	13	3	?	?	230
dehydrated, prepared w/whole milk	1 c	34	13	6	?	?	241
dehydrated, prepared w/whole milk	23.2 oz	86	34	16	?	?	602

■ BRAND NAME

A-1

Steak Sauce	1 T	?	0	?	?	?	12

	Portion	Chol (mg)	Total Fat(g)	Satur'd Fat(g)	Mono Fat(g)	Poly Fat(g)	Total Calor
Chun King							
mustard, brown	1 t	?	0	?	?	?	4
sauce/glaze mix for sweet 'n sour entree	3.8 oz	0	0	0	?	?	370
sweet & sour sauce	1.8 oz	?	0	?	?	?	60
Contadina Fresh Pasta & Cheese							
Italian sausage sauce	5 oz	15	6	1	?	<1	110
Bolognese meat sauce	5 oz	25	7	1	?	<1	130
plum tomato sauce w/basil	5 oz	5	4	<1	?	<1	80
garden vegetable sauce	5 oz	2	3	<1	?	<1	80
marinara sauce	5 oz	5	4	<1	?	<1	80
alfredo sauce	4 oz	100	34	20	?	2	350
pesto sauce	2⅓ oz	10	34	5	?	<1	350
four cheese sauce	4 oz	80	27	14	?	6	300
Escoffier							
Sauce Diable	1 T	?	0	?	?	?	20
Franco-American Gravies							
au jus	2 oz	?	0	?	?	?	10
beef	2 oz	?	1	?	?	?	25
chicken	2 oz	?	4	?	?	?	45
chicken giblet	2 oz	?	2	?	?	?	30
cream gravy	2 oz	?	2	?	?	?	35
mushroom	2 oz	?	1	?	?	?	25
pork	2 oz	?	3	?	?	?	40
turkey	2 oz	?	2	?	?	?	30
Fresh Chef							
Bolognese Sauce	4 oz	?	6	?	?	?	127
Pesto Sauce	4 oz	?	60	?	?	?	620
red clam sauce	4 oz	?	3	?	?	?	81
tomato sauce	4 oz	?	10	?	?	?	151
white clam sauce	4 oz	?	10	?	?	?	121
Grey Poupon							
dijon mustard	1 T	?	1	?	?	?	18
Hunt							
tomato sauce							
regular	4 oz	0	<1	?	?	?	30
special	4 oz	0	<1	?	?	?	35
herb flavored	4 oz	<1	2	?	?	?	70
Italian	4 oz	<1	2	1	?	1	60
w/onions	4 oz	0	<1	?	?	?	40
w/bits	4 oz	0	<1	?	?	?	30
w/garlic	4 oz	0	2	<1	?	1	70
no salt added	4 oz	0	<1	?	?	?	35
spaghetti sauce							
homestyle w/mushrooms	4 oz	0	1	<1	?	1	50
traditional	4 oz	0	2	<1	?	1	70
w/mushrooms	4 oz	0	2	<1	?	1	70
w/meat	4 oz	2	2	<1	?	1	70

	Portion	Chol (mg)	Total Fat(g)	Satur'd Fat(g)	Mono Fat(g)	Poly Fat(g)	Total Calor
chunky	4 oz	0	<1	?	?	?	50
homestyle	4 oz	0	2	<1	?	1	60
Kraft							
barbeque sauce							
regular	2 T	0	1	0	?	0	45
garlic	2 T	0	0	0	?	0	40
hickory smoke	2 T	0	1	0	?	0	45
hot	2 T	0	1	0	?	0	45
hot hickory smoke	2 T	0	1	0	?	0	45
Italian seasonings	2 T	0	1	0	?	0	50
Kansas City style	2 T	0	1	0	?	0	50
mesquite smoke	2 T	0	1	0	?	0	45
onion bits	2 T	0	1	0	?	0	50
thick 'n spicy w/honey	2 T	0	1	0	?	0	60
thick 'n spicy Kansas City style	2 T	0	1	0	?	0	60
thick 'n spicy mesquite smoke	2 T	0	1	0	?	0	50
thick 'n spicy original	2 T	0	1	0	?	0	50
Old El Paso							
chunky picante sauce (mild, medium or hot)	2 T	0	0	0	?	0	7
enchilada sauce							
mild	¼ c	0	1	?	?	?	25
hot	¼ c	0	1	?	?	?	30
green enchilada sauce	2 T	0	0	0	?	0	11
picante salsa (mild, medium or hot)	2 T	0	<1	?	?	?	10
taco sauce (can)	2 T	0	0	0	?	0	15
taco sauce (jar) (mild, medium or hot)	2 T	0	<1	?	?	?	10
thick 'n chunky green chili salsa	2 T	0	0	0	?	0	3
thick 'n chunky salsa (mild, medium or hot)	2 T	0	<1	?	?	?	6
thick 'n chunky salsa verde	2 T	0	<1	0	?	0	10
tomatoes & green chilis	¼ c	0	<1	?	?	?	14
Ortega							
green chile salsa							
medium	1 oz	0	0	0	?	?	12
mild	1 oz	0	0	0	?	?	8
hot	1 oz	0	0	0	?	?	12
taco sauce							
hot thick & smooth	1 oz	0	0	0	?	?	16
medium thick & smooth	1 oz	0	0	0	?	?	16
mild thick & smooth	1 oz	0	0	0	?	?	16

	Portion	Chol (mg)	Total Fat(g)	Satur'd Fat(g)	Mono Fat(g)	Poly Fat(g)	Total Calor
Prego							
regular	4 oz	?	5	?	?	?	130
marinara	4 oz	?	6	?	?	?	100
meat flavored	4 oz	?	6	?	?	?	140
mushroom	4 oz	?	5	?	?	?	130
no salt added	4 oz	?	6	?	?	?	110
onion & garlic	4 oz	?	4	?	?	?	110
three cheese	4 oz	?	2	?	?	?	100
tomato & basil	4 oz	?	2	?	?	?	100
extra chunky garden combination	4 oz	?	2	?	?	?	80
extra chunky mushroom & onion	4 oz	?	4	?	?	?	100
extra chunky mushroom & tomato	4 oz	?	5	?	?	?	110
extra chunky mushroom w/extra spice	4 oz	?	3	?	?	?	100
extra chunky sausage & green pepper	4 oz	?	8	?	?	?	160
Progresso							
sauces							
spaghetti	½ c	2	5	1	?	2	110
meat flavored spaghetti	½ c	5	5	1	?	2	110
mushroom spaghetti	½ c	5	5	1	?	2	110
marinara	½ c	1	5	1	?	3	90
white clam	½ c	?	8	?	?	?	110
red clam	½ c	?	3	?	?	?	70
mixed seafood	½ c	11	6	<1	?	<1	110
authentic pasta sauces							
alfredo	½ c	95	30	19	?	1	340
bolognese	½ c	20	8	2	?	<1	150
seafood	½ c	95	15	9	?	<1	190
white clam	½ c	19	9	1	?	<1	130
marinara	½ c	4	6	1.5	?	<1	110
creamy primavera	½ c	54	17	10	?	1.4	190
Wolf							
chili hot dog sauce	about ⅙ c	?	2	?	?	?	44

❏ SEAFOOD & SEAFOOD PRODUCTS

See also DINNERS, FROZEN; ENTREES & MAIN COURSES, FROZEN

Finfish

ahi *See* TUNA, YELLOWFISH, below
aku *See* TUNA, SKIPJACK, below
anchovy, European

raw	3 oz	?	4	1	?	?	111

	Portion	Chol (mg)	Total Fat(g)	Satur'd Fat(g)	Mono Fat(g)	Poly Fat(g)	Total Calor
canned in oil, drained solids	5	?	2	tr	?	?	42
bass, freshwater							
mixed species, raw	3 oz	58	3	1	?	?	97
striped, raw	3 oz	68	2	tr	?	?	82
bluefish, raw	3 oz	50	4	1	?	?	105
carp							
raw	3 oz	56	5	1	?	?	108
baked, broiled, microwaved	3 oz	72	6	1	?	?	138
catfish							
channel							
raw	3 oz	49	4	1	?	?	99
breaded & fried	3 oz	69	11	3	?	?	194
cod							
Atlantic							
raw	3 oz	37	1	tr	?	?	70
baked, broiled, microwaved	3 oz	47	1	tr	?	?	89
canned, solids & liquids	3 oz	47	1	tr	?	?	89
dried & salted	3 oz	129	2	tr	?	?	246
pacific, raw	3 oz	31	1	tr	?	?	70
croaker, Atlantic							
raw	3 oz	52	3	1	?	?	89
breaded & fried	3 oz	71	11	3	?	?	188
dogfish See SHARK, below							
dolphinfish, raw	3 oz	62	1	tr	?	?	73
drum, freshwater, raw	3 oz	54	4	1	?	?	101
flatfish							
raw	3 oz	41	1	tr	?	?	78
baked, broiled, microwaved	3 oz	58	1	tr	?	?	99
flounder See FLATFISH, above							
grouper, mixed species							
raw	3 oz	31	1	tr	?	?	78
baked, broiled, microwaved	3 oz	40	1	tr	?	?	100
haddock							
raw	3 oz	49	1	tr	?	?	74
baked, broiled, microwaved	3 oz	63	1	tr	?	?	95
smoked	3 oz	65	1	tr	?	?	99
hake See WHITING, below							
halibut							
Atlantic & Pacific							
raw	3 oz	27	2	tr	?	?	93
baked, broiled, microwaved	3 oz	35	2	tr	?	?	119
Greenland, raw	3 oz	39	12	2	?	?	158

	Portion	Chol (mg)	Total Fat(g)	Satur'd Fat(g)	Mono Fat(g)	Poly Fat(g)	Total Calor
herring							
Atlantic, raw	3 oz	51	8	2	?	?	134
baked, broiled, microwaved	3 oz	65	10	2	?	?	172
canned *See* SARDINE, ATLANTIC, below							
kippered	1.4 oz	33	5	1	?	?	87
pickled	½ oz	2	3	tr	?	?	39
lake *See* CISCO, above							
Pacific, raw	3 oz	65	12	3	?	?	166
ling, raw	3 oz	?	1	?	?	?	74
lox *See* SALMON, CHINOOK, SMOKED, below							
mackerel							
Atlantic							
raw	3 oz	60	12	3	?	?	174
baked, broiled, microwaved	3 oz	64	15	4	?	?	223
jack, canned, drained solids	1 c	150	12	3	?	?	296
king, raw	3 oz	45	2	tr	?	?	89
Pacific & jack, mixed species, raw	3 oz	40	7	2	?	?	133
Spanish, raw	3 oz	65	5	2	?	?	118
baked, broiled, microwaved	3 oz	62	5	2	?	?	134
mahimahi *See* DOLPHINFISH, above							
milkfish, raw	3 oz	44	6	?	?	?	126
monkfish, raw	3 oz	21	1	?	?	?	64
mullet							
raw, striped	3 oz	42	3	1	?	?	99
baked, broiled, microwaved	3 oz	54	4	1	?	?	127
ocean perch, Atlantic							
raw	3 oz	36	1	tr	?	?	80
baked, broiled, microwaved	3 oz	46	2	tr	?	?	103
perch, mixed species							
raw	3 oz	76	1	tr	?	?	77
baked, broiled, microwaved	3 oz	98	1	tr	?	?	99
pike							
northern							
raw	3 oz	33	1	tr	?	?	75
baked, broiled, microwaved	3 oz	43	1	tr	?	?	96
walleye							
raw	3 oz	73	1	tr	?	?	79
pollock							
Atlantic, raw	3 oz	60	1	tr	?	?	78
walleye							
raw	3 oz	61	1	tr	?	?	68

	Portion	Chol (mg)	Total Fat(g)	Satur'd Fat(g)	Mono Fat(g)	Poly Fat(g)	Total Calor
baked, broiled, microwaved	3 oz	82	1	tr	?	?	96
pompano, Florida							
raw	3 oz	43	8	3	?	?	140
baked, broiled, microwaved	3 oz	54	10	4	?	?	179
redfish *See* OCEAN PERCH, ATLANTIC, above							
rockfish, Pacific, mixed species							
raw	3 oz	29	1	tr	?	?	80
baked, broiled, microwaved	3 oz	38	2	tr	?	?	103
roughy, orange, raw	3 oz	17	6	tr	?	?	107
salmon							
Atlantic, raw	3 oz	47	5	1	?	?	121
chinook							
raw	3 oz	56	9	2	?	?	153
smoked	3 oz	20	4	1	?	?	99
chum							
raw	3 oz	63	3	1	?	?	102
canned, drained solids w/bone	3 oz	33	5	1	?	?	120
canned, drained solids w/bone	13 oz	144	20	5	?	?	521
coho							
raw	3 oz	33	5	1	?	?	124
boiled, poached, steamed	3 oz	42	6	1	?	?	157
pink							
raw	3 oz	44	3	tr	?	?	99
red *See* SOCKEYE, below							
sockeye							
raw	3 oz	53	7	1	?	?	143
baked, broiled, or microwaved	3 oz	74	9	2	?	?	183
sardine							
Atlantic, canned in oil, drained solids w/bone	2 sardines pr 0.8 oz	34	3	tr	?	?	50
Atlantic, canned in oil, drained solids w/bone	3.2 oz	131	11	1	?	?	192
Pacific, canned in tomato sauce, drained solids w/bone	1 sardine or 1.3 oz	23	5	1	?	?	68
Pacific, canned in tomato sauce, drained solids w/bone	13 oz	225	44	11	?	?	658
scrod *See* COD, ATLANTIC, above							

	Portion	Chol (mg)	Total Fat(g)	Satur'd Fat(g)	Mono Fat(g)	Poly Fat(g)	Total Calor
sea bass, mixed species							
raw	3 oz	35	2	tr	?	?	82
baked, broiled, microwaved	3 oz	45	2	1	?	?	105
sea trout, mixed species, raw	3 oz	71	3	1	?	?	88
shad, American, raw	3 oz	?	12	?	?	?	167
shark, mixed species							
raw	3 oz	43	4	1	?	?	111
batter-dipped & fried	3 oz	50	12	3	?	?	194
sheepshead							
raw	3 oz	?	2	1	?	?	92
baked, broiled, microwaved	3 oz	?	1	tr	?	?	107
smelt, rainbow							
raw	3 oz	60	2	tr	?	?	83
baked, broiled, microwaved	3 oz	76	3	tr	?	?	106
snapper, mixed species							
raw	3 oz	31	1	tr	?	?	85
baked, broiled, microwaved	3 oz	40	1	tr	?	?	109
sole See FLATFISH, above							
sturgeon, mixed species							
raw	3 oz	?	3	1	?	?	90
baked, broiled, microwaved	3 oz	?	4	1	?	?	115
smoked	3 oz	?	4	1	?	?	147
sucker, white, raw	3 oz	35	2	tr	?	?	79
sunfish, pumpkinseed, raw	3 oz	57	1	tr	?	?	76
swordfish							
raw	3 oz	33	3	1	?	?	103
baked, broiled, microwaved	3 oz	43	4	1	?	?	132
tilefish							
raw	3 oz	?	2	tr	?	?	81
baked, broiled, microwaved	3 oz	?	4	1	?	?	125
trout							
mixed species, raw	3 oz	49	6	1	?	?	126
rainbow, raw	3 oz	48	3	1	?	?	100
baked, broiled, microwaved	3 oz	62	4	1	?	?	129
tuna							
bluefin, fresh							
raw	3 oz	32	4	1	?	?	122
baked, broiled, microwaved	3 oz	42	5	1	?	?	157

	Portion	Chol (mg)	Total Fat(g)	Satur'd Fat(g)	Mono Fat(g)	Poly Fat(g)	Total Calor
tuna							
light, canned in soybean oil, drained solids	3 oz	15	7	1	?	?	169
canned in soybean oil, drained solids	6 oz	30	14	3	?	?	339
canned in water, drained solids	3 oz	?	tr	tr	?	?	111
canned in water, drained solids	5.8 oz	?	1	tr	?	?	216
white							
canned in soybean oil, drained solids	3 oz	26	7	?	?	?	158
canned in water, drained solids	3 oz	35	2	1	?	?	116
skipjack, fresh, raw	3 oz	40	1	tr	?	?	88
yellowfin, fresh, raw	3 oz	38	1	tr	?	?	92
turbot							
domestic See HALIBUT, GREENLAND, above							
European, raw	3 oz	?	3	?	?	?	81
whitefish, mixed species							
raw	3 oz	51	5	1	?	?	114
smoked	3 oz	28	1	tr	?	?	92
whiting, mixed species							
raw	3 oz	57	1	tr	?	?	77
baked, broiled, microwaved	3 oz	71	1	tr	?	?	98
wolffish, Atlantic, raw	3 oz	39	2	tr	?	?	82
yellowtail, mixed species, raw	3 oz	?	4	?	?	?	124

Shellfish

	Portion	Chol (mg)	Total Fat(g)	Satur'd Fat(g)	Mono Fat(g)	Poly Fat(g)	Total Calor
abalone, mixed species							
raw	3 oz	72	1	tr	?	?	89
fried	3 oz	80	6	1	?	?	161
clams, mixed species							
raw	3 oz	29	1	tr	?	?	63
raw	9 large or 20 small clams	60	2	tr	?	?	133
boiled, poached, steamed	3 oz	57	2	tr	?	?	126
boiled, poached, steamed	20 small	60	2	tr	?	?	133
breaded & fried	3 oz	52	9	2	?	?	171
breaded & fried	20 small	115	21	5	?	?	379
canned, drained solids	3 oz	57	2	tr	?	?	126
canned, drained solids	1 c	107	3	tr	?	?	236
canned, liquid	3 fl oz	?	tr	?	?	?	2
canned, liquid	1 c	?	tr	?	?	?	6

	Portion	Chol (mg)	Total Fat(g)	Satur'd Fat(g)	Mono Fat(g)	Poly Fat(g)	Total Calor
crab							
Alaska king							
raw	3 oz	35	1	?	?	?	71
raw	1 leg 1 lb	72	1	?	?	?	144
boiled, poached, steamed	3 oz	45	1	tr	?	?	82
boiled, poached, steamed	1 leg 1 lb	72	2	tr	?	?	129
blue							
raw	1 crab = 1/3 lb	16	tr	tr	?	?	18
raw	3 oz	66	1	tr	?	?	74
boiled, poached, steamed	3 oz	85	2	tr	?	?	87
boiled, poached, steamed	1 c not packed	135	2	tr	?	?	138
canned, dry pack or drained solids of wet pack	3 oz	76	1	tr	?	?	84
canned, dry pack or drained solids of wet pack	1 c not packed	120	2	tr	?	?	133
Dungeness, raw	3 oz	50	1	tr	?	?	73
Dungeness, raw	1 crab = 1½ lb	97	2	tr	?	?	140
queen, raw	3 oz	47	1	tr	?	?	76
crayfish, mixed species							
raw	3 oz	118	1	tr	?	?	76
boiled, poached, steamed	3 oz	151	1	tr	?	?	97
cuttlefish, mixed species, raw	3 oz	95	1	tr	?	?	67
lobster, northern							
raw	3 oz	81	1	?	?	?	77
raw	1 lobster = 1½ lb	143	1	?	?	?	136
boiled, poached, steamed	3 oz	61	1	tr	?	?	83
boiled, poached, steamed	1 c	104	1	tr	?	?	142
mussels, blue							
raw	3 oz	24	2	tr	?	?	73
raw	1 c	42	3	1	?	?	129
boiled, poached, steamed	3 oz	48	4	1	?	?	147
octopus, common, raw	3 oz	41	1	tr	?	?	70
oysters							
eastern							
raw	6 medium oysters (70/qt)	46	2	1	?	?	58
raw	1 c	136	6	2	?	?	170

	Portion	Chol (mg)	Total Fat(g)	Satur'd Fat(g)	Mono Fat(g)	Poly Fat(g)	Total Calor
boiled, poached, steamed	6 medium oysters (70 per qt)	46	2	1	?	?	58
boiled, poached, steamed	3 oz	93	4	1	?	?	117
cooked, breaded & fried	3 oz	69	11	3	?	?	167
cooked, breaded & fried	6 medium (70/qt)	72	11	3	?	?	173
canned, solids & liquids	3 oz	46	2	1	?	?	58
canned, solids & liquids	1 c	136	6	2	?	?	170
Pacific, raw	1 medium oyster (20/qt)	?	1	tr	?	?	41
pacific, raw	3 oz	?	2	tr	?	?	69
scallops, mixed species							
raw	2 large (30/lb) or 5 small (75/lb)	10	tr	tr	?	?	26
raw	3 oz	28	1	tr	?	?	75
breaded & fried	2 large (30/lb)	19	3	1	?	?	67
shrimp, mixed species							
raw	4 large (32/lb)	43	tr	tr	?	?	30
raw	3 oz	130	1	tr	?	?	90
boiled, poached, steamed	4 large (32/lb)	43	tr	tr	?	?	22
boiled, poached, steamed	3 oz	166	1	tr	?	?	84
breaded & fried	4 large (32/lb)	53	4	1	?	?	73
breaded & fried	3 oz	150	10	2	?	?	206
canned, dry pack or drained solids of wet pack	3 oz	147	2	tr	?	?	102
canned, dry pack or drained solids of wet pack	1 c	222	3	tr	?	?	154
snails, sea See WHELK, below							
spiny lobster, mixed species, raw	3 oz	60	1	tr	?	?	95
spiny lobster, mixed species, raw	1 lobster = 2 lb	146	3	tr	?	?	233
squid, mixed species							
raw	3 oz	198	1	tr	?	?	78
fried	3 oz	221	6	2	?	?	149

	Portion	Chol (mg)	Total Fat(g)	Satur'd Fat(g)	Mono Fat(g)	Poly Fat(g)	Total Calor
whelk							
raw	3 oz	55	tr	tr	?	?	117
boiled, poached, steamed	3 oz	110	1	tr	?	?	233

Seafood Products

	Portion	Chol (mg)	Total Fat(g)	Satur'd Fat(g)	Mono Fat(g)	Poly Fat(g)	Total Calor
caviar, black & red, granular	1 oz	165	5	?	?	?	71
crab cakes (blue crab)	1 cake	90	6	1	?	?	93
fish sticks, frozen (walleye pollock), reheated	1 stick = 1 oz	31	3	1	?	?	76
gefilte fish, commercial, sweet recipe w/broth	1 piece = 1½ oz	12	1	tr	?	?	35
ocean *See* WOLFFISH, below							
roe, mixed species, raw	1 oz	105	2	tr	?	?	39
surimi (processed from walleye, pollock)	1 oz	8	tr	?	?	?	28
surimi (processed from walleye, pollock)	3 oz	25	1	?	?	?	84
tuna salad	3 oz	11	8	1	?	?	159
imitation seafood made from surimi							
crab, Alaska king	3 oz	17	1	?	?	?	87
scallops, mixed species	3 oz	18	tr	?	?	?	84
shrimp, mixed species	3 oz	31	1	?	?	?	86

■ BRAND NAME

Rokeach

	Portion	Chol (mg)	Total Fat(g)	Satur'd Fat(g)	Mono Fat(g)	Poly Fat(g)	Total Calor
natural broth gefilte fish	1.7 oz	22	2	?	1	1	47
old Vienna gefilte fish	1.86 oz	26	3	1	1	0	50
whitefish & pike gefilte fish	3.9 oz	64	4	1	2	1	80
whitefish & pike gefilte fish in jellied broth	1.9 oz	18	1	1	1	<1	45

Underwood

	Portion	Chol (mg)	Total Fat(g)	Satur'd Fat(g)	Mono Fat(g)	Poly Fat(g)	Total Calor
sardines							
in mustard sauce	3.75 oz	?	16	?	?	?	220
in sild oil	3.75 oz	?	42	?	?	?	460
in soya oil	3 oz	?	18	?	?	?	230
w/Tabasco brand pepper sauce	3 oz	?	16	?	?	?	220
in tomato sauce	3.25 oz	?	16	?	?	?	220
brisling in olive oil	3.75 oz	?	20	?	?	?	260

	Portion	Chol (mg)	Total Fat(g)	Satur'd Fat(g)	Mono Fat(g)	Poly Fat(g)	Total Calor

❏ SEASONINGS

See also BREADCRUMBS, CROUTONS, STUFFINGS, & SEASONED COATINGS

Most spices & herbs for which values are available contain <½ g of fat, no chol., & <10 cal/t. The following are exceptions.

	Portion	Chol (mg)	Total Fat(g)	Satur'd Fat(g)	Mono Fat(g)	Poly Fat(g)	Total Calor
mace, ground	1 t	0	1	tr	?	?	8
mustard powder	1 t	0	1	?	?	?	9
mustard seed, yellow	1 t	0	1	tr	?	?	15
nutmeg, ground	1 t	0	1	1	?	?	12
poppyseed	1 t	0	1	tr	?	?	15

■ BRAND NAME

Old El Paso
seasoning mix

	Portion	Chol (mg)	Total Fat(g)	Satur'd Fat(g)	Mono Fat(g)	Poly Fat(g)	Total Calor
chili	⅕ pkg	0	1	?	?	?	21
enchilada	1/18 pkg	0	0	0	?	0	6
taco	1/12 pkg	0	<1	?	?	?	8
burrito	⅛ pkg	0	0	0	?	0	17
fijita marinade	⅛ jar	0	0	0	?	0	14
guacamole	1/7 pkg	0	0	0	?	0	7

Ortega

	Portion	Chol (mg)	Total Fat(g)	Satur'd Fat(g)	Mono Fat(g)	Poly Fat(g)	Total Calor
mild taco meat seasoning	1 oz	0	1	0	?	?	90

Shake 'n Bake Seasoning Mixture

	Portion	Chol (mg)	Total Fat(g)	Satur'd Fat(g)	Mono Fat(g)	Poly Fat(g)	Total Calor
Italian herb recipe	¼ pouch	0	1	?	?	?	80
original recipe							
for chicken	¼ pouch	0	2	?	?	?	80
for fish	¼ pouch	0	1	?	?	?	70
for pork	¼ pouch	0	1	?	?	?	40
for chicken barbeque	¼ pouch	0	2	?	?	?	90
for pork barbeque	¼ pouch	0	2	?	?	?	80
Country mild recipe	¼ pouch	0	4	?	?	?	80

❏ SEEDS & SEED-BASED BUTTERS, FLOURS, & MEALS

See also NUTS & NUT-BASED BUTTERS, FLOURS, MEALS, MILKS, PASTES, & POWDERS

	Portion	Chol (mg)	Total Fat(g)	Satur'd Fat(g)	Mono Fat(g)	Poly Fat(g)	Total Calor
alfalfa seeds, sprouted, raw	1 c	0	tr	tr	?	?	10
chia seeds, dried	1 oz	0	7	3	?	?	134

	Portion	Chol (mg)	Total Fat(g)	Satur'd Fat(g)	Mono Fat(g)	Poly Fat(g)	Total Calor
cottonseed							
kernels, roasted	1 T	0	4	1	?	?	51
flour							
low-fat	1 oz	0	tr	tr	?	?	94
partially defatted	1 T	0	tr	tr	?	?	18
meal, partially defatted	1 oz	0	1	tr	?	?	104
pumpkin & squash seeds							
whole, roasted	1 oz	0	6	1	?	?	127
kernels							
dried	1 oz	0	13	2	?	?	154
roasted	1 oz	0	12	2	?	?	148
safflower seed							
kernels, dried	1 oz	0	11	1	?	?	147
meal, partially defatted	1 oz	0	1	tr	?	?	97
sesame seeds							
whole							
dried	1 T	0	4	1	?	?	52
roasted & toasted	1 oz	0	14	2	?	?	161
kernels							
dried	1 T	0	4	1	?	?	47
toasted	1 oz	0	14	2	?	?	161
sesame butter							
paste	1 T	0	8	1	?	?	95
tahini							
from raw & stone ground kernels	1 T	0	7	1	?	?	86
from roasted & toasted kernels	1 T	0	8	1	?	?	89
from unroasted kernels	1 oz	0	16	2	?	?	173
from unroasted kernels	1 T	0	8	1	?	?	85
sesame flour							
high-fat	1 oz	0	11	1	?	?	149
partially defatted	1 oz	0	3	tr	?	?	109
low-fat	1 oz	0	1	tr	?	?	95
sesame meal, partially defatted	1 oz	0	14	2	?	?	161
squash seeds See PUMPKIN & SQUASH SEEDS, above							
sunflower seed kernels							
dried	1 oz	0	14	1	?	?	162
dry roasted	1 oz	0	14	1	?	?	165
oil roasted	1 oz	0	16	2	?	?	175
toasted	1 oz	0	16	2	?	?	176
sunflower seed butter	1 T	0	8	1	?	?	93
sunflower seed flour, partially defatted	1 T	0	tr	tr	?	?	16
sunflower seed flour, partially defatted	1 c	0	1	tr	?	?	261
tahini See SESAME BUTTER, TAHINI, above							

	Portion	Chol (mg)	Total Fat(g)	Satur'd Fat(g)	Mono Fat(g)	Poly Fat(g)	Total Calor
watermelon seed kernels, dried	1 oz	0	13	3	?	?	158
watermelon seed kernels, dried	1 c	0	51	11	?	?	602

▪ BRAND NAME

Arrowhead Mills
alfalfa seeds, sprouted	1 c	0	1	?	?	?	40
amaranth seeds	2 oz	0	3	?	?	?	200
flax seeds	1 oz	0	10	?	?	?	140
sesame seeds							
hulled	1 oz	0	14	?	?	?	160
whole	1 oz	0	14	?	?	?	160
sesame tahini, chemical-free	1 oz	0	17	?	?	?	170
sunflower seeds, hulled	1 oz	0	13	?	?	?	160

Planters
sunflower seeds	1 oz	0	14	2	?	?	160

❏ SHERBETS *See* DESSERTS, FROZEN

❏ SHORTENINGS *See* FATS, OILS, & SHORTENINGS

❏ SNACKS
See also CRACKERS

cheese puffs	1 oz	1	10	?	?	?	159
cheese straws	4	?	7	?	?	?	109
corn chips	1 oz	0	9	1	?	?	155
popcorn							
air-popped	1 c	0	tr	tr	?	?	30
popped in vegetable oil	1 c	0	3	1	?	?	55
sugar-sugar coated	1 c	0	1	tr	?	?	135
potato chips	10	0	7	2	?	?	105
made from dried potatoes	1 oz	0	13	4	?	?	164
potato sticks	1 oz	0	10	3	?	?	148
pretzels							
stick	10	0	tr	tr	?	?	10
twisted dutch	1	0	1	tr	?	?	65
twisted thin	10	0	2	tr	?	?	240
tortilla chips	1 oz	0	7	?	?	?	139

	Portion	Chol (mg)	Total Fat(g)	Satur'd Fat(g)	Mono Fat(g)	Poly Fat(g)	Total Calor

■ **BRAND NAME**

Arrowhead Mills

	Portion	Chol (mg)	Total Fat(g)	Satur'd Fat(g)	Mono Fat(g)	Poly Fat(g)	Total Calor
popcorn, unpopped	2 oz	0	3	?	?	?	210

Bugles

plain	1 oz	?	8	?	?	?	150
nacho cheese	1 oz	?	9	?	?	?	160
ranch flavor	1 oz	?	9	?	?	?	150

Cheerios-to-Go

apple cinnamon cheerios	1 oz pouch	0	2	?	?	?	110
cheerios	¾ pouch	0	2	?	?	?	80
honey nut cheerios	1 oz pouch	0	1	?	?	?	110

Frito Lay

CHEETOS

crunchy	26	0	9	?	?	?	150
curls	15	0	9	?	?	?	150
light	38	0	6	?	?	?	140
paws	16	0	10	?	?	?	160
puffs	33	0	9	?	?	?	160
puffed ball	38	0	10	?	?	?	160
cheddar valley	26	0	9	?	?	?	150
flamin' hot	26	0	9	?	?	?	150

DORITOS

taco	approx. 16	0	7	?	?	?	140
salsa rio	approx. 16	0	7	?	?	?	140
cool ranch	approx. 16	170	7	?	?	?	140
toasted corn	approx. 16	80	7	?	?	?	140
nacho cheese	approx. 16	160	7	?	?	?	140
jumpin' jack	approx. 16	220	0	?	?	?	140
light cool ranch	approx. 16	220	0	?	?	?	130
light nacho ranch	approx. 16	230	0	?	?	?	120

RUFFLES

original	approx. 17-20	0	10	?	?	?	150
light	approx. 17-20	0	6	?	?	?	130
ranch	approx. 17-20	0	10	?	?	?	160
cheddar & sour cream	approx. 17-20	0	10	?	?	?	160
mesquite grill bar b-q	approx. 17-20	0	10	?	?	?	160
sour cream & onion	approx. 17-20	0	10	?	?	?	160

	Portion	Chol (mg)	Total Fat(g)	Satur'd Fat(g)	Mono Fat(g)	Poly Fat(g)	Total Calor
light sour cream & onion	approx. 17-20	0	6	?	?	?	130
Monterey jack cheese flavor cheese attack	approx. 17-20	0	10	?	?	?	160
SANTITAS							
tortilla chips	1 oz	0	7	?	?	?	140
tortilla strips	1 oz	0	7	?	?	?	140
cantina style	1 oz	0	6	?	?	?	140
fajita flavored cantina style	1 oz	0	7	?	?	?	140
TOSTITOS							
traditional	11	0	8	?	?	?	140
bite size	16	0	8	?	?	?	150
white corn restaurant style	7	0	6	?	?	?	130
ROLD GOLD PRETZELS							
Bavarian	3	0	2	?	?	?	120
rods	3	0	2	?	?	?	110
sticks	50	0	2	?	?	?	110
tint twist	15	0	1	?	?	?	110
pretzel twist	10	0	1	?	?	?	110
unsalted	1 oz	0	1	?	?	?	110
LAY'S							
original	approx. 15-20	0	10	?	?	?	150
unsalted	approx. 15-20	0	10	?	?	?	150
bar b-q	approx. 15-20	0	15	?	?	?	150
tangy ranch	approx. 15-20	0	10	?	?	?	160
cheddar cheese	approx. 15-20	0	10	?	?	?	150
flamin' hot	approx. 15-20	0	9	?	?	?	150
salt & vinegar	approx. 15-20	0	10	?	?	?	150
sour cream & onion	approx. 15-20	0	10	?	?	?	160
Kansas style bar b-q	approx. 15-20	0	9	?	?	?	150
crunch tators							
original	approx. 16	0	8	?	?	?	150
hoppin' jalapeño	approx. 16	0	7	?	?	?	140
mighty mesquite	approx. 16	0	8	?	?	?	150
amaz' cajun	approx. 16	150	8	?	?	?	150
supreme sour cream	approx. 16	180	8	?	?	?	150

	Portion	Chol (mg)	Total Fat(g)	Satur'd Fat(g)	Mono Fat(g)	Poly Fat(g)	Total Calor
DELTA GOLD							
potato chips	28	0	10	?	?	?	160
dip style	18	0	10	?	?	?	160
mesquite flavored bar b-q	26	0	10	?	?	?	160
FRITOS							
original	34	0	10	?	?	?	150
dip size	13	0	10	?	?	?	150
wild 'n mild	32	0	9	?	?	?	160
crisp 'n thin	18	0	10	?	?	?	160
chili cheese	34	0	10	?	?	?	160
rowdy rustlers bar-b-q	34	0	9	?	?	?	150
non-stop nacho cheese	34	0	9	?	?	?	150
Hain							
carrot chips							
regular	1 oz	?	9	?	?	?	150
no salt added	1 oz	0	7	?	?	?	150
barbeque	1 oz	?	8	?	?	?	140
sesame tortilla chips							
regular	1 oz	0	7	?	?	?	140
cheese	1 oz	<5	8	?	?	?	160
no salt added	1 oz	0	7	?	?	?	140
taco style tortilla chips	1 oz	<5	11	?	?	?	160
Health Valley							
CHIPS							
carrot lites	17	0	1	?	?	?	70
cheddar lites							
regular or no salt	17	tr	2	?	?	?	40
w/green onion	17	0	1	?	?	?	40
Nabisco							
DOO DADS SNACKS							
original	1 oz = ½ c	?	6	?	?	?	140
cheddar 'n herb	1 oz = ½ c	?	6	?	?	?	140
zesty cheese	1 oz = ½ c	?	6	?	?	?	140
GREAT CRISPS! BAKED CRISPY SNACKS							
cheese 'n chive	9	?	4	?	?	?	70
French onion	7	?	4	?	?	?	70
Italian	9	?	4	?	?	?	70
nacho	8	?	4	?	?	?	70
real bacon	9	?	4	?	?	?	70
savory garlic	8	?	3	?	?	?	70
sesame	9	?	4	?	?	?	70
sour cream & onion	8	?	4	?	?	?	70
tomato & celery	9	?	4	?	?	?	70

	Portion	Chol (mg)	Total Fat(g)	Satur'd Fat(g)	Mono Fat(g)	Poly Fat(g)	Total Calor
CHEESE NIPS							
real cheddar cheese	13	?	3	?	?	?	70
pizza	20	?	3	?	?	?	70
taco	14	?	4	?	?	?	70
Nature Valley							
granola bars							
cinnamon	1	0	5	1	3	1	120
oat bran/honey graham	1	0	4	<1	3	1	110
oats 'n honey	1	0	5	1	3	1	120
peanut butter	1 oz	0	6	1	4	1	120
rice bran/cinnamon graham	1	0	4	<1	2	<1	90
Orville Redenbacher's Gourmet Popping Corn							
microwave							
caramel	2.5 c	<1	14	3	?	1	240
nacho	3 c	<1	8	2	?	<1	120
light natural	3 c	0	1	<1	?	<1	50
butter toffee	2.5 c	<1	12	3	?	1	210
light butter	3 c	0	1	<1	?	<1	50
natural	3 c	0	5	1	?	<1	80
butter	3 c	0	5	1	?	<1	80
salt free natural	3 c	0	5	1	?	<1	90
salt free butter	3 c	0	5	1	?	<1	90
cheddar cheese	3 c	2	8	2	?	<1	130
sour cream 'n onion	3 c	2	9	2	?	1	130
frozen microwave							
butter flavor	3 c	0	5	1	?	<1	80
natural flavor	3 c	0	5	1	?	<1	80
original	3 c	0	4	?	?	?	80
white	3 c	0	<1	?	?	?	40
hot air	3 c	0	?	?	?	?	40
Pepperidge Farm							
tiny goldfish crackers							
smoked flavor cheddar cheese	45 crackers	?	5	?	?	?	130
cheddar cheese	1 oz	5	4	1	2	2	120
parmesan cheese	1 oz	<5	4	1	2	0	120
original	1 oz	0	5	1	3	0	130
pretzel	1 oz	0	3	0	2	0	110
low salt cheddar cheese	1 oz	8	4	1	2	0	120
pizza flavored	1 oz	<5	5	1	2	0	130
distinctive crackers							
cheese goldfish thins	4 crackers	0	2	0	1	0	50
symphony cracker assortment							
*data available for each cracker variety							
butter flavored thins	4 crackers	<5	3	1	1	0	70
English wafer biscuits	4 crackers	0	1	0	1	0	70
sesame	4 crackers	0	4	1	2	0	80
hearty wheat	4 crackers	0	5	1	2	0	100
cracked wheat	3 crackers	0	4	1	2	0	100

	Portion	Chol (mg)	Total Fat(g)	Satur'd Fat(g)	Mono Fat(g)	Poly Fat(g)	Total Calor
toasted wheat w/onion	4 crackers	0	3	1	2	0	80
three cracker assortment							
*data available for each cracker variety							
snack sticks							
pumpernickel	8 crackers	0	6	1	3	1	140
sesame	8 crackers	0	5	1	2	2	140
cheese	8 crackers	0	5	2	1	1	130
pretzel	8 crackers	0	3	0	1	1	120
flutters							
golden sesame	3/4 oz	0	5	1	3	1	110
original butter	3/4 oz	5	4	1	2	0	100
garden herb	3/4 oz	0	4	1	3	0	100
toasted wheat	3/4 oz	0	5	1	4	0	110
snack mix							
classic	1 oz	0	8	1	4	1	140
lightly smoked	1 oz	0	9	1	5	2	150
spicey	1 oz	<5	8	2	4	2	140
wholesome crackers							
crispy graham	4 crackers	0	2	0	0	1	70
multi grain	4 crackers	0	2	0	0	1	70
garden vegetable	5 crackers	0	2	0	1	0	60
toasted rice	4 crackers	0	2	0	1	0	60
Ralston							
chex mix							
barbeque flavor	1 oz	0	5	?	?	?	130
golden cheddar	1 oz	0	5	?	?	?	130
cool sour cream & onion	1 oz	0	5	?	?	?	130
traditional	1 oz	0	5	?	?	?	120
Weight Watchers							
popcorn							
microwave	1 oz	?	1	?	?	?	100
ready-to-eat							
lightly salted	.66 oz	?	4	?	?	?	80
white cheddar cheese	.66 oz	?	6	?	?	?	100
corn snackers							
lightly salted	.5 oz	?	2	?	?	?	60
nacho cheese flavor	.5 oz	?	2	?	?	?	60
great snackers							
cheddar cheese	.5 oz	?	3	?	?	?	60
barbeque	.5 oz	?	3	?	?	?	60
toasted onion	.5 oz	?	3	?	?	?	60
fruit snacks							
apple chips	.75 oz	?	?	?	?	?	70
apple snacks	.5 oz	?	<1	?	?	?	50
cinnamon flavor fruit snacks	.5 oz	?	<1	?	?	?	50
strawberry flavor fruit snacks	.5 oz	?	<1	?	?	?	50
peach flavor fruit snacks	.5 oz	?	<1	?	?	?	50

	Portion	Chol (mg)	Total Fat(g)	Satur'd Fat(g)	Mono Fat(g)	Poly Fat(g)	Total Calor

❏ SOUPS, PREPARED

Canned

	Portion	Chol (mg)	Total Fat(g)	Satur'd Fat(g)	Mono Fat(g)	Poly Fat(g)	Total Calor
asparagus, cream of, condensed	1 can = 10¾ oz	12	10	3	?	?	210
prepared w/water	1 c	5	4	1	?	?	87
prepared w/whole milk	1 c	22	8	3	?	?	161
prepared w/whole milk	1 can	54	20	8	?	?	392
bean, black, condensed	1 can = 11 oz	0	4	1	?	?	285
prepared w/water	1 c	0	2	tr	?	?	116
bean w/bacon, condensed	1 can = 11½ oz	6	14	4	?	?	420
prepared w/water	1 c	3	6	2	?	?	173
bean & frankfurter, condensed	1 can = 11¼ oz	29	17	5	?	?	454
prepared w/water	1 c	12	7	2	?	?	187
bean w/ham, chunky, ready to serve	1 c	22	9	3	?	?	231
bean w/ham, chunky, ready to serve	1 can = 19¼ oz	49	19	7	?	?	519
beef broth or bouillon, ready to serve	1 c	tr	1	tr	?	?	16
beef broth or bouillon, ready to serve	1 can = 14 oz	1	1	tr	?	?	27
beef, chunky, ready to serve	1 c	14	5	3	?	?	171
beef, chunky, ready to serve	1 can = 19 oz	32	12	6	?	?	383
beef mushroom, condensed	1 can = 10¾ oz	15	7	4	?	?	?
prepared w/water	1 c	7	3	1	?	?	?
beef noodle, condensed	1 can = 10¾ oz	12	7	3	?	?	204
prepared w/water	1 c	5	3	1	?	?	84
celery, cream of, condensed	1 can = 10¾ oz	34	14	3	?	?	219
prepared w/water	1 c	15	6	1	?	?	90
prepared w/whole milk	1 c	32	10	4	?	?	165
prepared w/whole milk	1 can	78	24	10	?	?	400
cheese, condensed	1 can = 11 oz	72	25	16	?	?	377
prepared w/water	1 c	30	10	7	?	?	155
prepared w/whole milk	1 c	48	15	9	?	?	230
prepared w/whole milk	1 can	116	35	22	?	?	558
chicken, chunky, ready to serve	1 c	30	7	2	?	?	178

	Portion	Chol (mg)	Total Fat(g)	Satur'd Fat(g)	Mono Fat(g)	Poly Fat(g)	Total Calor
chicken, chunky, ready to serve	1 can = 10¾ oz	37	8	2	?	?	216
chicken, cream of, condensed	1 can = 10¾ oz	24	18	5	?	?	283
prepared w/water	1 c	10	7	2	?	?	116
prepared w/whole milk	1 c	27	11	5	?	?	191
prepared w/whole milk	1 can	66	28	11	?	?	464
chicken & dumplings, condensed	1 can = 10½ oz	80	13	3	?	?	236
prepared w/water	1 c	34	6	1	?	?	97
chicken broth, condensed	1 can = 10¾ oz	3	3	1	?	?	94
prepared w/water	1 c	1	1	tr	?	?	39
chicken gumbo, condensed	1 can = 10¾ oz	9	3	1	?	?	137
prepared w/water	1 c	5	1	tr	?	?	56
chicken mushroom, condensed	1 can = 10¾ oz	24	22	6	?	?	?
prepared w/water	1 c	10	9	2	?	?	?
chicken noodle							
chunky, ready to serve	1 c	18	6	1	?	?	?
chunky, ready to serve	1 can = 19 fl oz	40	13	3	?	?	?
condensed	1 can = 10½ oz	15	6	1	?	?	182
prepared w/water	1 c	7	2	1	?	?	75
chicken noodle w/meatballs, ready to serve	1 c	10	4	1	?	?	99
chicken noodle w/meatballs, ready to serve	1 can = 20 oz	23	8	2	?	?	227
chicken rice							
chunky, ready to serve	1 c	12	3	1	?	?	127
chunky, ready to serve	1 can = 19 oz	27	7	2	?	?	286
condensed	1 can = 10½ oz	15	5	1	?	?	146
prepared w/water	1 c	7	2	tr	?	?	60
chicken vegetable							
chunky, ready to serve	1 c	17	5	1	?	?	167
chunky, ready to serve	1 can = 19 oz	38	11	3	?	?	374
condensed	1 can = 10½ oz	21	7	2	?	?	181
prepared w/water	1 c	10	3	1	?	?	74
chili beef, condensed	1 can = 11¼ oz	32	16	8	?	?	411
prepared w/water	1 c	12	7	3	?	?	169

	Portion	Chol (mg)	Total Fat (g)	Satur'd Fat (g)	Mono Fat (g)	Poly Fat (g)	Total Calor
clam chowder (Manhattan)							
chunky, ready to serve	1 c	14	3	2	?	?	133
chunky, ready to serve	1 can = 19 oz	32	8	5	?	?	299
condensed	1 can = 10¾ oz	6	5	1	?	?	187
prepared w/water	1 c	2	2	tr	?	?	78
clam chowder (new England), condensed	1 can = 10¾ oz	12	6	1	?	?	214
prepared w/water	1 c	5	3	tr	?	?	95
prepared w/whole milk	1 c	22	7	3	?	?	163
prepared w/whole milk	1 can	54	16	7	?	?	396
consommé w/gelatin, condensed	1 can = 10½ oz	0	0	0	?	?	71
prepared w/water	1 c	0	0	0	?	?	29
crab, ready to serve	1 c	10	2	tr	?	?	76
crab, ready to serve	1 can = 13 oz	10	2	1	?	?	114
escarole, ready to serve	1 c	2	2	1	?	?	27
escarole, ready to serve	1 can = 19½ oz	6	4	1	?	?	61
gazpacho, ready to serve	1 c	0	2	tr	?	?	57
gazpacho, ready to serve	1 can = 13 oz	0	3	tr	?	?	87
lentil w/ham, ready to serve	1 c	7	3	1	?	?	140
lentil w/ham, ready to serve	1 can = 20 oz	17	6	3	?	?	320
minestrone							
chunky, ready to serve	1 c	5	3	1	?	?	127
chunky, ready to serve	1 can = 19 oz	11	6	3	?	?	285
condensed	1 can = 10½ oz	3	6	1	?	?	202
prepared w/water	1 c	2	3	1	?	?	83
mushroom, cream of, condensed	1 can = 10¾ oz	3	23	6	?	?	313
prepared w/water	1 c	2	9	2	?	?	129
prepared w/whole milk	1 c	20	14	5	?	?	203
prepared w/whole milk	1 can =	48	33	12	?	?	494
mushroom barley, condensed	1 can = 10¾ oz	0	5	1	?	?	?
prepared w/water	1 c	0	2	tr	?	?	?
mushroom w/beef stock, condensed	1 can = 10¾ oz	18	10	4	?	?	208
prepared w/water	1 c	7	4	2	?	?	85
onion, condensed	1 can = 10½ oz	0	4	1	?	?	138
prepared w/water	1 c	0	2	tr	?	?	57

	Portion	Chol (mg)	Total Fat(g)	Satur'd Fat(g)	Mono Fat(g)	Poly Fat(g)	Total Calor
onion, cream of, condensed	1 can = 10¾ oz	37	13	4	?	?	?
prepared w/water	1 c	15	5	1	?	?	?
prepared w/whole milk	1 c	32	9	4	?	?	?
prepared w/whole milk	1 can	78	23	10	?	?	?
oyster stew, condensed	1 can = 10½ oz	33	9	6	?	?	144
prepared w/water	1 c	14	4	3	?	?	59
prepared w/whole milk	1 c	32	8	5	?	?	134
prepared w/whole milk	1 can	77	19	12	?	?	325
pea, green, condensed	1 can = 11¼ oz	0	7	3	?	?	398
prepared w/water	1 c	0	3	1	?	?	164
prepared w/whole milk	1 c	18	7	4	?	?	239
prepared w/whole milk	1 can	43	17	10	?	?	579
pea, split, w/ham chunky, ready to serve	1 c	7	4	2	?	?	184
chunky, ready to serve	1 can = 19 oz	16	9	4	?	?	413
condensed	1 can = 11½ oz	20	11	4	?	?	459
prepared w/water	1 c	8	4	2	?	?	189
pepperpot, condensed	1 can = 10½ oz	24	11	5	?	?	251
prepared w/water	1 c	10	5	2	?	?	103
potato, cream of, condensed	1 can = 10¾ oz	15	6	3	?	?	178
prepared w/water	1 c	5	2	1	?	?	73
prepared w/whole milk	1 c	22	6	4	?	?	148
prepared w/whole milk	1 can	54	16	9	?	?	360
scotch broth, condensed	1 can = 10½ oz	12	6	3	?	?	195
prepared w/water	1 c	5	3	1	?	?	80
shrimp, cream of, condensed	1 can = 10¾ oz	40	13	8	?	?	219
prepared w/water	1 c	17	5	3	?	?	90
prepared w/whole milk	1 c	35	9	6	?	?	165
prepared w/whole milk	1 can	84	23	14	?	?	400
stockpot, condensed	1 can = 11 oz	9	9	2	?	?	242
prepared w/water	1 c	5	4	1	?	?	100
tomato, condensed	1 can = 10¾ oz	0	5	1	?	?	208
prepared w/water	1 c	0	2	tr	?	?	86
prepared w/whole milk	1 c	17	6	3	?	?	160
prepared w/whole milk	1 can	42	15	7	?	?	389
tomato beef w/noodle, condensed	1 can = 10¾ oz	9	10	4	?	?	341
prepared w/water	1 c	5	4	2	?	?	140
tomato bisque, condensed	1 can = 11 oz	11	6	1	?	?	300

	Portion	Chol (mg)	Total Fat(g)	Satur'd Fat(g)	Mono Fat(g)	Poly Fat(g)	Total Calor
prepared w/water	1 c	4	3	1	?	?	123
prepared w/whole milk	1 c	22	7	3	?	?	198
prepared w/whole milk	1 can	53	16	8	?	?	481
tomato rice, condensed	1 can = 11 oz	3	7	1	?	?	291
prepared w/water	1 c	2	3	1	?	?	120
turkey, chunky, ready to serve	1 c	9	4	1	?	?	136
turkey, chunky, ready to serve	1 can = 18¾ oz	21	10	3	?	?	306
turkey noodle, condensed	1 can = 10¾ oz	12	5	1	?	?	168
prepared w/water	1 c	5	2	1	?	?	69
turkey vegetable, condensed	1 can = 10½ oz	3	7	2	?	?	179
prepared w/water	1 c	2	3	1	?	?	74
vegetable, chunky, ready to serve	1 c	0	4	1	?	?	122
vegetable, chunky, ready to serve	1 can = 19 oz	0	8	1	?	?	274
vegetable, vegetarian, condensed	1 can = 10½ oz	0	5	1	?	?	176
prepared w/water	1 c	0	2	tr	?	?	72
vegetable w/beef, condensed	1 can = 10¾ oz	12	5	2	?	?	192
prepared w/water	1 c	5	2	1	?	?	79
vegetable w/beef broth, condensed	1 can = 10½ oz	6	5	1	?	?	197
prepared w/water	1 c	2	2	tr	?	?	81

Dehydrated

	Portion	Chol (mg)	Total Fat(g)	Satur'd Fat(g)	Mono Fat(g)	Poly Fat(g)	Total Calor
asparagus, cream of, prepared w/water	1 c	tr	2	tr	?	?	59
asparagus, cream of, prepared w/water	39.7 oz	1	8	1	?	?	265
bean w/bacon, prepared w/water	1 c	3	2	1	?	?	105
beef broth or bouillon cubed	1 cube = 0.1 oz	tr	tr	tr	?	?	6
prepared w/water	1 c	1	1	tr	?	?	19
prepared w/water	6 fl oz	tr	1	tr	?	?	14
beef noodle, prepared w/water	1 c	2	1	tr	?	?	41
beef noodle, prepared w/water	6 fl oz	1	1	tr	?	?	30
cauliflower, prepared w/water	1 c	tr	2	tr	?	?	68
celery, cream of, prepared w/water	1 c	1	2	tr	?	?	63

	Portion	Chol (mg)	Total Fat(g)	Satur'd Fat(g)	Mono Fat(g)	Poly Fat(g)	Total Calor
chicken, cream of, prepared w/water	1 c	3	5	3	?	?	107
chicken, cream of, prepared w/water	6 fl oz	2	4	3	?	?	80
chicken broth or bouillon							
cubed	1 cube = 0.2 oz	1	tr	tr	?	?	9
prepared w/water	1 c	1	1	tr	?	?	21
prepared w/water	6 fl oz	1	1	tr	?	?	16
chicken noodle	1 pkt = 2.6 oz	10	6	1	?	?	257
chicken noodle	1 pkt = 0.4 oz	2	1	tr	?	?	38
prepared w/water	1 c	3	1	tr	?	?	53
chicken rice, prepared w/water	1 c	3	1	tr	?	?	60
chicken vegetable, prepared w/water	1 c	3	1	tr	?	?	49
chicken vegetable, prepared w/water	6 fl oz	2	1	tr	?	?	37
clam chowder (Manhattan)	1 c	0	2	tr	?	?	65
clam chowder (New England)	1 c	1	4	1	?	?	95
consommé, w/gelatin added, prepared w/water	1 c	0	tr	tr	?	?	17
consommé, w/gelatin added, prepared w/water	39½ oz	0	tr	tr	?	?	77
leek, prepared w/water	1 c	3	2	1	?	?	71
minestrone, prepared w/water	1 c	3	2	1	?	?	79
mushroom	1 regular pkt = 2.6 oz	2	17	3	?	?	328
mushroom	1 instant pkt = 0.6 oz	0	4	1	?	?	74
prepared w/water	1 c	1	5	1	?	?	96
onion	1 pkt = 1.4 oz	2	2	1	?	?	115
onion	1 pkt = ½ oz	0	tr	tr	?	?	21
prepared w/water	1 c	0	1	tr	?	?	28
oxtail, prepared w/water	1 c	3	3	1	?	?	71
oxtail, prepared w/water	36 fl oz	11	11	6	?	?	318
pea, green or split	1 pkt = 4 oz	1	5	2	?	?	402

	Portion	Chol (mg)	Total Fat(g)	Satur'd Fat(g)	Mono Fat(g)	Poly Fat(g)	Total Calor
pea, green or split	1 pkt = 1 oz	0	1	tr	?	?	100
prepared w/water	1 c	3	2	tr	?	?	133
tomato (includes cream of tomato)	1 pkt = ¾ oz	1	2	1	?	?	77
prepared w/water	1 c	1	2	1	?	?	102
tomato vegetable (includes Italian vegetable & spring vegetable)	1 pkt = 1.4 oz	1	2	1	?	?	125
prepared w/water	1 c	tr	1	tr	?	?	55
vegetable, cream of, prepared w/water	1 c	0	6	1	?	?	105
vegetable beef, prepared w/water	1 c	1	1	1	?	?	53
vegetable beef, prepared w/water	1 pkt = 40 oz	5	5	2	?	?	240

■ BRAND NAME

Campbell's

CHUNKY SOUPS (READY TO SERVE)

	Portion	Chol (mg)	Total Fat(g)	Satur'd Fat(g)	Mono Fat(g)	Poly Fat(g)	Total Calor
beef	10¾ oz	?	5	?	?	?	200
beef Stroganoff style	10¾ oz	?	16	?	?	?	320
chicken corn chowder	10¾ oz	?	21	?	?	?	340
chicken noodle	10¾ oz	?	7	?	?	?	200
chicken nuggets w/vegetables & noodles	10¾ oz	?	6	?	?	?	190
chili beef	11 oz	?	7	?	?	?	290
chili beef	9¾ oz	?	6	?	?	?	260
clam chowder (Manhattan style)	10¾ oz	?	4	?	?	?	160
clam chowder (New England style)	10¾ oz	?	17	?	?	?	290
creamy chicken mushroom	10½ oz	?	19	?	?	?	270
ham 'n butter bean	10½ oz	?	10	?	?	?	280
old fashioned bean w/ham	11 oz	?	9	?	?	?	290
old fashioned chicken	10¾ oz	?	5	?	?	?	180
old fashioned vegetable beef	10¾ oz	?	6	?	?	?	190
sirloin burger	10¾ oz	?	9	?	?	?	220
split pea 'n ham	10¾ oz	?	6	?	?	?	230
steak & potato	10¾ oz	?	5	?	?	?	200
vegetable	10¾ oz	?	4	?	?	?	160

CONDENSED SOUPS, AS PACKAGED

	Portion	Chol (mg)	Total Fat(g)	Satur'd Fat(g)	Mono Fat(g)	Poly Fat(g)	Total Calor
asparagus, cream of	4 oz	?	4	?	?	?	80

	Portion	Chol (mg)	Total Fat(g)	Satur'd Fat(g)	Mono Fat(g)	Poly Fat(g)	Total Calor
bean w/bacon	4 oz	?	4	?	?	?	140
bean, homestyle	4 oz	?	1	?	?	?	130
beef	4 oz	?	2	?	?	?	80
beef broth (bouillon)	4 oz	?	0	?	?	?	16
beef noodle	4 oz	?	3	?	?	?	70
beef noodle, homestyle	4 oz	?	4	?	?	?	80
beef mushroom	4 oz	?	3	?	?	?	60
broccoli, cream of	4 oz	?	5	?	?	?	80
prepared w/milk	4 oz	?	7	?	?	?	100
celery, cream of	4 oz	?	7	?	?	?	100
cheddar cheese	4 oz	?	6	?	?	?	110
chicken, cream of	4 oz	?	7	?	?	?	110
chicken alphabet	4 oz	?	3	?	?	?	80
chicken barley	4 oz	?	2	?	?	?	70
chicken broth	4 oz	?	2	?	?	?	30
chicken broth w/noodles	4 oz	?	1	?	?	?	45
chicken 'n dumplings	4 oz	?	3	?	?	?	80
chicken gumbo	4 oz	?	2	?	?	?	60
chicken mushroom, creamy	4 oz	?	8	?	?	?	120
chicken noodle	4 oz	?	2	?	?	?	60
chicken noodle, homestyle	4 oz	?	3	?	?	?	70
chicken noodle-o's	4 oz	?	2	?	?	?	70
chicken & stars	4 oz	?	2	?	?	?	60
chicken vegetable	4 oz	?	3	?	?	?	70
chicken w/rice	4 oz	?	3	?	?	?	60
chili beef	4 oz	?	5	?	?	?	140
clam chowder (Manhattan style)	4 oz	?	2	?	?	?	70
clam chowder (New England style)	4 oz	?	3	?	?	?	80
prepared w/whole milk	4 oz	?	7	?	?	?	150
consomme	4 oz	?	0	?	?	?	25
curly noodle w/chicken	4 oz	?	3	?	?	?	80
French onion	4 oz	?	2	?	?	?	60
green pea	4 oz	?	3	?	?	?	160
minestrone	4 oz	?	2	?	?	?	80
mushroom, cream of	4 oz	?	7	?	?	?	100
mushroom, golden	4 oz	?	3	?	?	?	70
nacho cheese	4 oz	?	8	?	?	?	110
prepared w/milk	4 oz	?	12	?	?	?	180
noodles & ground beef	4 oz	?	4	?	?	?	90
onion, cream of	4 oz	?	5	?	?	?	100
prepared w/whole milk & water	4 oz	?	7	?	?	?	140
oyster stew	4 oz	?	5	?	?	?	70
prepared w/whole milk	4 oz	?	9	?	?	?	140
pepper pot	4 oz	?	4	?	?	?	90
potato, cream of	4 oz	?	3	?	?	?	80

	Portion	Chol (mg)	Total Fat (g)	Satur'd Fat (g)	Mono Fat (g)	Poly Fat (g)	Total Calor
prepared w/whole milk & water	4 oz	?	4	?	?	?	120
scotch broth	4 oz	?	3	?	?	?	80
shrimp, cream of	4 oz	?	6	?	?	?	90
prepared w/whole milk	4 oz	?	10	?	?	?	160
split pea w/ham & bacon	4 oz	?	4	?	?	?	160
teddy bear	4 oz	?	2	?	?	?	70
tomato	4 oz	?	2	?	?	?	90
prepared w/whole milk	4 oz	?	4	?	?	?	150
tomato bisque	4 oz	?	3	?	?	?	120
tomato, homestyle, cream of	4 oz	?	3	?	?	?	110
prepared w/milk	4 oz	?	7	?	?	?	180
tomato rice, old fashioned	4 oz	?	2	?	?	?	110
tomato zesty	4 oz	?	2	?	?	?	100
turkey noodle	4 oz	?	2	?	?	?	70
turkey vegetable	4 oz	?	3	?	?	?	70
vegetable	4 oz	?	2	?	?	?	90
vegetable, homestyle	4 oz	?	2	?	?	?	60
vegetable, old fashioned	4 oz	?	2	?	?	?	60
vegetable, vegetarian	4 oz	?	2	?	?	?	80
vegetable beef	4 oz	?	2	?	?	?	70
won ton	4 oz	?	1	?	?	?	40

DRY SOUP MIXES, AS PACKAGED

	Portion	Chol (mg)	Total Fat (g)	Satur'd Fat (g)	Mono Fat (g)	Poly Fat (g)	Total Calor
chicken noodle	.9 oz	?	2	?	?	?	100
chicken noodle w/white meat	.80 oz	?	2	?	?	?	90
creamy chicken w/white meat	.90 oz	?	4	?	?	?	90
hearty noodle	.9 oz	?	1	?	?	?	90
noodle	1 oz	?	2	?	?	?	110
noodle w/chicken broth	.90 oz	?	2	?	?	?	90
onion	.55 oz	?	0	?	?	?	30

HOME COOKIN' SOUPS (READY TO SERVE)

	Portion	Chol (mg)	Total Fat (g)	Satur'd Fat (g)	Mono Fat (g)	Poly Fat (g)	Total Calor
bean & ham	10¾ oz	?	4	?	?	?	210
beef w/vegetables	10¾ oz	?	2	?	?	?	140
chicken gumbo w/sausage	10¾ oz	?	4	?	?	?	140
chicken minestrone	10¾ oz	?	6	?	?	?	180
chicken rice	10¾ oz	?	6	?	?	?	150
chicken w/noodles	10¾ oz	?	4	?	?	?	140
country vegetable	10¾ oz	?	2	?	?	?	120
hearty lentil	10¾ oz	?	2	?	?	?	170
minestrone	10¾ oz	?	3	?	?	?	140
split pea w/ham	10¾ oz	?	1	?	?	?	230
tomato garden	10¾ oz	?	3	?	?	?	150
vegetable beef	10¾ oz	?	3	?	?	?	140

	Portion	Chol (mg)	Total Fat(g)	Satur'd Fat(g)	Mono Fat(g)	Poly Fat(g)	Total Calor
LOW-SODIUM SOUPS (READY TO SERVE)							
chicken broth	10½ oz	?	1	?	?	?	30
chicken w/noodles	10¾ oz	?	5	?	?	?	170
chunky vegetable w/beef	10¾ oz	?	5	?	?	?	180
mushroom, cream of	10½ oz	?	14	?	?	?	210
split pea	10¾ oz	?	4	?	?	?	230
tomato w/tomato pieces	10½ oz	?	6	?	?	?	190
MICROWAVE SOUPS							
beef flavor noodle	1.35 oz	?	2	?	?	?	130
chicken flavor noodle	1.35 oz	?	3	?	?	?	140
hearty noodle w/vegetables	1.70 oz	?	2	?	?	?	180
noodle soup w/chicken broth	1.35 oz	?	2	?	?	?	130
bean w/bacon 'n ham	7½ oz	?	5	?	?	?	230
chicken noodle	7½ oz	?	4	?	?	?	100
chicken w/rice	7½ oz	?	4	?	?	?	100
chili beef	7½ oz	?	4	?	?	?	190
vegetable beef	7½ oz	?	2	?	?	?	100
RAMEN SOUPS							
cup-a-ramen							
beef flavor w/vegetables	2.20 oz	?	10	?	?	?	270
chicken flavor w/vegetables	2.20 oz	?	10	?	?	?	270
oriental flavor w/vegetables	2.20 oz	?	10	?	?	?	270
shrimp flavor w/vegetables	2.20 oz	?	10	?	?	?	280
lowfat cup-a-ramen							
beef flavor w/vegetables	2 oz	?	2	?	?	?	220
chicken flavor w/vegetables	2.15 oz	?	2	?	?	?	220
oriental flavor w/vegetables	2 oz	?	2	?	?	?	220
shrimp flavor w/vegetables	2.20 oz	?	2	?	?	?	230
lowfat block ramen noodle soup							
beef flavor	1½ oz	?	1	?	?	?	160
chicken flavor	1½ oz	?	1	?	?	?	160
oriental flavor	1.6 oz	?	1	?	?	?	150
pork flavor	1½ oz	?	1	?	?	?	150
ramen noodle soup							
beef flavor	1½ oz	?	8	?	?	?	190
chicken flavor	1½ oz	?	8	?	?	?	190
oriental flavor	1½ oz	?	8	?	?	?	190
pork flavor	1½ oz	?	8	?	?	?	200

	Portion	Chol (mg)	Total Fat(g)	Satur'd Fat(g)	Mono Fat(g)	Poly Fat(g)	Total Calor
College Inn							
chicken broth	½ can	5	3	1	?	?	35
lower salt	½ can	5	2	1	?	?	20
beef broth	½ can	0	0	0	?	?	16
Hain							
CANNED							
chicken broth	8¾ oz	5	6	?	?	?	70
no salt added	8¾ oz	5	5	?	?	?	60
chicken noodle soup	9½ oz	20	4	?	?	?	120
no salt added	9½ oz	25	4	?	?	?	120
creamy mushroom	9¼ oz	15	4	?	?	?	110
Italian vege-pasta	9½ oz	20	5	?	?	?	160
low sodium	9½ oz	20	6	?	?	?	140
minestrone	9½ oz	0	2	?	?	?	170
no salt added	9½ oz	0	4	?	?	?	160
mushroom barley	9½ oz	10	2	?	?	?	100
New England clam chowder	9¼ oz	25	4	?	?	?	180
turkey rice	9½ oz	20	3	?	?	?	100
no salt added	9½ oz	15	4	?	?	?	120
vegetable chicken	9½ oz	15	4	?	?	?	120
no salt added	9½ oz	20	4	?	?	?	130
vegetarian lentil	9½ oz	5	3	?	?	?	160
no salt added	9½ oz	5	3	?	?	?	160
split pea	9½ oz	0	1	?	?	?	170
no salt added	9½ oz	0	1	?	?	?	170
vegetarian vegetable	9½ oz	0	4	?	?	?	140
no salt added	9½ oz	0	5	?	?	?	150
vegetarian broth	9½ oz	0	0	?	?	?	45
low sodium	9½ oz	0	<1	?	?	?	40
vegetarian split pea	9½ oz	0	1	?	?	?	170
no salt	9½ oz	0	1	?	?	?	170
MIXES							
cheese & broccoli soup recipe	¾ C	?	22	?	?	?	310
cheese savory soup & sauce	¾ C	?	16	?	?	?	250
lentil savory	¾ C	?	2	?	?	?	130
minestrone savory	¾ C	?	1	?	?	?	110
mushroom savory soup & recipe	¾ C	?	15	?	?	?	210
no salt added	¾ C	?	20	?	?	?	250
onion savory soup, dip & recipe	¾ C	?	2	?	?	?	50
no salt added	¾ C	?	1	?	?	?	50
potato leek savory	¾ C	?	18	?	?	?	260
split pea savory	¾ C	?	10	?	?	?	310
tomato savory soup & recipe	¾ C	?	14	?	?	?	220

	Portion	Chol (mg)	Total Fat(g)	Satur'd Fat(g)	Mono Fat(g)	Poly Fat(g)	Total Calor
vegetable savory	¾ C	?	1	?	?	?	80
no salt added	¾ C	?	1	?	?	?	80
Health Valley							
black bean	4 oz	0	3	?	?	?	115
lentil	4 oz	0	4	?	?	?	80
minestrone	4 oz	0	1	?	?	?	70
mushroom	4 oz	0	3	?	?	?	70
potato	4 oz	0	2	?	?	?	70
tomato	4 oz	0	2	?	?	?	60
vegetable	4 oz	0	4	?	?	?	80
fat free							
beef broth	1.9 oz	0	<1	?	?	?	10
black bean	7.5 oz	0	<1	?	?	?	70
chicken broth	6.9 oz	0	<1	?	?	?	20
country corn	7.5 oz	0	<1	?	?	?	60
5-bean vegetable	7.5 oz	0	<1	?	?	?	70
14 garden vegetable	7.5 oz	0	<1	?	?	?	50
lentil	7.5 oz	0	<1	?	?	?	70
split pea	7.5 oz	0	<1	?	?	?	80
tomato/vegetable	7.5 oz	0	<1	?	?	?	40
Nissin							
OODLES OF NOODLES/TOP RAMEN							
beef	?		1	18	?	?	?	390
chicken	?		1	18	?	?	?	400
CUP O' NOODLES							
beef	?	<1	14	?	?	?	290
beef onion	?	<1	12	?	?	?	280
chicken	?	<1	14	?	?	?	280
crab	?	<1	13	?	?	?	270
garden vegetable	?	<1	12	?	?	?	280
lobster	?	<1	13	?	?	?	290
pork	?	<1	12	?	?	?	280
spicy chicken	?	<1	12	?	?	?	290
CUP O' NOODLES (TWIN PACK)							
beef	?	<1	7	?	?	?	150
chicken	?	<1	6	?	?	?	150
HEARTY CUP O' NOODLES							
beef vegetable	?	8	13	?	?	?	290
chicken oriental	?	8	14	?	?	?	300
old fashioned vegetable	?	8	15	?	?	?	290
seafood chowder	?	8	15	?	?	?	300
shrimp chow mein	?	8	14	?	?	?	300
Progresso							
BEEF & PORK FLAVORED							
beef	10½ oz can	35	6	?	?	?	180
beef barley	10½ oz can	30	5	?	?	?	150

	Portion	Chol (mg)	Total Fat(g)	Satur'd Fat(g)	Mono Fat(g)	Poly Fat(g)	Total Calor
beef minestrone	10½ oz can	35	6	?	?	?	180
beef vegetable	10½ oz can	40	3	?	?	?	170
chickarina	9½ oz	20	5	?	?	?	130
ham & bean	9½ oz	10	2	?	?	?	140
hearty beef	9½ oz	35	4	<1	2	?	160
lentil w/sausage	9½ oz	20	8	?	?	?	170
split pea w/ham	10½ oz can	15	5	?	?	?	160
seasoned beef broth	4 oz	0	<1	?	?	?	10
CHICKEN FLAVORED							
chicken barley	9 oz	20	2	?	?	?	100
broth	4 oz	<5	0	?	?	?	8
chicken minestrone	10½ oz can	40	4	?	?	?	140
chicken noodle	10½ oz can	40	4	?	?	?	120
chicken rice	10½ oz can	25	4	?	?	?	120
cream of chicken	9.5 oz	35	11	?	?	?	190
hearty chicken	10½ oz can	30	4	?	?	?	130
homestyle chicken	9.5 oz	20	3	?	?	?	110
NON-MEAT FLAVORED							
corn chowder	9¼ oz	20	3	?	?	?	200
cream of mushroom	9¼ oz	15	10	?	?	?	160
creamy tortellini	9¼ oz	35	16	85	?	1	240
green split pea	10½ oz can	?	3	?	?	?	201
hearty minestrone	9¼ oz	<5	2	?	?	?	110
lentil	10½ oz can	0	4	?	?	?	140
Manhattan clam chowder	10½ oz can	10	2	?	?	?	120
minestrone	10½ oz can	0	3	?	?	?	120
New England style clam chowder	10½ oz can	20	12	?	?	?	220
tomato	9½ oz	0	3	?	?	?	120
tomato tortellini	9¼ oz	10	5	?	?	?	130
tortellini	9½ oz	10	3	?	?	?	90
vegetable	10½ oz can	<5	2	?	?	?	80
zesty minestrone	10½ oz can	10	8	?	?	?	150
Stouffer's Frozen Soups							
clam chowder (New England)	8 oz	?	9	?	?	?	180
spinach, cream of	8 oz	?	15	?	?	?	210

	Portion	Chol (mg)	Total Fat(g)	Satur'd Fat(g)	Mono Fat(g)	Poly Fat(g)	Total Calor
Swanson							
beef broth	7¼ oz	?	1	?	?	?	18
chicken broth	7¼ oz	?	2	?	?	?	30
natural goodness clear chicken broth	7¼ oz	?	1	?	?	?	20
Weight Watchers							
vegetable w/beef stock	10½ oz	?	2	?	?	?	90
turkey vegetable	10½ oz	?	2	?	?	?	70
chunky vegetarian vegetable	10½ oz	?	2	?	?	?	100
cream of mushroom	10½ oz	?	2	?	?	?	90
chicken noodle	10½ oz	?	2	?	?	?	80
instant broth mix							
beef	1 packet	?	?	?	?	?	8
chicken	1 packet	?	?	?	?	?	8

❑ **SOUR CREAM** *See* MILK, MILK SUBSTITUTES, & MILK PRODUCTS

❑ **SOYBEANS & SOYBEAN PRODUCTS**

Soybeans

boiled	½ c	0	8	1	?	?	149
dry roasted	½ c	0	19	3	?	?	387
roasted	½ c	0	22	3	?	?	405
green, boiled, drained	½ c	0	6	1	?	?	127
kernels, roasted & toasted	1 oz	0	7	1	?	?	129
kernels, roasted & toasted	1 c whole kernels	0	26	3	?	?	490
mature seeds, sprouted							
raw	½ c	0	2	tr	?	?	45
steamed	½ c	0	2	tr	?	?	38
stir fried	3½ oz	0	7	?	?	?	125

Soybean Products

fermented products							
miso	½ c	0	8	1	?	?	284
natto	½ c	0	10	1	?	?	187
tempeh	½ c	0	6	1	?	?	165
soy flour							
full-fat							
raw	½ c stirred	0	9	1	?	?	182
roasted	½ c stirred	0	9	1	?	?	184
low-fat	½ c stirred	0	3	tr	?	?	163
defatted	½ c stirred	0	1	tr	?	?	164

	Portion	Chol (mg)	Total Fat(g)	Satur'd Fat(g)	Mono Fat(g)	Poly Fat(g)	Total Calor
soy meal, defatted, raw	1/2 c	0	1	tr	?	?	206
soy milk, fluid	1 c	0	5	1	?	?	79
soy protein							
concentrate	1 oz	0	tr	tr	?	?	92
isolate	1 oz	0	1	tr	?	?	94
soy sauce							
ready to serve	1 T	0	0	0	?	?	11
ready to serve	1 fl oz	0	0	0	?	?	23
made from hydrolyzed vegetable protein	1 T	0	tr	tr	?	?	7
made from hydrolyzed vegetable protein	1/4 c	0	tr	tr	?	?	24
made from soy (tamari)	1 T	0	tr	tr	?	?	11
made from soy (tamari)	1/4 c	0	tr	tr	?	?	35
made from soy & wheat (shoyu)	1 T	0	tr	tr	?	?	9
made from soy & wheat (shoyu)	1/4 c	0	tr	tr	?	?	30
teriyaki sauce							
ready to serve	1 T	0	0	0	?	?	15
ready to serve	1 fl oz	0	0	0	?	?	30
dehydrated	1 pkt = 1.6 oz	0	1	tr	?	?	130
prepared w/water	1 c	0	1	tr	?	?	131
tofu							
raw							
regular	4.1 oz	0	6	1	?	?	88
regular	1/2 c	0	6	1	?	?	94
firm	2.9 oz	0	7	1	?	?	118
firm	1/2 c	0	11	2	?	?	183
dried-frozen (koyadofu)	0.6 oz	0	5	1	?	?	82
fried	1/2 oz	0	3	tr	?	?	35
okara	1/2 c	0	1	tr	?	?	47
salted & fermented (fuyu)	0.4 oz	0	1	tr	?	?	13

▪ BRAND NAME

Arrowhead Mills

	Portion	Chol (mg)	Total Fat(g)	Satur'd Fat(g)	Mono Fat(g)	Poly Fat(g)	Total Calor
soybean flakes	2 oz	0	11	?	?	?	250
soybeans	2 oz	0	10	?	?	?	230
soy flour	2 oz	0	11	?	?	?	250
Fearn							
lecithin							
liquid, regular	1 T	0	16	2	?	7	130
liquid, mint-flavored	1 T	0	12	2	?	7	113
granules	2 T, level	0	12	2	?	6	100
natural soya powder	1/4 c	?	5	?	?	?	100
soya granules	1/4 c	?	0	?	?	?	140
soya protein isolate	1/4 c	?	0	?	?	?	60

	Portion	Chol (mg)	Total Fat(g)	Satur'd Fat(g)	Mono Fat(g)	Poly Fat(g)	Total Calor
Health Valley							
Soy Moo soybean milk	8 fl oz	0	6	?	?	?	140
Kikkoman							
soy sauce							
regular	1 T	tr	tr	?	?	?	10
lite	1 T	tr	tr	?	?	?	10
stir-fry sauce	1 t	0	tr	?	?	?	6
sweet & sour sauce	1 T	0	tr	?	?	?	18
teriyaki sauce	1 T	tr	tr	?	?	?	15

❏ SPECIAL DIETARY FOODS

	Portion	Chol (mg)	Total Fat(g)	Satur'd Fat(g)	Mono Fat(g)	Poly Fat(g)	Total Calor
Carnation							
SLENDER							
instant							
Dutch chocolate	1 envelope	2	1	<1	<1	<1	110
chocolate	1 envelope	2	1	<1	<1	<1	110
French vanilla	1 envelope	3	<1	<1	<1	<1	110
liquid							
all flavors	10 oz	?	4	?	?	?	220
bars							
chocolate peanut butter	2 bars	0	15	5	9	1	270
chocolate	2 bars	0	14	5	9	1	270
chocolate chip	2 bars	0	14	5	8	0	270
vanilla	2 bars	0	15	6	9	0	270
Sego							
LIQUID DIET FOOD							
Sego lite							
chocolate	10 oz	5	3	?	?	?	150
Dutch chocolate	10 oz	5	3	?	?	?	150
French vanilla	10 oz	5	4	?	?	?	150
strawberry	10 oz	5	4	?	?	?	150
vanilla	10 oz	5	4	?	?	?	150
Sego very							
chocolate	10 oz	5	1	?	?	?	225
chocolate malt	10 oz	5	1	?	?	?	225
strawberry	10 oz	5	5	?	?	?	225
vanilla	10 oz	5	5	?	?	?	225

	Portion	Chol (mg)	Total Fat(g)	Satur'd Fat(g)	Mono Fat(g)	Poly Fat(g)	Total Calor

❏ **SPICES** *See* SEASONINGS

❏ **STUFFINGS** *See* BREADCRUMBS, CROUTONS, STUFFINGS, & SEASONED COATINGS

❏ **SUGARS & SWEETENERS: HONEY, MOLASSES, SUGAR, SUGAR SUBSTITUTES, SYRUP, & TREACLE**

Honey

	Portion	Chol (mg)	Total Fat(g)	Satur'd Fat(g)	Mono Fat(g)	Poly Fat(g)	Total Calor
honey	1 T	0	0	0	?	?	61

Molasses

	Portion	Chol (mg)	Total Fat(g)	Satur'd Fat(g)	Mono Fat(g)	Poly Fat(g)	Total Calor
first extraction, light	1 T	0	0	0	?	?	50
second extraction, medium	1 T	0	0	0	?	?	46
third extraction, blackstrap	1 T	0	0	0	?	?	43

Sugar

	Portion	Chol (mg)	Total Fat(g)	Satur'd Fat(g)	Mono Fat(g)	Poly Fat(g)	Total Calor
brown	1 T	0	0	0	?	?	52
maple	1 T	0	0	0	?	?	52
sugarcane juice	1 T	0	tr	?	?	?	16
white							
powdered	1 T	0	0	0	?	?	42
granular	1 cube	0	0	0	?	?	24
granular	1 t	0	0	0	?	?	16
granular	1 T	0	0	0	?	?	46
granular	½ c	0	0	0	?	?	385

Syrups

	Portion	Chol (mg)	Total Fat(g)	Satur'd Fat(g)	Mono Fat(g)	Poly Fat(g)	Total Calor
cane	1 T	0	0	0	?	?	53
corn	1 T	0	0	0	?	?	57
dark corn	1 T	0	0	0	?	?	60
maple	1 T	0	0	0	?	?	50
maple, imitation	1 T	0	0	0	?	?	55
sorghum, pancake	1 T	0	0	0	?	?	52
table blend, pancake							
cane & maple	1 T	0	0	0	?	?	50
mainly corn	1 T	0	0	0	?	?	57

	Portion	Chol (mg)	Total Fat(g)	Satur'd Fat(g)	Mono Fat(g)	Poly Fat(g)	Total Calor
Treacle							
black	1 T	0	0	0	?	?	53

■ **BRAND NAME**

	Portion	Chol (mg)	Total Fat(g)	Satur'd Fat(g)	Mono Fat(g)	Poly Fat(g)	Total Calor
Aunt Jemima							
syrup	1.4 fl oz	32	0	0	0	0	109
lite syrup	1 fl oz	92	.1	0	0	0	54
butter lite syrup	1 fl oz	88	0	0	0	0	53
Brer Rabbit							
molasses, light & dark	1 T	0	0	?	?	?	60
syrup, light or dark	1 T	0	0	?	?	?	60
Diamond Crystal							
sugar substitute	1 pkg	0	0	0	?	?	1
Equal							
sugar substitute	1 pkg	0	0	0	?	?	4
Grandma's							
molasses, gold & green	1 T	0	0	0	?	?	70
Golden Griddle							
syrup	1 T	0	0	0	?	?	50
Karo							
dark corn syrup	1 T	0	0	0	?	?	60
light corn syrup	1 T	0	0	0	?	?	60
pancake syrup	1 T	0	0	0	?	?	60
Log Cabin							
pancake or waffle syrup	1 fl oz	0	0	?	?	?	100
Country Kitchen syrup	1 fl oz	0	0	?	?	?	100
lite	1 fl oz	0	0	?	?	?	50
NutraSweet							
sugar substitute	1 pkt	0	0	0	?	?	4
Sugartwin							
sugar substitute							
white	1 pkg	0	0	0	?	?	3
white/brown	1 t	0	0	0	?	?	1
Sweet & Low							
sugar substitute	1 pkg	0	0	0	?	?	4
Sweet 10							
sugar substitute	⅛ t	0	0	0	?	?	0

❏ **SYRUP** *See* SUGARS & SWEETENERS

❏ **SYRUP, DESSERT** *See* DESSERT SAUCES, SYRUPS, & TOPPINGS

	Portion	Chol (mg)	Total Fat(g)	Satur'd Fat(g)	Mono Fat(g)	Poly Fat(g)	Total Calor

❏ **TOFU, FROZEN** *See* DESSERTS, FROZEN

❏ **TREACLE** *See* SUGARS & SWEETENERS

❏ **TURKEY** *See* POULTRY, FRESH & PROCESSED; PROCESSED MEAT & POULTRY PRODUCTS

❏ **VEAL** *See* LAMB, VEAL, & MISCELLANEOUS MEATS

❏ **VEGETABLES, PLAIN & PREPARED**
See also LEGUMES & LEGUME PRODUCTS
See also PICKLES, OLIVES, RELISHES, & CHUTNEYS
See also RICE & GRAINS, PLAIN & PREPARED

	Portion	Chol (mg)	Total Fat(g)	Satur'd Fat(g)	Mono Fat(g)	Poly Fat(g)	Total Calor
amaranth							
raw	1 c	0	tr	tr	?	?	7
boiled, drained	½ c	0	tr	tr	?	?	14
artichokes, Globe & French varieties							
boiled	1 medium = 4.2 oz	0	tr	tr	?	?	53
boiled	½ c hearts	0	tr	tr	?	?	37
frozen, boiled, drained	9 oz pkg	0	1	tr	?	?	108
artichokes, Jerusalem *See* JERUSALEM ARTICHOKES, below							
asparagus, cuts & spears							
raw	4 spears = 2 oz	0	tr	tr	?	?	13
boiled	4 spears = 2.1 oz	0	tr	tr	?	?	15
canned							
drained solids	½ c	0	1	tr	?	?	24
canned, solids & liquids	½ c	0	tr	tr	?	?	17
frozen, boiled, drained	10 oz pkg	0	1	tr	?	?	82
frozen, boiled, drained	4 spears = 2.1 oz	0	tr	tr	?	?	17
asparagus beans *See* YARDLONG BEANS, under LEGUMES & LEGUME PRODUCTS							
bamboo shoots							
raw	½ c	0	tr	tr	?	?	21

	Portion	Chol (mg)	Total Fat(g)	Satur'd Fat(g)	Mono Fat(g)	Poly Fat(g)	Total Calor
boiled, drained	1 c	0	tr	tr	?	?	15
canned, drained	1 c	0	1	tr	?	?	25
basella *See* VINESPINACH, below							
beans, lima *See* LEGUMES & LEGUME PRODUCTS							
beans, mung *See* LEGUMES & LEGUME PRODUCTS							
beans, pinto *See* LEGUMES & LEGUME PRODUCTS							
beans, shellie, canned, solids & liquids	½ c	0	tr	tr	?	?	37
beans, snap							
raw	½ c	0	tr	tr	?	?	17
boiled, drained	½ c	0	tr	tr	?	?	22
canned							
drained solids	½ c	0	tr	tr	?	?	13
solids & liquids	½ c	0	tr	tr	?	?	18
solids & liquids, seasoned	½ c	0	tr	tr	?	?	18
frozen, boiled, drained	½ c	0	tr	tr	?	?	18
beet greens							
raw	½ c	0	tr	tr	?	?	4
boiled, drained	½ c	0	tr	tr	?	?	20
beets							
raw	½ c sliced	0	tr	tr	?	?	30
boiled, drained	½ c sliced	0	tr	tr	?	?	26
canned							
drained solids	½ c sliced	0	tr	tr	?	?	27
solids & liquid	½ c	0	tr	tr	?	?	36
pickled, canned, solids & liquids	½ c	0	tr	tr	?	?	75
beets, Harvard, canned, solids & liquids	½ c sliced	0	tr	tr	?	?	89
bok choy *See* CABBAGE, CHINESE, below							
borage							
raw	½ c	0	tr	?	?	?	9
boiled, drained	3½ oz	0	1	?	?	?	25
broad beans *See* LEGUMES & LEGUME PRODUCTS							
broccoli							
raw	1 spear = 5.3 oz	0	1	tr	?	?	42
boiled, drained	½ c	0	tr	tr	?	?	23
boiled, drained	1 spear = 6.3 oz	0	1	tr	?	?	53
frozen, boiled, drained	½ c chopped	0	tr	tr	?	?	25
frozen, boiled, drained	½ c spears	0	tr	tr	?	?	69
frozen, boiled, drained	10 oz pkg spears	0	tr	tr	?	?	25
brussel sprouts							
boiled, drained	0.73 oz	0	tr	tr	?	?	8
boiled, drained	½ c	0	tr	tr	?	?	30
frozen, boiled, drained	½ c	0	tr	tr	?	?	33

	Portion	Chol (mg)	Total Fat(g)	Satur'd Fat(g)	Mono Fat(g)	Poly Fat(g)	Total Calor
burdock root							
raw	1 c	0	tr	?	?	?	85
boiled, drained	1 c	0	tr	?	?	?	110
cabbage							
raw	½ c shredded	0	tr	tr	?	?	8
boiled, drained	½ c shredded	0	tr	tr	?	?	16
cabbage, Chinese							
bok choy							
raw	½ c shredded	0	tr	tr	?	?	5
drained	½ c shredded	0	tr	tr	?	?	10
pe-tsai							
raw	½ c shredded	0	tr	tr	?	?	6
boiled, drained	1 c shredded	0	tr	tr	?	?	16
cabbage, red							
raw	½ c shredded	0	tr	tr	?	?	10
boiled, drained	½ c shredded	0	tr	tr	?	?	16
cabbage, savoy							
raw	½ c shredded	0	tr	tr	?	?	10
boiled, drained	½ c shredded	0	tr	tr	?	?	18
cardoon, raw	½ c shredded	0	tr	tr	?	?	18
carrots							
raw	½ c	0	tr	tr	?	?	24
boiled, drained	½ c sliced	0	tr	tr	?	?	35
canned							
drained solids	½ c sliced	0	tr	tr	?	?	17
solids & liquids	½ c sliced	0	tr	tr	?	?	28
frozen, boiled, drained	½ c sliced	0	tr	tr	?	?	26
cassava, raw	3½ oz	0	tr	tr	?	?	120
cauliflower							
raw	½ c	0	tr	tr	?	?	12
boiled, drained	½ c	0	tr	tr	?	?	15
frozen, boiled, drained	½ c	0	tr	tr	?	?	17
celeriac							
raw	½ c	0	tr	tr	?	?	31
boiled, drained	3½ oz	0	tr	?	?	?	25
celery							
raw	1 stalk = 1.4 oz	0	tr	tr	?	?	6
raw	½ c diced	0	tr	tr	?	?	9
boiled, drained	½ c dices	0	tr	tr	?	?	11

	Portion	Chol (mg)	Total Fat(g)	Satur'd Fat(g)	Mono Fat(g)	Poly Fat(g)	Total Calor
celtuce, raw	1 leaf = 0.3 oz	0	tr	?	?	?	2
chard, Swiss							
raw	½ c chopped	0	tr	?	?	?	3
boiled, drained	½ c chopped	0	tr	?	?	?	18
chicory, raw							
greens	½ c chopped	0	tr	tr	?	?	21
roots	½ c 1" pieces	0	tr	tr	?	?	33
witloof	½ c	0	tr	tr	?	?	7
Chinese parsley *See* CORIANDER, below							
Chinese preserving melon *See* WAX GOURD, below							
chives							
raw	1 T	0	tr	tr	?	?	1
freeze-dried	1 T	0	tr	tr	?	?	1
collards							
raw	½ c chopped	0	tr	?	?	?	18
boiled, drained	½ c chopped	0	tr	?	?	?	13
frozen, boiled, drained	½ c chopped	0	tr	?	?	?	31
coriander (cilantro), raw	¼ c	0	tr	?	?	?	1
corn, sweet							
raw	½ c kernels	0	1	tr	?	?	66
boiled, drained	½ c kernels	0	1	tr	?	?	89
canned							
drained solids	½ c kernels	0	1	tr	?	?	66
solids & liquid	½ c kernels	0	1	tr	?	?	79
cream style	½ c	0	1	tr	?	?	93
vacuum pack	½ c	0	1	tr	?	?	83
w/red green peppers, solids & liquid	½ c	0	1	tr	?	?	86
frozen, boiled, drained	½ c kernels off cob	0	tr	tr	?	?	67
corn pudding	1 c	230	13	6	?	?	271
cowpeas *See* LEGUMES & LEGUME PRODUCTS							
cress, garden							
raw	½ c	0	tr	tr	?	?	8
boiled, drained	½ c	0	tr	tr	?	?	16
cucumber, raw	½ c sliced	0	tr	tr	?	?	7
daikon *See* RADISHES, ORIENTAL, below							

	Portion	Chol (mg)	Total Fat(g)	Satur'd Fat(g)	Mono Fat(g)	Poly Fat(g)	Total Calor
dandelion greens							
raw	½ c chopped	0	tr	?	?	?	13
boiled, drained	½ c chopped	0	tr	?	?	?	17
dasheen *See* TARO, below							
dock							
raw	½ c chopped	0	tr	?	?	?	15
boiled, drained	3½ oz	0	1	?	?	?	20
eggplant, boiled, drained	1 c 1″ cubes	0	tr	tr	?	?	27
endive, raw	½ c chopped	0	tr	tr	?	?	4
endive, Belgian *See* CHICKORY, WITLOOF, above							
escarole *See* ENDIVE, above							
garlic, raw	1 clove = 0.1 oz	0	tr	tr	?	?	4
ginger root, raw	0.4 oz	0	tr	tr	?	?	8
ginger root, raw	¼ c sliced	0	tr	tr	?	?	17
horseradish-tree leafy tips							
raw	½ c chopped	0	tr	?	?	?	6
boiled, drained	½ c chopped	0	tr	?	?	?	13
pods							
raw	1 = 0.4 oz	0	tr	?	?	?	4
boiled, drained	½ c sliced	0	tr	?	?	?	21
hyacinth beans *See* LEGUMES & LEGUME PRODUCTS							
Jerusalem-artichokes, raw	½ c sliced	0	tr	0	?	?	57
jicama *See* YAM BEAN, below							
kale							
raw	½ c chopped	0	tr	tr	?	?	17
boiled, drained	½ c chopped	0	tr	tr	?	?	21
frozen, boiled, drained	½ c chopped	0	tr	tr	?	?	20
kale, Scotch							
raw	½ c chopped	0	tr	tr	?	?	14
boiled, drained	½ c chopped	0	tr	tr	?	?	18
kohlrabi							
raw	½ c sliced	0	tr	tr	?	?	19
boiled, drained	½ c sliced	0	tr	tr	?	?	24
leeks							
raw	¼ c chopped	0	tr	tr	?	?	16

	Portion	Chol (mg)	Total Fat(g)	Satur'd Fat(g)	Mono Fat(g)	Poly Fat(g)	Total Calor
boiled, drained	¼ c chopped	0	tr	tr	?	?	8
freeze-dried	1 T	0	0	0	?	?	1
lentils *See* LEGUMES & LEGUME PRODUCTS							
lettuce, raw							
butterhead (includes Boston & Bibb types)	2 leaves = ½ oz	0	tr	tr	?	?	2
butterhead (includes Boston & Bibb types)	1 head = 5.7 oz	0	tr	tr	?	?	21
cos or romaine	1 inner leaf = 0.35 oz	0	tr	tr	?	?	2
cos or romaine	½ c shredded	0	tr	tr	?	?	4
iceberg	1 leaf = 0.7 oz	0	tr	tr	?	?	3
iceberg	1 head = 1 lb 3 oz	0	1	tr	?	?	70
looseleaf	1 leaf = 0.35 oz	0	tr	tr	?	?	2
looseleaf	½ c shredded	0	tr	tr	?	?	5
lima beans *See* LEGUMES & LEGUME PRODUCTS							
manioc *See* CASSAVA, above							
mountain yam, hawaii, steamed	½ c	0	tr	tr	?	?	59
mung beans *See* LEGUMES & LEGUME PRODUCTS							
mushrooms							
raw	½ c pieces	0	tr	tr	?	?	9
boiled, drained	½ c pieces	0	tr	tr	?	?	21
canned, drained solids	½ c	0	tr	tr	?	?	19
mushrooms, shitake							
dried	0.1 oz	0	tr	tr	?	?	11
cooked	½ oz	0	tr	tr	?	?	40
mustard greens							
raw	½ c chopped	0	tr	tr	?	?	7
boiled, drained	½ c chopped	0	tr	tr	?	?	11
frozen, boiled, drained	½ c chopped	0	tr	tr	?	?	14
mustard spinach							
raw	½ c chopped	0	tr	?	?	?	17
boiled, spinach	½ c chopped	0	tr	?	?	?	14
New Zealand spinach							
raw	½ c chopped	0	tr	tr	?	?	4
boiled, drained	½ c chopped	0	tr	tr	?	?	11

	Portion	Chol (mg)	Total Fat(g)	Satur'd Fat(g)	Mono Fat(g)	Poly Fat(g)	Total Calor
okra							
boiled, drained	½ c sliced	0	tr	tr	?	?	25
frozen, boiled, drained	½ c sliced	0	tr	tr	?	?	34
onion rings, frozen, heated in oven	0.7 oz	0	5	2	?	?	81
onions							
raw	1 T chopped	0	tr	tr	?	?	3
raw	½ c chopped	0	tr	tr	?	?	27
boiled, drained	1 T chopped	0	tr	tr	?	?	4
boiled, drained	½ c chopped	0	tr	tr	?	?	29
canned, solids & liquids	2.2 oz	0	tr	tr	?	?	12
dehydrated flakes	1 T	0	tr	tr	?	?	16
frozen, boiled, drained	1 T chopped	0	tr	tr	?	?	4
frozen, boiled, drained	½ c chopped	0	tr	tr	?	?	30
onions, spring, raw	1 T chopped	0	tr	tr	?	?	2
onions, spring, raw	½ c chopped	0	tr	tr	?	?	13
onions, Welsh, raw	3½ oz	0	tr	tr	?	?	34
oysterplant See SALSIFY, below							
parsley							
raw	10 sprigs = 0.35 oz	0	tr	?	?	?	3
raw	½ c chopped	0	tr	?	?	?	10
freeze-dried	1 T	0	tr	?	?	?	1
parsnips							
raw	½ c sliced	0	tr	tr	?	?	50
boiled, drained	½ c sliced	0	tr	tr	?	?	63
peas, edible pods							
raw	½ c	0	tr	tr	?	?	30
boiled, drained	½ c	0	tr	tr	?	?	34
frozen, boiled, drained	½ c	0	tr	tr	?	?	42
frozen, boiled, drained	10 oz pkg	0	1	tr	?	?	132
peas, green							
raw	½ c	0	tr	tr	?	?	63
boiled, drained	½ c	0	tr	tr	?	?	67
canned							
drained solids	½ c	0	tr	tr	?	?	59
solids & liquids	½ c	0	tr	tr	?	?	61
solids & liquids, seasoned	½ c	0	tr	tr	?	?	57
frozen, boiled, drained	½ c	0	tr	tr	?	?	63

	Portion	Chol (mg)	Total Fat(g)	Satur'd Fat(g)	Mono Fat(g)	Poly Fat(g)	Total Calor
mature seeds, sprouted							
raw	½ c	0	tr	tr	?	?	77
boiled, drained	3½ oz	0	1	tr	?	?	118
peas, split *See* LEGUMES & LEGUME PRODUCTS							
peas & carrots							
canned, solids & liquids	½ c	0	tr	tr	?	?	48
frozen, boiled, drained	½ c	0	tr	tr	?	?	38
frozen, boiled, drained	10 oz pkg	0	1	tr	?	?	133
peas & onions							
canned, solids & liquids	½ c	0	tr	tr	?	?	30
frozen, boiled, drained	½ c	0	tr	tr	?	?	40
peppers							
hot chili							
raw	1 pepper = 1.6 oz	0	tr	tr	?	?	18
raw	½ c chopped	0	tr	tr	?	?	30
canned, solids & liquids	1 pepper = 2.6 oz	0	tr	tr	?	?	18
canned, solids & liquids	½ c chopped	0	tr	tr	?	?	17
jalapeño, canned, solids & liquids	½ c chopped	0	tr	tr	?	?	17
sweet							
raw	1 pepper = 2.6 oz	0	tr	tr	?	?	18
raw	½ c chopped	0	tr	tr	?	?	12
boiled, drained	1 pepper = 2.6 oz	0	tr	tr	?	?	13
boiled, drained	½ c chopped	0	tr	tr	?	?	12
canned, solids & liquids	½ c halves	0	tr	tr	?	?	13
freeze-dried	1 T	0	tr	tr	?	?	1
freeze-dried	¼ c	0	tr	tr	?	?	5
frozen, unprepared	10 oz pkg chopped	0	1	tr	?	?	58
frozen, boiled, drained	3½ oz chopped	0	tr	tr	?	?	18
pigeon peas *See* LEGUMES & LEGUME PRODUCTS							
pimentos *See* PICKLES, OLIVES, RELISHES, & CHUTNEYS							
pinto beans *See* LEGUMES & LEGUME PRODUCTS							
poi	½ c	0	tr	tr	?	?	134
potato chips & sticks *See* SNACKS							
potato flour *See* FLOURS & CORNMEALS							
potato pancakes	1	93	13	3	?	?	495
potato puffs, frozen, prepared	1	0	1	tr	?	?	16

	Portion	Chol (mg)	Total Fat(g)	Satur'd Fat(g)	Mono Fat(g)	Poly Fat(g)	Total Calor
potato salad	½ c	86	10	2	?	?	179
potatoes							
raw							
flesh	3.9 oz	0	tr	tr	?	?	88
skin	1.3 oz	0	tr	tr	?	?	22
baked							
flesh & skin	7.1 oz	0	tr	tr	?	?	220
flesh	5½ oz	0	tr	tr	?	?	145
skin	2 oz	0	tr	tr	?	?	115
boiled in skin							
flesh	4.8 oz	0	tr	tr	?	?	119
skin	1.2 oz	0	tr	tr	?	?	27
boiled w/out skin, flesh	4.8 oz	0	tr	tr	?	?	116
microwaved in skin							
flesh & skin	7.1 oz	0	tr	tr	?	?	212
flesh	5½ oz	0	tr	tr	?	?	156
skin	2 oz	0	tr	tr	?	?	77
canned							
drained solids	1.2 oz	0	tr	tr	?	?	21
solids & liquids	1 c	0	tr	tr	?	?	120
frozen, whole							
unprepared	½ c	0	tr	tr	?	?	71
French fried							
frozen, fried in animal fat & vegetable oil	1.8 oz	6	8	3	?	?	158
fried in vegetable oil	1.8 oz	0	8	3	?	?	158
heated in oven	1.8 oz	0	4	2	?	?	111
cottage-cut, heated in oven	1.8 oz	0	4	2	?	?	109
extruded, heated in oven	1.8 oz	0	9	4	?	?	163
potatoes, au gratin							
dry mix, prepared	5½ oz pkg	?	34	21	?	?	764
homemade	½ c	29	9	6	?	?	160
potatoes, hashed brown							
frozen, plain, prepared	½ c	?	9	4	?	?	170
frozen, in butter sauce, unprepared	6 oz pkg	?	11	4	?	?	229
homemade prepared in vegetable oil	½ c	?	11	4	?	?	163
potatoes, mashed							
dehydrated flakes, prepared (whole milk & butter added)	½ c	15	6	4	?	?	118
granules w/milk, prepared	½ c	2	2	1	?	?	83
granules w/out milk, prepared (whole milk & butter added)	½ c	18	7	1	?	?	137
homemade	½ c	2	4	1	?	?	111
homemade	½ c	2	1	tr	?	?	81

	Portion	Chol (mg)	Total Fat(g)	Satur'd Fat(g)	Mono Fat(g)	Poly Fat(g)	Total Calor
potatoes, O'Brien							
frozen, prepared	3½ oz	?	13	3	?	?	204
homemade	1 c	7	2	2	?	?	157
potatoes, scalloped							
dry mix, prepared w/whole milk & butter	5½ oz pkg	?	35	22	?	?	764
homemade	½ c	14	4	3	?	?	105
pumpkin							
boiled, drained	½ c mashed	0	tr	tr	?	?	24
canned	½ c	0	tr	tr	?	?	41
pumpkin flowers							
raw	1 c	0	tr	tr	?	?	5
boiled, drained	½ c	0	tr	tr	?	?	10
pumpkin leaves, boiled, drained	½ c	0	tr	tr	?	?	7
radishes, raw	10 radishes = 1.6 oz	0	tr	tr	?	?	7
Oriental							
raw	½ c	0	tr	tr	?	?	8
boiled, drained	½ c sliced	0	tr	tr	?	?	13
dried	½ c	0	tr	tr	?	?	157
white icicle, raw	½ c sliced	0	tr	tr	?	?	7
radish seeds, sprouted, raw	½ c	0	tr	tr	?	?	8
rutabagas							
raw	½ c cubed	0	tr	tr	?	?	25
boiled, drained	½ c cubed	0	tr	tr	?	?	29
boiled, drained	½ c mashed	0	tr	tr	?	?	41
salsify							
raw	½ c sliced	0	tr	?	?	?	55
boiled, drained	½ c sliced	0	tr	?	?	?	46
sauerkraut, canned, solids & liquids	½ c	0	tr	tr	?	?	22
seaweed							
agar, raw	3½ oz	0	tr	tr	?	?	26
kelp, raw	3½ oz	0	1	tr	?	?	43
laver, raw	3½ oz	0	tr	tr	?	?	35
spirulina, raw	3½ oz	0	tr	tr	?	?	26
dried	3½ oz	0	8	3	?	?	290
wakame, raw	3½ oz	0	1	tr	?	?	45
shallots							
raw	1 T chopped	0	tr	tr	?	?	7
freeze-dried	1 T	0	tr	tr	?	?	3

snow peas *See* PEAS, EDIBLE PODS, above
soybeans *See* SOYBEANS & SOYBEAN PRODUCTS

	Portion	Chol (mg)	Total Fat(g)	Satur'd Fat(g)	Mono Fat(g)	Poly Fat(g)	Total Calor
spinach							
raw	½ c chopped	0	tr	tr	?	?	6
boiled, drained	½ c	0	tr	tr	?	?	21
canned							
drained solids	½ c	0	1	tr	?	?	25
solids & liquids	½ c	0	tr	tr	?	?	22
frozen, boiled, drained	½ c	0	tr	tr	?	?	27
frozen, boiled, drained	10 oz pkg	0	tr	tr	?	?	63
spinach, mustard *See* MUSTARD SPINACH, above							
spinach, New Zealand *See* NEW ZEALAND SPINACH, above							
spinach soufflé	1 c	184	18	7	?	?	218
sprouts *See* PLANT NAME (ALFALFA, MUNG BEAN, ETC.) above							
squash, summer							
all varieties							
raw	½ c sliced	0	tr	tr	?	?	13
boiled, drained	½ c sliced	0	tr	tr	?	?	18
crookneck							
raw	½ c sliced	0	tr	tr	?	?	12
boiled, drained	½ c sliced	0	tr	tr	?	?	18
canned, drained solids	½ c sliced	0	tr	tr	?	?	14
frozen, boiled, drained	½ c sliced	0	tr	tr	?	?	24
scallop							
raw	½ c sliced	0	tr	tr	?	?	12
boiled, drained	½ c sliced	0	tr	tr	?	?	14
zucchini							
raw	½ c sliced	0	tr	tr	?	?	9
boiled, drained	½ c sliced	0	tr	tr	?	?	14
canned, Italian style, in tomato sauce	½ c	0	tr	tr	?	?	33
frozen, boiled, drained	½ c	0	tr	tr	?	?	19
squash, winter							
all varieties							
raw	½ c cubed	0	tr	tr	?	?	21
baked	½ c cubed	0	1	tr	?	?	39
acorn							
baked	½ c cubed	0	tr	tr	?	?	57
boiled	½ c mashed	0	tr	tr	?	?	41
butternut							
baked	½ c cubed	0	tr	tr	?	?	41
frozen, boiled	½ c mashed	0	tr	tr	?	?	47
hubbard							
baked	½ c cubed	0	1	tr	?	?	51
boiled	½ c mashed	0	tr	tr	?	?	35
spaghetti, boiled, drained, or baked	½ c	0	tr	tr	?	?	23
string beans *See* BEANS, SNAP, above							

	Portion	Chol (mg)	Total Fat(g)	Satur'd Fat(g)	Mono Fat(g)	Poly Fat(g)	Total Calor
succotash							
boiled, drained	½ c	0	1	tr	?	?	111
canned, w/cream style corn	½ c	0	1	tr	?	?	102
canned, w/whole kernel corn, solids & liquids	½ c	0	1	tr	?	?	81
frozen, boiled, drained	½ c	0	1	tr	?	?	79
swamp cabbage							
raw	1 c chopped	0	tr	?	?	?	11
boiled, drained	1 c chopped	0	tr	?	?	?	20
sweet potato leaves							
raw	1 c	0	tr	tr	?	?	12
steamed	1 c	0	tr	tr	?	?	22
sweet potatoes							
baked in skin	½ c mashed	0	tr	tr	?	?	103
baked in skin	1 sweet potato = 4 oz	0	tr	tr	?	?	118
boiled w/out skin	½ c mashed	0	tr	tr	?	?	172
candied	3.7 oz	8	3	1	?	?	144
canned							
in syrup, drained solids	1 c	0	1	tr	?	?	213
in syrup, solids & liquids	1 c	0	tr	tr	?	?	202
mashed	1 c	0	1	tr	?	?	258
vacuum packed	1 c pieces	0	tr	tr	?	?	183
vacuum packed	1 c mashed	0	1	tr	?	?	233
frozen, baked	½ c cubed	0	tr	tr	?	?	88
swiss chard *See* CHARD, SWISS, above							
taro							
raw	½ c sliced	0	tr	tr	?	?	56
cooked	½ c sliced	0	tr	tr	?	?	94
taro chips	10 chips = 0.8 oz	0	6	2	?	?	110
taro leaves							
raw	1 c	0	tr	tr	?	?	12
steamed	1 c	0	1	tr	?	?	35
taro shoots							
raw	1 shoot = 2.9 oz	0	tr	tr	?	?	9
cooked	½ c sliced	0	tr	tr	?	?	10
taro, Tahitian							
raw	½ c sliced	0	1	tr	?	?	25
cooked	½ c sliced	0	tr	tr	?	?	30

	Portion	Chol (mg)	Total Fat(g)	Satur'd Fat(g)	Mono Fat(g)	Poly Fat(g)	Total Calor
tomatoes, green, raw	1 tomato = 4.3 oz	0	tr	tr	?	?	30
tomatoes, red, ripe							
raw	1 tomato = 4.3 oz	0	tr	tr	?	?	24
boiled	½ c	0	tr	tr	?	?	30
canned							
stewed	½ c	0	tr	tr	?	?	34
wedges in juice	½ c	0	tr	tr	?	?	34
whole	½ c	0	tr	tr	?	?	24
w/green chilies	½ c	0	tr	tr	?	?	18
stewed	1 c	0	2	tr	?	?	59
tomato paste, canned	½ c	0	1	tr	?	?	110
tomato puree, canned	1 c	0	tr	tr	?	?	102
tomato sauce *See* SAUCES, GRAVIES, & CONDIMENTS							
towel gourd *See* GOURD, DISHCLOTH, above							
tree fern, cooked	½ c chopped	?	tr	?	?	?	28
turnips							
raw	½ c cubed	0	tr	tr	?	?	18
boiled, drained	½ c cubed	0	tr	tr	?	?	14
frozen, boiled, drained	3½ oz	0	tr	tr	?	?	23
turnip greens							
raw	½ c chopped	0	tr	tr	?	?	7
boiled, drained	½ c	0	tr	tr	?	?	15
canned, solids & liquids	½ c	0	tr	tr	?	?	17
frozen, boiled, drained	½ c	0	tr	tr	?	?	24
turnip greens & turnips, frozen, boiled, drained	3½ oz	0	tr	tr	?	?	17
vegetables, mixed							
canned							
drained solids	½ c	0	tr	tr	?	?	39
solids & liquids	½ c	0	tr	tr	?	?	44
frozen, boiled, drained	½ c	0	tr	tr	?	?	54
frozen, boiled, drained	10 oz pkg	0	tr	tr	?	?	163
vinespinach, raw	3½ oz	0	tr	?	?	?	19
water chestnuts, Chinese							
raw	1¼ oz	0	tr	?	?	?	38
canned, solids & liquids	1 oz	0	tr	?	?	?	14
watercress, raw	½ c chopped	0	tr	tr	?	?	2
wax beans *See* BEANS, SNAP, above							
wax gourd (Chinese preserving melon) boiled, drained	½ c	0	tr	tr	?	?	11
winged beans *See* LEGUMES & LEGUME PRODUCTS							
yam, baked or boiled	½ c cubed	0	tr	tr	?	?	79

	Portion	Chol (mg)	Total Fat(g)	Satur'd Fat(g)	Mono Fat(g)	Poly Fat(g)	Total Calor
yambean, tuber only							
raw	1 c sliced	0	tr	?	?	?	49
boiled, drained	3½ oz	0	tr	?	?	?	46
yardlong beans See LEGUMES & LEGUME PRODUCTS							

■ BRAND NAME

Betty Crocker
POTATO MIXES

	Portion	Chol (mg)	Total Fat(g)	Satur'd Fat(g)	Mono Fat(g)	Poly Fat(g)	Total Calor
au gratin (+ ⅙ of added ingredients)	⅙ pkg (½ c)	?	5	?	?	?	140
cheddar 'n bacon (+ ⅙ of added ingredients)	⅙ pkg (½ c)	?	5	?	?	?	140
hash browns (+ ⅙ of added ingredients)	⅙ pkg (½ c)	?	6	?	?	?	160
julienne (+ ⅙ of added ingredients)	⅙ pkg (½ c)	?	5	?	?	?	130
potato buds (+ ⅛ of added ingredients)	⅓ c flakes (½ c)	?	6	?	?	?	130
scalloped (+ ⅙ of added ingredients	⅙ pkg (½ c)	?	5	?	?	?	140
scalloped potatoes & ham (+ ⅕ of added ingredients	⅕ pkg (½ c)	?	6	?	?	?	160
smokey cheddar (+ ⅙ of added ingredients)	⅙ pkg (½ c)	?	5	?	?	?	140

TWICE BAKED POTATOES

	Portion	Chol (mg)	Total Fat(g)	Satur'd Fat(g)	Mono Fat(g)	Poly Fat(g)	Total Calor
bacon & cheddar (+ ⅙ of added ingredients)	⅙ pkg (½ c)	?	11	?	?	?	210
herbed butter (+ ⅙ of added ingredients)	⅙ pkg (½ c)	?	13	?	?	?	220
mild cheddar w/onion (+ ⅙ of added ingredients)	⅙ pkg (½ c)	?	10	?	?	?	190
sour cream & chive (+ ⅙ of added ingredients)	⅙ pkg (½ c)	?	11	?	?	?	200

HOMESTYLE POTATOES

	Portion	Chol (mg)	Total Fat(g)	Satur'd Fat(g)	Mono Fat(g)	Poly Fat(g)	Total Calor
American cheese (+ ⅙ of added ingredients)	⅙ pkg (½ c	?	5	?	?	?	140
broccoli au gratin (+ ⅙ of added ingredients)	⅙ pkg (½ c)	?	5	?	?	?	130

	Portion	Chol (mg)	Total Fat(g)	Satur'd Fat(g)	Mono Fat(g)	Poly Fat(g)	Total Calor
Birds Eye Frozen Vegetables							
all Regular, Deluxe, & Farm Fresh Frozen vegetables	1 serving	0	0–1	0–1	?	?	?
CHEESE SAUCE COMBINATION							
baby brussels sprouts w/cheese sauce	4½ oz	5	7	?	?	?	130
broccoli w/cheese sauce	5 oz	10	7	?	?	?	130
broccoli, cauliflower and carrots w/cheese sauce	4½ oz	5	5	?	?	?	110
cauliflower w/cheese sauce	5 oz	10	7	?	?	?	130
peas & pearl onions w/cheese sauce	5 oz	5	5	?	?	?	140
COMBINATION							
creamed spinach	3 oz	0	4	?	?	?	60
French green beans w/toasted almonds	3 oz	0	2	?	?	?	50
green peas & pearl onions	3.3 oz	0	0	0	?	?	70
green peas & potatoes w/cream sauce	5 oz	0	12	?	?	?	190
small onions w/cream sauce	5 oz	0	10	?	?	?	140
CUSTOM CUISINE							
chow mein vegetables in oriental sauce	4.6 oz	0	2	?	?	?	80
pasta & vegetables in creamy stroganoff sauce	4.6 oz	30	5	?	?	?	120
vegetables w/authentic oriental sauce for beef	4.6 oz	0	4	?	?	?	90
vegetables w/creamy mushroom sauce for beef	4.6 oz	5	2	?	?	?	60
vegetables w/delicate herb sauce for chicken or shrimp	4.6 oz	0	5	?	?	?	90
vegetables w/Dijon mustard sauce for chicken or shrimp	4.6 oz	5	3	?	?	?	70
vegetables w/savory tomato basil sauce for chicken	4.6 oz	0	3	?	?	?	110

	Portion	Chol (mg)	Total Fat(g)	Satur'd Fat(g)	Mono Fat(g)	Poly Fat(g)	Total Calor
FOR ONE							
broccoli, cauliflower and carrots in cheese sauce	5 oz	5	5	?	?	?	110
cheese tortellini in tomato sauce	5.5 oz	30	5	?	?	?	210
potatoes au gratin	5.5 oz	30	13	?	?	?	240
rice & broccoli au gratin	5.75 oz	5	6	?	?	?	180
INTERNATIONAL RECIPES							
Bavarian Style	3.3 oz	10	5	?	?	?	100
Italian Style	3.3 oz	0	5	?	?	?	100
Japanese Style	3.3 oz	0	5	?	?	?	90
New England Style	3.3 oz	0	7	?	?	?	130
oriental style	3.3 oz	0	4	?	?	?	70
Pasta Primavera Style	3.3 oz	5	5	?	?	?	120
San Francisco Style	3.3 oz	0	5	?	?	?	100
PORTION PACK							
broccoli cuts	3 oz	0	0	?	?	?	20
cut green beans	3 oz	0	0	?	?	?	25
green peas	3 oz	0	0	?	?	?	70
leaf spinach	3.2 oz	0	0	?	?	?	20
mixed vegetables	3.2 oz	0	0	?	?	?	50
whole kernel cut corn	3.2 oz	0	1	?	?	?	70
SAUCE COMBINATION VEGETABLES							
broccoli, cauliflower & carrots in butter sauce	3.3 oz	5	2	?	?	?	45
broccoli spears in butter sauce	3.3 oz	5	2	?	?	?	45
STIR-FRY							
Chinese Style	3.3 oz	0	0	0	?	?	35
Japanese Style	3.3 oz	0	0	0	?	?	30
Chun King							
bamboo shoots	2 oz	?	0	?	?	?	16
bean sprouts	4 oz	?	0	?	?	?	40
chow mein vegetables	4 oz	?	0	?	?	?	35
water chestnuts (whole, sliced)	2 oz	?	0	?	?	?	45
Claussen							
sauerkraut	½ c	?	tr	tr	?	?	22
Kraft							
POTATOES & CHEESE							
au gratin	½ c	40	5	2	?	0	130
broccoli au gratin	½ c	40	5	2	?	0	150
scalloped	½ c	25	5	2	?	0	140

	Portion	Chol (mg)	Total Fat(g)	Satur'd Fat(g)	Mono Fat(g)	Poly Fat(g)	Total Calor
scalloped w/ham	½ c	15	5	2	?	1	150
sour cream w/chives	½ c	10	5	2	?	0	150
2-cheese	½ c	10	4	2	?	0	130
Mrs Paul's Prepared Vegetables							
candied sweet potato	4 oz	?	1	?	?	?	170
corn fritters	2	?	9	?	?	?	240
eggplant parmigiana	5 oz	?	16	?	?	?	240
crispy onion rings	2½ oz	?	12	?	?	?	190
Ortega							
green chiles, whole, diced, strips, sliced	1 oz	?	0	?	?	?	10
hot peppers, whole, diced	1 oz	?	0	?	?	?	8
jalapeño peppers, whole, diced	1 oz	?	0	?	?	?	10
tomatoes & jalapeños	1 oz	?	0	?	?	?	8
Progresso							
PEPPERS							
roasted	½ c	0	<1	<1	?	<1	20
sweet fried	½ jar	0	3	<1	?	<1	37
hot cherry	½ c	0	20	3	?	8	190
pickled	½ c	0	12	2	?	6	130
piccalilli	½ c	0	20	3	?	8	190
tuscan	½ c	0	0	0	?	0	20
eggplant (caponata)	½ can	0	4	?	?	?	70
Stouffer							
corn soufflé	4 oz	?	7	?	?	?	160
creamed spinach	4 oz	?	14	?	?	?	170
green bean mushroom casserole	4¾ oz	?	11	?	?	?	160
potatoes au gratin	⅓ of 11½ oz pkg	?	6	?	?	?	110
scalloped potatoes	4 oz	?	4	?	?	?	90
spinach soufflé	4 oz	?	9	?	?	?	140

❏ **VINEGAR** *See* SALAD DRESSINGS, MAYONNAISE, VINEGAR, & DIPS

❏ **WHEY** *See* MILK, MILK SUBSTITUTES, & MILK PRODUCTS

❏ **YOGURT** *See* MILK, MILK SUBSTITUTES, & MILK PRODUCTS

❏ **YOGURT, FROZEN** *See* DESSERTS, FROZEN